D1236753

Germfree Life
and
Gnotobiology

Observations relatives à la Note précédente de M. Duclaux; *par* M. **Pasteur**.

« Je prends la liberté, en presentant cette Note de M. Duclaux, de lui suggérer l'idée d'un travail auquel le préparent non seulement celui que je dépose, en son nom, à l'Académie, mais les travaux non moins distingués qu'il a déjà produits sur le rôle des microbes dans la digestion.

» Souvent, dans nos causeries du laboratoire, depuis bien des années, j'ai parlé, aux jeunes savants qui m'entouraient, de l'intérêt qu'il y aurait à nourrir un jeune animal (lapin, cobaye, chien, poulet), dès sa naissance, avec des matières nutritives *pures*. Par cette dernière expression, j'entends désigner des produits alimentaires qu'on priverait artificiellement et complètement des microbes communs.

» Sans vouloir rien affirmer, je ne cache pas que j'entreprendrais cette étude, si j'en avais le temps, avec la pensée préconçue que la .ie, dans ces conditions, deviendrait impossible.

» Si ces genres de travaux se simplifiaient par leur développement même, on pourrait peut-être tenter l'étude de la digestion par l'addition systématique, aux matières nutritives *pures* dont je parle, de tel ou tel microbe simple ou de microbes divers associés bien déterminés.

» L'œuf de poule se prêterait sans difficulté sérieuse à cette nature d'expériences. Privé extérieurement au préalable de toute poussière vivante au moment où le petit poulet va sortir, mis aussitôt après dans un espace sans germes quelconques de microbes, espace où se renouvellerait un air *pur*, on fournirait facilement du dehors au jeune poulet des aliments *purs* (eau, lait, grains).

» Que le résultat soit positif et confirme la vue préconçue que je mets en avant ou qu'il soit négatif et même en sens inverse, c'est-à-dire, que la vie soit plus facile et plus active, il y aurait un grand intérêt à tenter l'expérience. »

GERMFREE LIFE
AND
GNOTOBIOLOGY

by

THOMAS D. LUCKEY

Department of Biochemistry
University of Missouri School of Medicine
Columbia, Missouri

ACADEMIC PRESS, New York and London
1963

ACADEMIC PRESS INC.
111 Fifth Avenue, New York 3, New York

United Kingdom Edition published by
ACADEMIC PRESS INC. (LONDON) LTD.
Berkeley Square House, London W.1

LIBRARY OF CONGRESS CATALOG CARD NUMBER: 63-13105

PRINTED IN THE UNITED STATES OF AMERICA

Dedicated to the scientists and friends of science who helped establish germfree research as a new biological tool.

PREFACE

During the past decade the use of the techniques of germfree research has increased to such an extent that now is the appropriate time for the appearance of this comprehensive review of the whole field of germfree research and gnotobiology. The last detailed review, written in German, is that of Glimstedt (1936). Several brief reviews which have appeared since then are mentioned in Chapter 2; the most recent of these is that of Mickelsen (1962).

This volume treats the theory and general aspects of germfree research and provides a summary of germfree work in all phyla, thus presenting an over-all picture of the subject. The chapters on methods and nutrition are sufficiently detailed to serve as guides for experimental work. Germfree vertebrates are characterized from available data on morphology, biochemistry, nutrition, serology, and physiology. The final chapter reviews exploratory research concerned with the inoculation of germfree animals with known kinds of microorganisms.

The phylogenetic approach has been used in order to give perspective to the work with any given species, to emphasize areas needing further research, and to provide a broad enough survey to facilitate evaluation of gnotobiotics by workers in peripheral fields. Certain aspects have been discussed within more than one context in the book in order to develop the subject fully enough so that the reader will not be burdened by the need for undue cross-reference to other sections.

New terms have been introduced to describe new concepts and to provide precise communication. For the convenience of the reader there is a glossary in the appendix section. Also included in the appendix is a chronology which gives some idea of the extent to which various people, laboratories, and nations have been involved in germfree research.

The extensive bibliography will serve as a guide to the literature in the field. Where a specific reference is not given for data in the text the implication is that the source can be found in references listed under the author's name or under Reyniers *et al.* (with the author as a collaborator); in some cases data are from the author's unpublished work.

This volume has been planned for those who are engaged in germ-free research, those just entering the field of gnotobiology, those in related fields who need to incorporate the concepts of gnotobiology into their own thinking and practice, and who wish to apply the techniques in their own work, and those who are interested in the progress of science in our time. The monograph will also provide a background for many practical aspects: the maintenance and supply of specific pathogen-free and gnotobiotic laboratory animals, techniques in experimental surgery, modification of hospital procedures, the developing industry of raising disease-free pigs, and biological problems in space exploration.

Personal conversations or correspondence with most of the current investigators in germfree research have enriched this manuscript. The trust evidenced in their helpful responses has had a sobering and humbling influence.

T. D. LUCKEY

April, 1963

Acknowledgments

The unpublished work was done with financial aid of the Office of Naval Research at the University of Notre Dame, and the National Science Foundation at the University of Missouri. Collaborators at the University of Notre Dame were J. A. Reyniers, R. F. Ervin, M. Wagner, Dr. H. A. Gordon, R. Meeks, Dr. T. Mende, J. Pleasants, and B. A. Teah. The technical assistance of Mrs. Akrevy Mauer, Mrs. Margaret Beaver, Mrs. Lou McAllister, Mrs. Nancy Conbere, A. Lorance, and D. Donalek is gratefully acknowledged. Dr. H. T. Miller has been of special assistance in the work with the germfree room at the University of Missouri and also in the preparation of this manuscript. A special contribution to the work described in this monograph was the provision of five germfree mice, by the University of Notre Dame through Dr. R. E. Thorsen, F. X. Bradley, and Dr. H. A. Gordon.

Credit or reference is given with each photograph excepting those by the author. Acknowledgment is given for permission to duplicate material from the publishers of the following journals: *Annals of the New York Academy of Sciences, Journal of Dental Research, Journal of Nutrition, Lobund Reports, Texas Reports of Biology and Medicine, and The Journal of Experimental Medicine.*

Special thanks are expressed to those who translated literature: Drs. G. J. Mannering, S. Landry, H. A. Gordon, H. T. Miller, Fun Sun Chu, and Mrs. Leida Piip. Drs. M. Miyakawa and J. Tanami introduced me to the Japanese research and literature. Dr. J. J. Landry was helpful in allowing use of material on sterile surgery and pig operations. I am especially indebted to Dr. Victor Cabelli for critical reading of the manuscript, to Morris Wagner for reviewing the methods on testing for sterility, and to Mrs. Pauline Luckey for final proofreading. While all have helped make this document presentable, the author assumes full responsibility for errors and omissions.

Contents

PREFACE vii

ACKNOWLEDGMENTS ix

1

Theory and General Aspects of Germfree Life and Gnotobiology

Biological Isolation as the Basis of Germfree Life 1
Germfree Conditions in Nature 4
Essential Elements in Germfree Research 8
Biological Significance of Germfree Research 19
Relationship to Other Enclosed Systems 24
Gnotobiology 25
Nomenclature and Terminology 27
Summary 31

2

Phylogenetic Development of Germfree Research

Early Concepts 34
Sterile Plants 36
Germfree Culture of Tissues 41
Germfree Invertebrates 43
Germfree Vertebrates 60
Summary 96

3

Germfree Animal Techniques

Cages 99
Sterilization 143
Obtaining Germfree Animals 171
Microbial Testing 179
Summary of Methods 188
Production, Maintenance, and Repair Problems 201
Decontamination 206
Summary 210

4

Nutrition of Germfree Animals

General Considerations 213
Intestinal Synthesis Theory 214
Diet and Microorganisms 216
Diet Changes during Sterilization 218

Contents

The First Colony of Germfree Mammals 225
Diets and Feeding 242
Nutritional Requirements 250
Summary 280

5

Characteristics of Germfree Animals

Introduction 283
General Characteristics 286
Systems, Organs, and Tissues 291
Defense Mechanisms 368
Abnormalities in Form and Function 381
Reparative Processes 388
Summary 391

6

Gnotophoric Animals

Introduction 398
Methods 400
Bacteria-Host Gnotobiotes 402
Virus-Host Gnotobiotes 419
Protozoa-Host Gnotobiotes 422
Invertebrate-Host Gnotobiotes 424
Conventionalization 425
Summary 428

REFERENCES 430

APPENDICES

I. Chronology 476
II. Glossary 485
III. Diets for Germfree Animals 489

INDEX 497

Germfree Life
and
Gnotobiology

CHAPTER 1

Theory and General Aspects
of Germfree Life and Gnotobiology

Biological Isolation as the Basis of Germfree Life

Complete isolation, a state which has more philosophical than practical importance, is not easily attained. A small fraction of the air we breathe was in the lungs of Christ, Mohammed, and Buddha. The complete biological isolation of any but the first living organism is denied by the ontogenetic law. No organism is entirely alone; the phylogeny of the individual transcends species barriers. Living cells are born of other living organisms. Plants use carbon dioxide from animals to build their substance; and animals must rely upon the photosynthetic activity of plants for fuel and specific organic nutrients without which animals would soon perish. Autotrophic bacteria and some plants can survive on inorganic substances, but even they use biologically formed organic molecules on most occasions.

Since experimentation with complete biological isolation is not practical with present day limitations, the most strict definition of pure culture may be ignored. More pertinent is a consideration of a usable definition of *germfree* with the concomitant development of a detection system for any and all living contaminants and the relegation of viruses to an acceptable and practical category for future experimental work. Classically, germfree animals, sterile plants, and axenic invertebrates are each defined as a single species isolated from all other demonstrable *living* microorganisms. Theoretically, germfree research is an extension of the pure culture concept of bacteriology. This concept began in the early days of taxonomy and may be traced back to Aristotle. It gathered strength from the theory of the immutability of species, was tarnished by the theory of evolution, and finally was crystallized by the work of Koch (and Lister) who isolated single microbial cells to give assurance of a pure culture according to the

1

cell theory of biology. The weakness of the identification of biological isolation procedures and of germfree research with the pure culture concept is that inherent in the cell theory of life itself.

As Hughes (1959) points out, the cell is a convenient mechanical unit for the basis of life but not the ultimate one. The individuality of the cell is less fundamental than is usually portrayed. Consider cells which harbor intracellular parasites, cells such as striated muscle with more than one nucleus, bacteria without well defined nuclei, or living organisms without cell walls such as the slime mold *Physarum polycephalum*. Corliss (1957) briefly reviewed the complexity of protozoa whether considered as cells or individuals. Blood has many characteristics of living tissue without being strictly cellular. Mature red blood cells are cellular and respire, but the absence of nuclear material precludes them from being called living. Viruses obviously do not fit into the cell theory; they are analogous to only one part of a cell—a fragment of a chromosome. If such a contaminant is part of the genetic apparatus, Reyniers (1959c) suggests it may be eliminated by following appropriate breeding patterns or by finding a strain of the same species which does not carry the contaminant. The occult or nonsymptomatic virus becomes of real importance in the definition of the individuality of the cell or the organism. Is it really a stranger when it has occupied a regular place in the chromosomal pattern? If viruses are considered to be living and if a regular place in a chromosome is occupied by viral nucleic acids, no organism can be completely gnotobiotic. Infectious nucleic acids must be considered in similar concept. Practically, the definitions of germfree and gnotobiosis must include the term "detectable living forms."

Dmochowski (1961) emphasizes the fact that living organisms should be defined neither in terms of cell morphology nor of cellular constituents. The cell is a useful biological compartment which allows concentration of bioconstituents for the reactions of growth, organization, and reproduction characterizing living organisms. The cell is a characteristic unit of living organisms, but this unit is of little importance as a characteristic of life. An organism has the same number and kinds of cells immediately after death as it had as a living organism; placement of the cells is similar; form is little changed; and most of the bioconstituents are present in concentrations characteristic of life. Only the reactions are different; the energy equilibria have shifted. Life must ultimately be defined only as it can be understood, in biochemical and biophysical concepts. The detection of unwanted living organisms must ultimately be based upon life as a process characterized by acceptable morphologic, chemical, and physiological criteria. The importance of this view to the theory of germfree research will become apparent in the testing for contaminants. This view suggests that the ultimate test for living organisms cannot rest entirely upon the presence of cells or other morphologic characteristics, but it must include the biochemical and thermodynamic characteristics of life.

Of the many possible approaches to define life, a descriptive definition in physical and chemical concepts might be the most useful for the detection of unwanted living forms which may or may not be known forms. Life is the consummate activity of specially organized systems (usually cellular organisms) in which material is processed and energy is continually expended for: (1) synthesis of more system(s) through growth and reproduction; (2) increased assurance of survival by variation via adaptation and mutation; and (3) maintenance of the effectiveness and internal integrity of the system(s) to prevent disability, disorder, and death. The advantage of using such a definition is that it will not only fit the classical living systems for which tests have been routine, but it also asks for new and improved methods for examination and suggests that there are broader views of life than is usually seen in laboratory testing. For example, the synthesis of more system(s), or the increase of total mass through growth and reproduction, includes the nutritive requirements and the "physiology" of microorganisms usually considered in differentiation between one species and another. Respiration and metabolism are needed for each item considered, but they are more easily examined by activities associated with the first point. The second point emphasizes that growth and reproduction alone are not enough for a general criterion of life; mutation is a means for variation on a grand scale and adaptation allows for variation by the individual. Both are essential for the continuity and survival of life. The third point, the continuous victory of life over randomness, could be explored as a means for detecting life in an unknown area, or for finding new systems which actually are living according to the general definition but would not otherwise be recognized as living. Captured matter and energy are incorporated into the metastable complex required for the equilibrium and *further development* of delicate catalytic and coupled reactions without net energy loss to increased randomness. It is suggested that cybernetic mechanisms of life will differ in complexity if not in quality from those of nonliving systems. The third criterion suggests that one way to distinguish a living system from a nonliving system is to subject the system to a destructive stress: the living system(s) will have reactions built into it to preserve its integrity. Gnotobiotic monitoring must include methods to detect states of decreased or suspended animation of viable systems. Hibernating animals, dormant seeds, spores, and crystalline viruses represent special cases in which the potential of full life may be retained during periods of stress. The continuity of the central theme of life, reproduction with variation, becomes evolution and indicates the direction of life. From this viewpoint life is the activity of a diverse holobiota to continuously evolve more efficient means (both chemical and physical) to incorporate energy and matter into intricate, orderly systems.

Germfree Conditions in Nature

The existence of one or more species in an environment separate from another given species is frequently seen in nature. This separation may be as infinite as life on planets a million light-years apart, or as intimate as commensalism. However, biological isolation in which a single species exists free from all others in a separate environment is rare; organisms usually exist in intimate contact with many species of microorganisms. Bacteria, yeasts, mold, and protozoa comprise the billion inhabitants of the gastrointestinal tract of every human and of large animals.

The cells of many of our own tissues are in direct contact with cells of other living species. However, as Pasteur noted, blood and urine do not "ferment" if drawn aseptically. It is generally believed that tissues of healthy individuals are *bacteriologically* sterile. Perry *et al.* (1955) found human blood and portal blood to be sterile while canine liver was sometimes contaminated. Kassel and Rottino (1955) found no diphtheroids in the blood when germfree techniques were used in the study. Transient showers of bacteria may be found in the blood following chewing during which infections of any weakened tissue may occur. These organisms are normally eliminated by phagocytosis and other mechanisms of defense. However, some individuals carry diseased tissue throughout life; some infections are passed *in utero*, i.e., *Salmonella pullorum*. Modern evidence favors the concept of Chienne and Ewart (1878), who found sterile tissues when they improved the original technique of Tiegel (1874). This concept was confirmed by Babes (1882) and Dowdeswell (1884). Bulloch (1938) reviews much of the early work.

Examples wherein single species may exist alone or with a limited number of other species in the immediate environment can be discussed as phenomena of natural occurrence, medical practice, and experimental science. The phenomenon of a single living species existing alone must have occurred about 2 billion years ago when life was first brought forth on the earth. Depending upon our definition of life, several primordial species probably struggled into oblivion before one or more organisms struck the chord of reproductive continuity. This biochemical phenomenon must have occurred on thousands of other planets during eons past. On each, the first living form was alone. Such thinking is reflected in the "sterile" techniques used to prepare rockets to be sent to the moon or other planets. Some biologists argue that we should not contaminate another heavenly body with earth species before identification of the "native" flora and fauna. It takes little effort to combine the thoughts of the purists who would ensure that space vehicles do not contaminate another planet, with the suggestion of Williams (1959) that there is the possibility of raising our children without germs. Imagine a future planet populated with germfree people! Microbial decontamination techniques will need to be perfected in order that "conventional guests" from contaminated earth may visit.

Partial isolation of organisms in "nature" is found where the environment is detrimental to all except specialized organisms. *Thiobacillus thiooxidans* is one of the few organisms known to grow in 5% H_2SO_4. *Lactobacillus bifidus* is the predominant (99.9% pure) organism in the gastrointestinal tract of infants fed only colostrum. Other places where "pure cultures" of organisms occur are hot springs, several meters underground, and the inside of a colony of microorganisms where the colony via antibiosis has eliminated effective growth of other species. Confined areas exist both in time and in space where one species dominates to the partial extinction of other species. The ecological balance can be dramatically affected by variation in the nutrients present, the amount of water, pH, osmotic pressure, eH, oxygen tension, CO_2 tension, light, heat, radiation, and harmful compounds. A less effective means of isolation is the development of special adaptations by species for the use of air, land, or water masses. Once developed, the specialization often has proceeded with other changes which prevent that species from effectively using all three areas. Ecology has many illustrations of the partial isolation of one or more species from others due to physical barriers. The early spring algae in each small lake and *Tigriopus* in coastal splash pools live with few competitors as compared to the usual variety of species. Allen (1952) notes that blue-green algae are the first organisms to invade sterile volcanic soils.

The ovum, refractive after fertilization, effectively denies from the immediate environment of the new creature-to-be not only other sperm but also all other organisms except highly invasive pathogens. Thus, the fertile egg from a healthy chicken has no bacteria or other microorganisms within the shell. The best evidence for this is the routine procurement of germfree chicks and cells and/or extracts for tissue culture. In eggs from disease-free flocks the healthy embryo develops within a miniature world containing no other living organism. This isolation can be broken by contamination or inoculation during the course of embryological development and is normally broken when the hatching chick breaks the multi-layered shell, its main barrier against invading microorganisms. Similarly, the fetus *in utero* is completely isolated from all detectable living organisms other than its mother and sometimes its twin or other sibs. The uterine cavity and placental barrier are most effective against most invading microorganisms. Of hundreds of Cesarean-born rats taken into germfree cages, only one dam had young which were infected *in utero* according to the bacteriological tests of M. Wagner. The isolation barrier remains unbroken in mammals until the moment of birth. The initial shock of multiple contamination is apparently not of a magnitude comparable to that of the many other changes at birth borne by the baby. Yet this microbial shock will routinely kill older mammals which are maintained germfree for part of their lives before being exposed to contamination. The newborn has special powers of resistance and receives such special material in colostrum that it is not often harmed by infection.

Both the embryo in the egg and that *in utero* are of more than theoretical interest; both have been used experimentally as source material for germfree research. Woolpert (1952) has reviewed microbial work using embryos *in utero*. Others have used it to study digestion, morphology, and serology in the unborn. Studies on the embryonated egg are commonplace.

A naturally occurring system of especial interest is that of intracellular parasites. Here, one organism lives within the environment of a cell of another species. The biological rigidity of this relationship makes it comparable to that of organisms in germfree conditions with the exception that the cellular environment of the host is necessarily present. Intracellular parasites often exist in a constant environment free from other species excepting the host. This concept includes helminths, protozoa, bacteria, rickettsia, and viruses. Extracellular parasites live in an environment which greatly limits the kinds of microorganisms which can survive in it; the host again is present. Some parasites exist free of contaminants: tissue parasites are routinely obtained in sterile culture from the host by simple aseptic operation. Cesarean-born pups delivered into germfree chambers were found to harbor filarial worms without microbial contaminants —they were "germfree but not wormfree."

The early literature on the microflora of the gastrointestinal tract of Arctic animals indicated that these animals had either sterile tracts or very few organisms. This lead was actively pursued by bacteriologists because it was believed that important inferences could be made from such data relating to the importance of intestinal microorganisms in digestion. Later literature partially refutes this idea and suggests that some Arctic animals have a relatively "normal" population in their stomach and intestines. Levin (1899) found some Arctic animals (such as sharks, eider ducks, and penguins) to be bacteria free; in others (one polar bear and two seals) he found a bacterium similar to *E. coli*; and others (white winged gulls and marine invertebrates) had many microorganisms in their intestines. Ekelof (1908) found no growth in bacteriological media with several samples of intestine of Antarctic birds. Hesse (1914) found one snipe, one guillemot, and one eider duck to be free from bacteria and one snipe with bacteria. He reported that during the 1902–1903 South Polar Expedition Gazert found seals to be infected while terns, stormy petrels, and penguins had "sterile" intestinal contents. Hesse also reported that H. Pirie found both sterile and infected animals in the 1902–1904 Antarctic expedition. Since later workers have found bacteria in reduced numbers in Arctic animals (excepting Bunt, 1955), it seems possible as Glimstedt suggested that the media used were incomplete. Seiburth (1959) suggests the combination of the reports of "bacteriological sterility" may be explained by such factors as the antibacterial activity of dietary material, sea water phytoplankton, and serum. He found no "bacteriologically sterile" birds.

It is known that different foods, vitamins, and antibiotics change the predominating organisms in the intestinal tract. It is reasonable to expect that the differences in digestive juices (compare the spider, cat, sheep and, shark with that of man) would provide a *milieu* in which some organisms would flourish whereas others could not survive. It should be emphasized that aerobic microorganisms do not flourish in the intestinal tract. Most significant work has been reported with insects. Portier (1905) found that the intestinal canal of some caterpillars (*Tinea, Lithocolletis,* and *Nepticula*) is always free of bacteria. Couvreur (1906) found that the bacteria disappear during the pupal stage of a silk-spinning insect. E. Metchnikoff (1909) and his wife found that alligators, parrots, and bats had few bacteria in their intestinal canals while *Galleria, Tinea,* and scorpions had sterile intestinal contents. These findings were not adequate to admit a positive answer to the major microbial question of that time: is life possible without bacteria?

Essential Elements in Germfree Research

Philosophic Considerations

The essence of germfree research is isolation. Isolation must be attained mechanically, proven scientifically, and understood philosophically. As mentioned previously, practical biological limitations in the continuity of life prevent the absolute aloneness of any individual. In the sense that we can never know life completely, we can never define the complete biological isolation of one species. This is the basis of one criticism of the term, *gnotobiotic,* which means literally to know life completely. The criticism was met by limiting the concept when the new word was derived. *Gnotobiota,* a word denoting that the flora and fauna are completely known, is a more acceptable word for the base (Trexler, 1960c).

The concept of life free from all demonstrable living microorganisms suggests that the ultimate in biological research would be the complete isolation of the animals from any organisms living or dead and from products of organisms which retain their species identity. However, this state has not been achieved in the past nor is it likely to be achieved in the immediate future. The extent to which one approaches the ideal is dependent upon available methods and procedures, and the specific use to which animals are put, for example, in studying problems of innate immunity the presence of dead bacteria in the food may confound the result.

Individuals of the same species are not considered trespassers in germfree work. Similarly, a germfree rat may be in the same cage with a germfree mouse, rabbit, or chicken without violating the connotation of germfree. Presumably, there is little biological effect of any of these species upon another. The existence of germfree lice on chickens, or worms in germfree dogs presents biological implications that would seem to distort the germfree concept. Since the term *germfree* is defined in terms of microbes a more exclusive term is required. The term *monobiotic* is defined more generally and excludes all other forms of life which have a direct *intimate* effect on the animal.

The presence of the operator has thus far been ignored in germfree theory. Yet the animal must sense and react to the man even though he is seen only through a porthole. The handling of the animal with sterile gloves obviously has tremendous biological implications (Ruegamer *et al.*, 1954). This consideration must be extended to the presence of a man in a sterile suit inside a germfree room. From the animal viewpoint, the only principal characteristic of man which is missing would seem to be man odor.

The presence of dead microbes in the food, water, and air (dust) of the germfree animal has not been enough "contamination" to dissuade the use of the term germfree. These dead microorganisms of the diet may be present in great numbers when part of the food is of bacterial origin. The oral inoculation of germfree animals with dead bacteria does produce antigenic reactions and lymphatic development. Presumably this source of antigen could be prevented by providing antigen-free air, water, diets, and cages. The *antigen-free* animal would be more useful for many studies and provide a more standardized biological tool than the germfree animal with its variable antigenic experience. Animals in the two categories should differ in certain morphological and chemical aspects and should not be considered together in concept. Since no antigen-free animals have been reared, they will not be considered in detail.

In practice, viable microorganisms may be present in the germfree cage without actually contributing to the immediate environment of the germfree animal. A singular example of such a phenomenon occurred during a test run of germfree rats in the "big tank" (see Chapter 3, section on cages). Routine tests of the tank wall, air, food, rats, etc., indicated the germfree status of the experiment until one rat escaped from its cage into the relative freedom of the big tank. When captured, this occupant was found to be contaminated while the caged rats continued to show no contamination. Another example is found in germfree chick work. The mercuric chloride left on the egg shell is not a completely effective germicide. Neutralization of this germistatic compound will often reveal the presence of organisms which have remained dormant indefinitely in the dried germicide on the egg shell within the germfree cage. A drop of water on the shell would reactivate the germicide to kill any germinating spores. If a germfree chick eats shells inoculated with *Bacillus subtilis* which have 1% $HgCl_2$ on them, the chick remains germfree although the organism can be recovered from the shell (Miller, 1962).

Viruses are presently disturbing the germfree concept. Symptomatic viruses are routinely excluded in germfree research by the simple expediency of not using abnormal animals. Occult viruses present a problem which will take years to resolve. Their status as living organisms is questionable (Weidel and Dmochowski, 1961). They are not free living; they are obligate parasites to specific hosts and are really little different from a part of a chromosome or a chromatin granule. However, their infectivity combined with a remarkable reproductive capacity with variation equivalent to genetic mutation, makes them continue to be considered as equivalent to living organisms in the concepts and work presented herein. Further discussions of this problem are presented later.

The germfree concept is one of special isolation conditions; it is far from adequate and not entirely consistent. It is a useful concept to define one grade of purity of biological material. The concept of germfreeness has been a goal which stimulated much research and will contribute to a greater understanding of biological isolation.

Mechanical Considerations

Although the exact concept of germfree animals may fluctuate with time, it still demands that germfree animals be considered separately from the usual laboratory animals in their need for a microbial barrier. While this germ curtain may consist of a variety of physical agents, the completeness of the barrier is essential. Obviously the barrier must encompass the animal, food, water, air, adequate living space, and usually some equipment for the work to be performed (which must include adequate procedures to establish the absence of all microbial species). Reyniers (1959a) suggests the most desired quality in the barrier or isolator to be dependability. As discussed in some detail in the chapter on cages, the barrier may be steel, plastic, glass, rubber, cotton, glass-wool, germicidal liquids, or sometimes simply sterile air going through an opening.

The sterile system must have a means of introducing the species under study. This may be as simple as a germicidal bath for eggs, seeds, or spores, or as complicated as a separate operating cage for the Cesarean birth of microbe-free young. The enclosed system usually has a means of introducing material needed during an experiment; i.e., sterile food, water, media, or instruments. These are sometimes sterilized during the intake procedure, i.e., steam sterilized in a clave attached to the side of the cage. Animals may need to be transferred from one cage to another; the same device used to bring material in may be used for transfer. For example, Gustafsson (1959b) sometimes transferred rats from one cage to another by sealing them in a small container (glass jar) and taking this out through the attached germicidal trap (dunk tank) and into the new germfree cage via the dunk trap before the air in the container was exhausted.

The last major item of importance under mechanical considerations is the manipulation of material or animals. This can be accomplished in a limited manner using gravity or sudden movement of the entire cage, or through the walls of a pliable cage; more effective are mechanical devices. Miyakawa (1959c) uses mechanical arms and fingers of the type familiar to workers with radioactive materials. Gloves attached as a component part of the germfree cage are most useful if the system is of appropriate size. Large cages and rooms require a man in a sterile suit for practical work.

Miscellaneous items to be considered include provision for air exchange, viewing the interior, proper heating or cooling, humidity, bedding, and photographic records. The term bedding includes water for fish, snails, etc., nesting material for mammals, and sand or agar for insects to deposit eggs.

Food

Germfree animals must be provided with sterile food adequate for growth, maintenance, and/or reproduction, depending upon the requirements of the work to be done. The fact that this has been accomplished shows that some animals can be nurtured without contribution from the myriad microorganisms in the gastrointestinal tract.

Obviously, the food changes during its sterilization; therefore, sterile food must be fed to control animals in order to test its character. One exception to this is the use of food grown aseptically. The use of such food will have much more consideration in the future than it has had in the past. Unless specifically stated otherwise, control animals were always fed diets sterilized in the same manner as those fed to germ-free animals.

It should be noted that, to date, germfree animals have not been fed bacteria-free diets. Diets used have contained microbial cells and débris killed and acted upon by the sterilization process but still active as antigens and probably in other ways. Antigen-free diets have been considered, but no experiments with antigen-free animals have been performed and reported.

It is axiomatic that synthetic (chemically defined) diets can fulfill their main function only in gnotobiotic animals. When eaten by a conventional (also called *classic* herein) animal, the first thing which happens is the food is intimately mixed with the myriad microorganisms of the saliva, gastric, and intestinal juices. Although no one knows the changes wrought by microorganisms in this environment, students of rumen digestion know something of the complications of *in vivo* fermentation. The assumption that digestion in nonruminants is less complicated is shattered by the finding of Johnson *et al.* (1960) that classic rats metabolized about 30% of the C^{14} cellulose fed to them. Thus one does not know what materials are transferred via the intestinal mucosa when a synthetic diet is fed to a classic animal. The feeding of a chemically defined diet to a germfree animal would be an important step to a thorough understanding of digestion.

Animal Background

Research with a variety of germfree animals was made possible by practices other than medicine and science. Invaluable to the animal experimentation era of the twentieth century science are centuries of experience in keeping animals in zoos. The use of methods and concepts learned since the time of the zoological garden of Aristotle makes the evaluation of this contribution very difficult. Methods of obtaining housing and feeding a variety of animals had already been learned when science needed a new species. The large number of mammals which zoologists had already characterized was most helpful in the evaluation of animals for germfree research. Nuttall and Thierfelder (1896b) did not need to develop a new experimental animal for mammalian research; they chose the guinea pig because its known characteristics fitted their need.

Germfree research resembles other new areas of investigation in that the pioneers in this work borrowed methods from related disciplines to establish major concepts and techniques, but had relatively little success in application of the new tool. During the half-century lag period (1897–1947), a few men expended great energy to gradually improve the procedures used. The decade 1950–1960 introduced wider use of the tool and commercial development of different types of apparatus. The next decade appears to be the one which will firmly entrench germfree techniques as an essential tool in the repertory of biological science. The small laboratory animals have proven the most valuable for germfree work where space and time are at a premium.

The first problem approached in the thinking and work with germfree animals was posed by Pasteur in 1885 (see Frontispiece). Is life possible in the absence of bacteria? Pasteur admitted that if he were younger, he would approach the problem with the preconceived idea that animals could not live without the intestinal microorganisms to help provide nutriment. Evolutionary considerations suggested that animals had developed in the presence of the myriad microorganisms in their gastrointestinal tract; it seemed a plausible argument that the host animal had not only adapted to their presence but might also have become dependent upon their activity for the digestion of food or the production of one or more compounds essential for life. Nencki (1886) disagreed. This chemist, who first unraveled the complex chemistry of the ptomaines, understood the unique action and source of these compounds. He suggested that the absence of the microorganisms which produce such toxic compounds as indole and skatole would be beneficial to the animal, and that animals without bacteria should be more healthy and grow faster. *This is the argument which launched the first two decades of germfree research.* Metchnikoff, the head of the Pasteur Institute, believed that the beneficial organisms in Bulgarian buttermilk (Yoghurt) promoted longevity by counteracting the numbers and effect of the putrefactive bacteria in the tract. Since he thought that the fewer bacteria present the better, he must have despaired with each report by his wife, Olga Metchnikoff, of failure to rear germfree tadpoles. Wollman (1913) and Cohendy (1912a) had shown that the life of tadpoles and chicks respectively was not only possible but that the animals actually grew in the absence of bacteria. This view is now amply confirmed by reproduction in germfree chickens, rats, mice, guinea pigs, and rabbits.

The biological individuality of animals is obscured by their long association with microbes. According to the current theory of evolution, multicellular species developed from unicellular organisms. The development of animal species in the presence of the ubiquitous microbes and their intimate association through a million centuries gave ample opportunity for evolutionary changes to occur. Some of these could have made the hosts dependent upon the microbes. Such is clearly the case for ruminants. What other groups are dependent upon the microbial association? Are all animals partially dependent upon the microbes for stimulus of defense mechanisms? Only the germfree animal and inoculated gnotobiotes can give clear answers to such questions. The biological purity of the individual cannot be appreciated until the extent of its dependence upon its microbes has been determined. A high degree of biological isolation for the study of the isolated "normal" individual cannot be attained until all essential functions usually contributed by microbes are provided in their absence. This may include material to reduce cecal distention, to stimulate lymphatic development, and to develop active phagocytes. Such work will help the role of the microorganism in the ecology and economy of animals to be better understood. The elaboration of physiological diseases and aging without a microbial vector should lead to benefits through an understanding of the uncomplicated syndromes.

Procurement of Germfree Material

Germfree animals in a variety of ages or sizes may be obtained from one of several colonies as are other laboratory animals with the exceptions that the cages are most special and there are few commercial suppliers. One must be prepared to use the animals without allowing contamination. However, there must be a beginning other than the reproduction of germfree animals in a stock colony. For the egg-laying species, the fertile egg is sterilized in germicide and the embryo allowed to hatch into a sterile environment. If the interior of the egg is sterile and no contamination occurs during the transfer and incubation period, the individual will be germfree. Since some diseases are transmitted through the egg, stock free from those particular diseases must be used. Thus, chicks obtained from hens harboring *Salmonella*

pullorum are expected to contain at least one microbial contaminant—
actually, experiments designed to support this supposition have occurred in the author's experience as accidents but have not been
reported. Germfree mammals are usually obtained by Cesarean section. The chapter on nutrition presents details of the long, tedious,
hand-feeding job to be accomplished (if a germfree foster mother is
not available) before germfree rats or mice are weaned and ready for
most experimental work. Foster mothers are most useful for introducing different strains into the germfree world.

Some experiments, as those concerned with the nutrition of newborn mammals, can be performed directly upon Cesarean-born animals. A few experiments have used the unborn embryo as a source of
germfree material. And some progress has been made on the bacteriological decontamination of laboratory animals.

Any contamination of a germfree animal makes it of little value for
its original purpose. Experiments in which contamination is found are
usually discarded. However, sometimes only a single contaminant is
found and the work can be continued with recognition of the biological variable added. From a practical viewpoint, there is little difference between a germfree animal contaminated with one identified
strain of bacteria and a germfree animal inoculated with that same
strain. Theoretically, the latter case has less chance of having present
an unknown contaminant in addition to the known bacteria. Much
important gnotobiotic work with germfree animals which have been
inoculated with one or more microbes remains to be done. Germfree
animals are the base from which other gnotobiotic states may be
prepared (inoculation of a germfree animal with a single species of
microorganism would form a dibiotic system). Most gnotobiotic colonies could be used to form a "disease-free colony" or a specific
pathogen free colony for commercial as well as experimental use.

Testing

The value of all germfree work relies ultimately upon one's ability
to establish the absence of all microbial forms. Here the consideration
of time presents two problems. First, the ability of bacteriologists is
related to the state of microbial testing devices in a chronological
sense. New and better tests are devised as understanding of microbes
is increased. Each advance in understanding and technique modifies
the germfree concept. The salient point at present is the status of
occult viruses. In the past, germfree animals which showed no sign

of a virus infection were routinely considered to be virus free. This position was strengthened by the occasional attempts to uncover the viruses in germfree animals. As the tools of virology are sharpened, this complacence is being shaken. Second, time is a constant problem in germfree work because it actually takes more than 1 week for bacteriologists to carry out adequate cultural tests in their routine search for any "strangers" in the system. This means that on any given day the operator knows only that the animals were germfree 2 or more weeks previously, and he will not know until 2 or 3 weeks later what the "germ status" was on that day. In practice, some contaminants can be suspected more rapidly; some grow rapidly on culture media while others produce a changed odor of the outlet air. A fecal stench announces the presence of coliforms or a fecal organism and the "cornflakes for breakfast" odor is reliable for the lactics.

Standard bacteriological testing procedures are used routinely to evaluate the germfree state. But this standardization must be extended to include details of what to look for (bacteria, fungi, molds, algae, protozoa, helminths, and viruses), where samples for testing are to be procured (i.e., should the cecal contents be included in routine testing, should "whole animal" tests be resumed), and how and when the samples should be taken and incubated. This standardization is needed to help compare work from different laboratories. It is essential to define the tests before the nomenclature can be stabilized. Special principles should be applied to tests involving monoinoculated animals.

The germfree animal is itself a unique testing device for contamination. It continually collects samples from the air, food, water, surfaces of itself, the cage, and apparatus. It provides a good anaerobic culture medium in the gastrointestinal tract with constant temperature, frequent replenishing of food, and good waste disposal. Fastidious organisms or parasites have no competitors, and they catch the host with his defenses down. In spite of this some organisms are hard to detect.

Controls

The problem of a proper control for experiments involving germfree animals is not a simple one. At first thought, one would suggest the "normal" animal in the laboratory fed the sterilized diet. Kijanizin (1895) performed such experiments in the last century. In theory one would add water sterilized in the same kind of containers used for the germfree animals. In practice this is not always done. Should not the air also be sterilized? Then the control animals should be placed in a closed container to simulate conditions of the germfree group. Now the flow, dust, pressure, humidity, and composition of the air should be controlled. The temperature rise during simulated diet sterilization should be instituted for these animals as though they were germfree. Then one remembers the bacterial flora—these animals are in a "locked-flora" condition. What little data are available on such animals indicates that these are far from the "normal" control really needed. The locked bacterial flora tends to simplify itself. These animals have some characteristics more like the germfree animals than those of "normal" animals. Therefore, a daily visitor is introduced from the outside, allowed to stay 1 day, and exchanged the next day for another visitor from the outside world. Or should germfree animals be inoculated with different organisms for the "control?" Such questions explain why more than one control is often used in germfree work.

Such a series is noted in Lobund Report No. 3. Chicks in group A were germfree; group B contained chicks hatched from sterilized eggs, maintained in conventional brooders in an open laboratory and fed sterile diet and water in order to give an indication of the effect of autoclaving of the diet, group C chicks were hatched from unsterilized eggs, maintained as group B and fed nonsterile diet and water; group D was maintained as group B and fed farm diet in order to control and differentiate between it and the syntype diets used; group E was maintained under farm conditions with the farm diet; group F and group G were maintained in germfree cages with everything sterilized as if they were germfree. In addition group G chicks had a daily visitor chick from the conventional chicks in the brooder. The determination of the proper control depends upon the point of view. One control which is not yet available is the use of animals which had developed in the presence of microorganisms until the time of the experiment, then by decontamination they would be rendered bacteriologically sterile without destroying the microbic stimulated systems of the conventional animal.

The dilemma is dissolved when the germfree animal is considered the control and all others as experimental. The germfree animal has one less variable than all of the other groups considered—that of the microbial flora, and it has more than one less variable than most of the groups. Its environment can be defined and duplicated in terms of pressure, humidity, air exchange, dust sources, etc. With germfree animals as controls, the experimental animals can best be germfree animals inoculated with desired species of microbes; then the conventional animal presently used as a control assumes the rightful role of a polycontaminated, conglomerate, and biologically impure animal of indefinable state. Compare, if you will, the description of the intestinal flora of the "normal" animal by two or three different laboratories.

Men in Gnotobiotics

Men do not attempt this difficult biological technique without expecting to expend considerable time and effort on the mechanics of learning to keep, maintain, and evaluate germfree animals. The only easy experiments are those which can be performed on germfree material (animals, tissues, or residues) immediately after it is received from a germfree production group with assurance that it is actually germfree when shipped. One important job for all who do germfree research is to carry out the bacteriological tests. Since this takes considerable time, training, and material, most germfree research is done by a team where one man is responsible for routine microbial testing. The same is true to a lesser degree for the nutrition, the mechanical operation of the apparatus, the handling of the animals, and the administration. Classically the germfree team has varied from three to more than fifty people. In recent years, laboratories have begun to use germfree research systematically as a part of a graduate student training program. The tendency here is to let one person, the student, do all aspects of the work much as many of the original workers did in this field. As the general usage of these methods increases, the ease of operation will improve so the individual investigator has less time involved in the mechanics of keeping animals germfree and relatively more effort can be applied to the problem for which the technique is being used.

The research investigator and his technicians rightly receive emphasis because their scientific lives and ideas are most important ingredients of germfree research. Germfree research is costly in terms of time and energy. The energy expenditure is best illustrated by quoting Küster's (1915a) comments on his first experiment with germfree goats:

The care of the apparatus and the experimental animals required such an expenditure of effort that it was not possible for us and only through the unanimous cooperation of the entire personnel of the Institute of Health were we able to accomplish this work. Now I understand the observations of Nuttall and Thierfelder that they once had to give up their experiments on the rearing of germfree guinea pigs because of the exhaustion of the experimenters.

In this respect germfree and gnotobiotic research is no different from most of the modern techniques of science. Some work can be done with little money—a man can build the apparatus with his own hands. But the proper use of this technique is to facilitate the translation of ideas into experimental data.

Biological Significance of Germfree Research

Germfree research removes one veil to reveal the subject in full microbial naiveté. Here is the animal (or plant) developed to its full genetic potential in an environment with no subsidation, stimulus, fatigue, or retardation from living microorganisms. The first question raised was "Is life possible without bacteria?" Since this can generally be answered in the affirmative, subsequent questions center around the animal *per se*. Does morphogenesis proceed in the same fashion and to the same extent without microorganisms? Will animals grow larger or at a faster rate in a germfree environment? Can a germfree animal be considered normal? Can it digest natural foods? The germfree animal and gnotobiotics become a potent tool in research whenever the role of the microbial flora is questioned in problems of biology and medicine. They are stepping stones to both applications and refinements in isolation. Germfree animals are a source material for sterile tissues (particularly mucosal tissue), organs, and fluid sources to be used in tissue culture. Pat Neville, in the author's laboratory, is presently rearing sterile insects as a source of sterile hemolymph for insect tissue culture. Applications in the production of disease-free colonies and sterile surgical techniques have already been made, and extension to other species including man is foreseen. Refinements to virus free and/or antigen free states are forthcoming as the removal of one veil invites the lifting of the next.

Germfree research is important in theoretical biology because it eliminates the microbial variable from biological experimentation. The uncontrolled flora in the intestine have caused much concern from the viewpoint of the "intestinal synthesis" theory; no one knows the exact contribution of the intestinal microflora to the nutrition of the host. Infection is a damaging variable in much biological work where the animal is stressed or becomes weakened as in wound healing, hemorrhagic stress, heat stress, radiation sickness, chronic nutritional deficiencies, and certain genetic dyscrasias (such as agammaglobulinemia). Only with the germfree animals can these be studied as "pure" physiological diseases. The elimination of the microbial variable allows a more exact evaluation of other parameters (as genetic, social, or physical factors) in biological variation.

The lack of a proper base line has hampered antibody formation studies and prevented adequate understanding of natural antibodies and so called innate immunity. Germfree animals, and eventually antigen-free and/or virus-free animals, will open the door to a systematic study of the development of mechanisms of defense. Germfree animals will supply a source of uneducated phagocytes, underdeveloped lymphatic tissue, and other defense components useful in determining what specific compounds in the makeup of microorganisms will stimulate the production of inflammation, nonspecific γ-globulins, or specific antibody agglutinins, and what specific compounds are involved in eliciting phagocytic response. As is seen in the final chapter certain species of bacteria elicit very little response in one of these reactions and much response in another. A part of the intestinal flora problem is a specific factor(s) involved in the enlarged cecum and the compounds used to increase the muscle tonus of the intestinal wall.

Since germfree laboratory animals do develop and mature through several generations, they may be considered to be "normal" from an unsophisticated viewpoint. Other species might be most abnormal in the germfree state. It will be impossible to rear in germfree conditions many species carrying symbionts until the essential function of the symbiont is provided by other means. A striking illustration is presented by Buchner (1955). The findings of Poulson et al. (1961) confirm this work. Buchner noted that when mycetocytes invade the ovary of Stictococcus, nearby oocytes are invaded, but not others. Parthenogenic development of the eggs (normal for this genus) gives rise to females from infected eggs and males, with one lost chromosome, from the noninfected eggs. Since the presence of symbionts from different microorganisms prevents the loss of a chromosome, Buchner suggests that the effect is due to a nonspecific stimulus. Thus, an equally valid view of germfree research is to ask the importance of intimate microbial contact in metazoans. What does the intestinal microflora do? Is there a specific role for each specific microorganism, as is seen in nitrogen fixation in plants? Are there general symbiotic relationships in which a variety of microorganisms may fulfill a function, i.e., the development of defense mechanisms, or the development of tonus in the muscles of the cecal wall? This approach will bear fruit as the *in vivo* metabolism of microorganisms is studied with germfree animals inoculated with specific organisms.

Virus research has special problems which require germfree or gnotobiotic animals. The absence of microorganisms is important in order to detect asymptomatic virus, to study the virus etiology of cancer, and to experiment with the origin of viruses. Germfree animals offer opportunity to characterize pure virus diseases in the absence of bacterial competition and body defense mechanisms developed by microbial stimulation. Another question which could be approached includes this: will *in vivo* culture of bacteria enhance the development of phage or the resistance of the microorganism to phage?

Germfree research and gnotobiotics present a new dimension in studies of the interrelationships between the host and the specific microorganisms. The methods of germfree research can be used to maintain animals which have been inoculated with one or more species of microorganisms. While studies on the *in vivo* metabolism of microorganisms could be made, the emphasis of this work has centered upon the effect of specific microorganisms upon the host. Such work is reviewed in Chapter 6.

With slight changes in operation, the germfree cages may be used to prevent laboratory infections. The exhaust air must be sterilized, a slight negative pressure inside the cage is desirable, and the cage interior and all material must be sterilized before being opened. This use of gas tight enclosures has been presented by Gremillion (1960) and Walton (1958).

The germfree technique is also useful to show whether or not a disease is caused by specific microorganisms. Kassel and Rottino (1955) illustrated this principle by showing that the number of microorganisms associated with malignant disease appeared to decrease as techniques for isolation became more stringent. When germfree techniques were used, no microorganisms were found in the blood of patients having Hodgkins disease or lymphoma, or in the blood of mice which were carcinomatous.

Some of the more practical applications should be presented without undue speculation. One of the major applications of germfree research is the production of disease-free swine in the United States.

It is very possible that a similar industry will arise for disease-free chickens. The production of disease-free laboratory animals began about 1940; the recent growth of this industry is due in no small part to the application of germfree techniques (Foster, 1959). The extension of germfree techniques into experimental surgery can be foreseen; the complete elimination of extraneous microorganisms from a surgical area will allow extensive sterile operations to be performed. In addition to the complete absence of airborne germs, a major advantage of the enclosed surgery is the control of the immediate environment with respect to temperature, pressure, humidity, and air composition. The development of new isolators, new methods of air sterilization, and sterile rooms will allow modification of the isolation procedures used in hospitals and lead to better preparation of hospital rooms and patient areas. The multiplicity of cages already on the market indicates the wide variety of uses to which germfree techniques will be adapted.

Germfree research and gnotobiotics are directly applicable to the control of contamination of other planets and the sterilization of space vehicles. The microbial problems of a single mammal in an enclosed environment for any length of time have not been studied adequately. The problems discussed in this book on the locked flora give some indication of what can happen and ways to avoid any undesirable effects. If a single animal is in a closed environment with sterile food, water, and air for a few weeks, the flora becomes simplified to one or two species. When simple procedure for decontamination has been completed, it is within reason that a bacteriologically sterile man of the future could walk upon another planet without contaminating it with earth microorganisms. From data presented herein, it is obvious that care should be exercised in choosing the microorganism used to inoculate him prior to his landing upon a germ-laden planet.

One of the most intriguing uses of germfree techniques is the study of the origin of life. Pasteur effectively quieted all proponents of spontaneous generation, but in the last decade the biochemists have awakened to the possibilities of abiotic synthesis of organic compounds in nature. Since compounds which we consider to be typical of life can be synthesized without the help of any living forms, the next step is obviously that of trying to put together a system which resembles the mechanisms and nature of life. In this study, germfree techniques of the highest degree will be required in order to prove the point that the synthesis carried out and the organization obtained was not derived from living cells.

It is important to remember that the biological material presently available for germfree work has not been obtained by bacterial decontamination of conventional animals. The individual itself has developed from conception in an environment protected from all microbes. In the case of the chick, the egg is usually formed and ejected as a bacteriologically sterile package. The inside remains thus unless the surface is traumatized. The outside of the shell becomes contaminated upon first contact with the world outside the oviduct. The evagination of the oviduct during the expulsion of the egg decreases contamination with the cloacal flora and fauna. The developing mammalian fetus is sterile *in utero*. The function of the Cesarean operation is the aseptic transfer of bacteriologically sterile individuals from one sterile environment, the uterus, to another, the germfree rearing cage.

The bacteriological decontamination of conventional animals for germfree experiments is an operation significantly different from the relatively simple transfer of a germfree individual from one container to another. The little work done on this problem is reported later.

Germfree research gives a new parameter to the standardization of laboratory animals. Strains of rats, mice, and chickens have been standardized by inbreeding for many generations. Usually only two to six characteristics are used as the basis of selection, but in many problems in biology the most exacting work fails to resolve the question of the role of the bacteria and other microorganisms. The elimination of this variable is important progress in the standardization of experiment biology. Most other parameters can be controlled by well-established means: type of cage, diet composition and particle size, food intake, foreign antigens, exercise, water, coprophagy, air pressure, composition of respiratory gas, air flow, temperature, light, humidity, sound, motion, and even social conditions such as crowding. When they are controlled they should be specified in published reports to help standardize biological experimentation.

The ultimate biotron will control all physical factors and allow a standard set of conditions to be selected for each experiment. The phytotrons of Hendricks and Went (1958) are prototypes. The use of synthetic diets will be a necessary step for proper standardization. Then, with the microbes excluded, only one major variable remains— that of genetics. The use of litter mates and inbred strains is far from the exact control needed. The proper tool would be a line-bred colony of a species with identical sibs such as that produced by the furry armadillo. The use of germfree identical sibs fed a chemically defined diet in a properly engineered biotron will make biology comparable to the exact sciences. Experiments will be reproducible and results should become predictable.

Relationship to Other Enclosed Systems

Pioneers in germfree research borrowed heavily from bacteriology, animal respiration studies, and plant physiology; and a vigorous exchange of ideas, techniques, and apparatus continues between people in germfree work and those in related work. This concept should be apparent in subsequent chapters which are developed with a historical thread to give continuity both in time and among related sciences. The early work in the chemistry of gases required the complete separation of two environments. The bell jar of Priestly and Dumas and Gay-Lussac was easily adapted for the study of the respiratory exchange of animals by LaPlace and Lavoisier. Early plant physiologists reared sterile plants in simple flasks and bottles. Simple apparatus is adequate for invertebrates, but most vertebrate work requires special cages. The refinement of the bell jar of chemistry into the chemical hoods with controlled gas composition and dry boxes is paralleled by refinements made by the biologists to provide the plant growth chambers and the germfree cages of today. Such apparatus has, in turn, been used to control the atmosphere to study the survival of mammals in the absence of inert gas (MacHattie and Rahn, 1960). Many similarities are seen in concepts, problems, equipment, and manipulation of radioactive remote control systems, germfree systems, bacteriological safety cabinets, diving bells and suits, submarine work, and the present development of manned space vehicles.

Phillips and Hoffman (1960) have reviewed the problem of the contamination of celestial vehicles. However, the sterilization of a *man*-bearing space ship is not as simple as the procedures outlined, i.e., the use of noxious gases for final sterilization. The International Committee on Contamination by Extraterrestrial Exploration has recommended that the moon and other celestial bodies not be contaminated. Sampling of these bodies prior to contamination would give tremendously important information regarding the abiotic synthesis of organic compounds in nature (Sagan, 1959), the composition of rocks and occluded gases in the absence of photosynthesis (Garrison *et al.*, 1951) and respiration, and the origin of life. In answer to DeMent (1960), who suggested we would need germfree men to land on the planets, one could reply that this could be done mechanically by remote control apparatus or by decontaminated men (see Chapter 3).

Industry has adopted these concepts for sterile hoods, sterile rooms, and sterile areas. The pure culture concept of bacteriology which was the basis for rearing germfree animals has now gone full circle; germfree animal cages are now adapted for mass culture techniques in bioengineering, and microbiologists have adapted germfree cages and techniques for the protection of workers using virulent pathogens—the infected animals are maintained inside the cages with extra precautions taken to ensure that the pathogens used never get out alive.

The germfree system may also be used to study controlled states of biological complexity—a germfree animal may be inoculated with one or more strains of microorganism. This aspect of gnotobiotics is elaborated in Chapter 6 under the term, *gnotophoresis*. Further modification of the germfree concept by Young *et al.* (1959), Foster (1959), and others has led to innovations in two rapidly expanding industries: the production of disease-free stock in the swine industry and the use of specific pathogen-free laboratory animals for research.

Gnotobiology

The term *germfree* has occasionally been strained to the point of being meaningless. Obviously a germfree animal inoculated with a culture of microorganisms is no longer germfree. Of the many proposals suggested for a broader concept, *gnotobiotics* (the "g" is silent) has the most general acceptance. Gnotobiotics ("known life," from the Greek roots *gnoto* and *biota*) is defined as the field of investigation or work in which only known kinds (species) of living organisms are present. This ungainly word nicely includes all germfree work as well as that in which more than a single known species is present in the same environment. All the criticism of the word has not prevented it from becoming the only accepted term for the over-all technique. In concept, it can include work with antigen-free and virus-free organisms when these become available.

An example may clarify the concept of gnotobiology. A gnotobiotope containing only rats and chicks would contain two gnotobiotic species both of which would be called germfree animals. If that system were inoculated with *Lactobacillus acidophilus*, there would be no germfree animals and three kinds of gnotobiotes.

In both theory and practice the techniques of gnotobiology are very similar to those of germfree work. The added features when working with inoculated animals (or with animals carrying only known contaminants) are the means of introducing the microorganism and the added burden of proving bacteriologically that the only microorganisms present are those already known to be present. Since the techniques are so clearly related and because there has been little work in gnotobiotics other than germfree, the emphasis of this presentation must remain on germfree work. This does not imply that research with dibiotic systems is less important; the subject will be covered as fully as the limited amount of work permits. Exceptions are that a full review will not be attempted of work in virology, tissue culture, or sterile plants.

The major classes of gnotobiotic organisms include germfree and gnotophoric animals. Germfree animals are gnotobiotic by definition: an animal which is free of all demonstrable living microorganisms is one in which only known species are present. When a germfree animal is inoculated (or contaminated) by a single known species, i.e., *Streptococcus faecalis*, a monoflora may establish itself in the animal and each is a part of a dibiotic system. Since all species present are known, the system is gnotobiotic and each species may be considered to be a gnotobiote. Such reasoning could be extended to diflora animals, tribiotes; triflora animals, tetrabiotes, etc. The need for a name to designate this state is clearly indicated by the use of phrases such as "germfree" rats monocontaminated with *S. faecalis*. Animals bearing known species of microorganisms are obviously different from germfree animals. Such distinction is readily discerned by the introduction of the new term, *gnotophoric* from the Greek *gnoto* (known) and *phorein* (to bear). This is a shortened form of the more descriptive term *gnotobiophoric*. A *gnotophoric* animal carries one or more known forms of living organisms in intimate contact with it and no demonstrable living species which are not known to the investigator. The host could be called a *gnotophore;* this term is not appropriate for the microorganism unless one wishes to designate a microorganism carrying a virus. *Gnotophoresis* is defined as the state of existence of an animal bearing one or more known species in intimate contact with it, in the absence of all other demonstrable living organisms. Gnotophoric animals are a powerful tool with which to study infectious diseases and other phenomena. Judicious comparison of monoinoculated germfree animals to form a dibiotic system with germfree animals can be used to evaluate the effect of subclinical and clinical infections on the economy and well-being of the host. Inoculation of germfree animals with a single species (or two) of microorganism is being used to study such diverse areas as the etiology of dental caries, experimental endocarditis, intestinal synthesis, and the mode of action of antibiotics. Other uses include the evaluation of specific microorganisms as variables in biological research, the determination of which microorganisms best stimulate different components of the defense mechanism, variations in microbial virulence, and that which prompted Reyniers (1932) to enter germfree research, the use of germfree animals as a culture medium for fastidious microorganisms. The "inoculated germfree animal" (a *gnotophore*) will permit development of methods to detect species which cannot be cultivated *in vitro* and to study metabolism, physiology, and life cycles in fastidious microorganisms (both protista and micrometazoans). Germfree animals inoculated with either vitamin producing or B-vitamin requiring bacteria are being used to obtain direct evidence on intestinal synthesis (Miller and Luckey, 1962). Germfree ruminants offer a direct approach to many problems in rumen digestion. Only with germfree sheep and other ruminants inoculated with known microorganisms can the component microbial systems of the rumen be thoroughly studied. Fortunately, scientists at Ohio State University and Michigan State University are beginning serious study on germfree ruminants.

The germfree animal inoculated with microorganisms will open the door to the study of microbial reactions *in vivo*. Excepting tissue culture work, few studies have appeared which compare the metabolic reactions of pure cultures of microbes *in vitro* to those *in vivo*. Since this interesting field awaits future investigation it is premature to speculate upon the contribution of the host to the metabolism of the microbe.

Nomenclature and Terminology

The best things to be said for the term *germfree* are that it is easily understood, it has popular acceptance, and it is historically the term of importance. It is acceptable as long as it is used in the limited sense for which it was proposed. The early workers concerned only with animals reared in the complete absence of microorganisms found the term sufficient in several languages: *privé de germs, privé de microbes, aseptic, Keimfreie, Bakterienfreie, ohne Bakterien, sterile, axenic, gf, germfree, germ-free* and *germ free* are all essentially synonymous. Since symptomatic viruses are absent in most germfree work, and early attempts to search for nonsymptomatic viruses were generally unfruitful, it was thought that germfree animals were also virus free. This concept is questionable and depends upon the definition of latent viruses, the question of the *de novo* origin of viruses and attempts by competent virologists to examine germfree animals for the presence of viruses.

The word *germfree* and, to a greater extent, the word *sterile* both suffer by providing the ambiguous connotation that reproductive sterility is implied. In this respect neither is entirely acceptable to the uninitiated. The germfree state, designated "Gf," is defined as the existence of an organism(s) in the absence of intimate contact with demonstrable viable protista or metazoa. Dead microbial cells and debris, antigenic material, or occult viruses may be present. Terms which have been proposed as replacements or modifications of *germfree* are listed in Appendix I. As new concepts or improved methods of testing are developed, they may be used to provide a better understanding which will help to crystallize terminology in this new field. Although *sterile* is quite acceptable when applied to inanimate objects and has been consistently so applied to bacteria, plants, and sometimes invertebrates, it is not acceptable in general usage. The term *aseptic* or *in the absence of microorganisms (l'absence d'êtres microscopiques)* suffers from most of the shortcomings of germfree and sterile and has not been accepted generally for this work. *Aseptic* has a useful connotation of its own.

Germfree and *axenic* both suffer from the negative quality implied in each. Neither becomes a good base for a system intricate enough to define the interrelationship which can exist in gnotobiotic research. *Axenic* (meaning literally "free from strangers") could be equivalent to gnotobiotic, but it has thus far been equated to *germfree*. It has acceptance in the protozoa and the invertebrate areas with the simple connotation of "free from other species." As defined (Baker and Ferguson, 1942) axenic animals could well harbor virus since "axenic organisms are individuals of a species free from any demonstrable life apart from that produced by their own protoplasm." Both terms denote a condition that may never be known—one may never be sure that *no* other species exists within the experimental confines. Since knowledge of the absence of all other living forms is limited to the efficiency in detecting *all* other living organisms, little assurance can be given that the terms *germfree* and *axenic* will be stabilized in the near future without arbitrary action by workers in the field. This is not as deplorable as it may seem at first consideration. The definitions of both germfree and *axenic* allow for the limitation of the test. The simple and historically important definition of *germfree* implies the existence of no *detectable living microbial* forms. This concept, linked to the ability for detection of living microorganisms, varies some from one laboratory to another and has varied much from one decade to another. Therefore, the detection system needs to be standardized in order to stabilize the term. This will permit the introduction of new terms as new techniques for detection are used. The viruses may again be used as the pièce de résistance. To date the term *germfree* has included the connotation of freedom from symptomatic viruses. Although Balzam (1937) and Riback and Reyniers (1949) inoculated germfree chicks with virus, the term *germfree* has excluded occult viruses prior to 1958 (Ward, 1959), although the major investigators admit they have no good way to make a positive statement regarding the absence of nonsymptomatic viruses.

The term *germfree* is adequate to describe one level of existence: organisms with no demonstrable living microbes. The term *gnotobiotics* is acceptable to denote the techniques. There remain many quantitative biological relationships which need simple and exact description. Qualitative relationships are usually described by such terms as symbiotic, parasitic, mutualistic, and commensalistic. A system which describes the quantitative relationships presently known in gnotobiology and which has potential for growth as future relationships are elucidated is recommended. Many of the terms presented here have been discussed by Reyniers *et al.* (1949e), Dougherty (1953b), or Just (1959).

The base, *biologically pure,* acquired its heritage in the concept of Pasteur (1885), *air et aliments purs,* and acquired added stature from the pure culture concept and methods of bacteriology from whence germfree work was derived. *Biologically pure* means the state of an animal, strain, or species existing entirely separate from direct contact with all other species and their biologically distinct products. This is an ideal state which may never be realized. In order to keep the definition within practical possibilities of use, it is advisable to make exception to the observations and indirect manipulations of the experimenter. Biologically pure species would bear the letters "Bp" after their designation as shown in examples below. Phillips and Smith (1959) have pioneered in the use of letters to designate biological status. *Biologically pure* is a useful theoretical term. However, it may not be of practical use until the conflicts over the definition of life and the status of occult viruses are resolved.

The state close to that of biological purity would be that of antigen freeness. An antigen-free individual, strain, or species would exist entirely separate from direct contact with biologically distinct products of all other species. These antigen-free organisms too may or may not be free from occult viruses. Antigen-free species would be designated by "Af" following the name. This is a category for the future since no Af animals have been used in experimentation. Presumably the young of a germfree mammal would approach the antigen free state before they take in material other than their mother's milk; they may have natural antibodies or antibodies formed in response to occult viruses. Since germfree animals usually have had no contact with other living forms, the antigens they contact are either naturally inherent for the species, derived from dead material, or of nonbiological origin.

The designation "Vf" is appropriate to indicate species which are virus free. They may have, or have had, contact with other species or their biologically distinct products, e.g., antigens. Vf animals may have one or more bacterial species in them. At present it is premature to indicate the exact relationships between this state and the two presented above.

Germfree, virus free, or biologically pure species which have been inoculated or contaminated (followed by adequate determination of the kinds of contamination) form a special category. While the term "*mixed culture*" adequately describes this state and is used in microbiology, the more elegant term "dibiotic system" has been used in animal work. In gnotobiology the isolated individual is called a *monobiote*. Although proposed separately (Luckey, 1959c) this terminology may be considered to be a euphonious contraction of monognotobiote. In a dibiotic system each individual should be termed a *dibiote;* this can be extended to tribiote or polybiote, etc., and be familiar enough to be self-explanatory.

Workers in germfree research have had increasing difficulty in the designation of the usual laboratory animal with its myriad microbes. For some time it was called the control animal. This is frustrating when a germfree experiment is run with germfree controls. It is a misnomer when germfree and "control" animals are compared because the germfree animal is the more standardized and has fewer variables of the two. The next tendency was to use the term *normal control*. This compounds errors of intent because these animals may be far from normal (the experimental design may have actually prevented this), and this carries the connotation that the germfree animal is abnormal. For some years the usual polycontaminated animals were called conventional animals, contaminated animals, ordinary animals, or stock animals with general understanding of what was meant. Combinations (normal stock, etc.) have also been used but are not really useful. One of the few terms which fulfills this need is *xenbiote* or *xenote* from the Greek word *Xeno*, meaning stranger. Xenbiotic individuals are not gnotobiotic by definition. *Conventional* is one term used herein. *Classic* may become the preferred term.

Other terms for designating less exact biological relationships in experimental material are useful in laboratory and field work (Jenkins, 1960). *Specific pathogen free* (SPF) has been used following the extensive use of tested "pullorum free" chickens and eggs. These animals are free of the disease-causing agent as determined by laboratory examination; they may have other diseases not specified. The terms *pathogen-free* and/or *disease-free* are used to indicate the usual infectious diseases named in specific pathogen-free species; SPF is a better basis to use for this category. Trexler and Reynolds (1957) have suggested *alpha gnotobiote* for germfree animals having extensive testing to show germfreeness through more than one generation. *Beta gnotobiotes* have met similar microbiological standards but have not reproduced, and *gamma gnotobiotes* are maintained under conditions in which accidental contamination may occur. They fail to recognize the susceptibility of animals in beta (or alpha) conditions to become accidentally contaminated, or the possibility that a new test may show microorganisms in animals under gamma, beta, and alpha conditions.

Summary

Complete isolation of any individual is impossible since all organisms are related phylogenetically and share the same physical world. The obvious exceptions are the first living organisms on any given planet. *Gnotobiosis* is the existence of one or more individuals, strains, or species in an environment containing only species known to the investigator. The definition of *gnotobiotic* and *germfree* is limited by the ability to define life and to confine it to a simple cellular system. Within these limits and with the acknowledged exception of the actions of the experimenter, the theory of germfree research and gnotobiology are examined. Natural as well as man-made barriers allow separation of one species or strain from some others and on rare occasions from all the other active metabolizing species. It is notable that embryos *in utero* and often in seeds or eggs are "sterile" and sometimes used experimentally *in situ*. Aseptic delivery of these organisms into a sterile environment is technically a relatively simple operation. Bacteriological decontamination of an individual is not yet practical.

Germfree animal research developed from sterile plant work with generous contributions from respiration physiology, zoological practices, and isolation systems such as the bell jar and chemical hoods. These have been blended with bacteriological procedures and mechanical gadgetry to give the variety of approaches available today. As suggested by these statements, the apparatus, methods, and philosophy are similar and somewhat interchangeable for a variety of operations. These include germfree research, gnotobiotics other than germfree, sterile industrial processes, work with highly infectious human or animal pathogens, radioactive isotope studies, work in a chemical dry box, production of specific pathogen-free laboratory animals, disease-free swine, and exploration of space.

Except for germfree research, the parameters of biological isolation have not been well defined by experimental work. The effect of the proximity of the investigator, the use of antigen-free diets and environment, the possibility of having virus-free animals, and the presence of intracellular parasites have yet to be fully evaluated.

Essential elements in germfree research and gnotobiotics are germfree animals, adequate sterile diet, thorough microbiological examination, experienced operators, and proper environment. The sterile environment is circumscribed by a physical barrier which effectively prevents the entry of microbes. The size of the cage varies from a pint jar to a sterile room, and the material used varies from plastic or rubber to glass and steel. Sterile air, food, and water are introduced as needed. Light, a viewing system, and a means of introducing sterile equipment are normally provided in the system. Most germfree cages have a means for manipulating animals or material; this means may be gloves attached to the wall of the cage, remote control fingers, or a man in a sterile suit inside a sterile room. The remaining element is testing. Standard bacteriological procedures for culturing and direct observation indicate the presence or absence of bacteria, yeasts, molds, protozoa, worms, and sometimes viruses.

Problems in nomenclature are presented and certain new terms are introduced. These are further defined in the glossary.

CHAPTER 2

Phylogenetic Development
of Germfree Research

Early Concepts

The Chronology (Appendix I) outlines the multi-sided base from which developed the concepts of germfree research, the slow acceptance of the challenge presented by the difficult techniques, and the dramatic growth of this new tool of biological research during the past decade. Work is reviewed following a classification system similar to that of Spector (1956). The work on each vertebrate species is reviewed from the early attempts to obtain it germfree to the first success in obtaining growth, development, and reproduction. Details of nutritional problems and requirements of vertebrates constitute a separate chapter.

The foundations of germfree research and the pure culture concept lay in the early grasping at ideas about the etiology of infectious disease. A summary of the concepts and techniques needed for germfree research was gleaned from readily available histories of bacteriology, such as those by Dolley (1885), Bulloch (1938), Salle (1948), and Reddish (1954).

Primitive man dimly realized the action of microorganisms in the production of fermented beverages long before he developed written languages. Repeated association of infectious agents, *pestis*, miasms (or contagion) with sickness, and the value of isolation in infectious disease were noted long before microorganisms were actually seen by Leeuwenhoek (1677) or the germ theory of disease crystallized. Evidence from the microscope provided the basis for a permanent and consistent germ theory of disease. Continued development made the microscope an important instrument for the detection and identification of microorganisms.

While animal inoculation experiments had given pure cultures of pathogenic organisms by Coze and Feltz (1866), Davaine (1870), and Koch (1881), the development of different media from 1861 to 1881 gave impetus to workers to try to isolate the different forms of bacteria which had been studied and classified microscopically for a century (Muller, 1786). Klebs (1873) isolated pure strains of fast growing bacteria by repeated short term subculture. Salmonsen (1877) used blood clotted in capillary tubes to grow isolated colonies. Lister (1878) diluted samples with large amounts of sterile media to isolate single cells. Koch (1881, 1883) developed the streak and pour plate methods which produced isolated colonies. The development of newer methods of single cell isolation has been reviewed by Hildebrand (1938) and Wilson and Miles (1955).

Work with isolation and characterization continued with microorganisms other than bacteria. Pure cultures of a limited number of species of Myxomycophyta have been obtained recently (Bonner, 1959). Difficulties in nutrition are greater than mechanical problems in the maintenance of cultures of many species in this phylum. Fungi from lichens are obtained quite simply in pure culture for study of their metabolites (Ahmadjian and Reynolds, 1961). In the phylum Eumycophyta, Johnson (1957) found tetracyclines to be useful in the isolation of soil fungi; Goldberg (1959) reviewed the use of antibiotics in routine isolation of pathogenic fungi which are resistant to cycloheximide as well as bacterial antibiotics.

While all of the methods used to obtain pure cultures are important conceptually, those involving micromanipulation are more important to the theory, methodology, and results of germfree vertebrate research. The resemblance between these two techniques is particularly striking. Here is biological isolation in its simplest form. A single cell is separated from all other cells, picked from the media, and transferred to a sterile environment in which it is nurtured and studied. In principle this is the method of germfree research. Philosophic problems raised by the pure culture technique are equally important in germfree research. Is the single bacterium a complete individual? Pure culture of bacteria free of virus would represent the simplest "germfree" system until the day when rickettsia or virus can be grown *in vitro* without other living forms. Does the single isolated cell carry contaminants; i.e., a latent virus in its genetic structure? Is this individual different for having been isolated from benign and harmful neighbors? Not only are the concepts, apparatus, and methods of the pure culture of bacteria similar to those of germfree animal research, but even the questions raised are hauntingly similar. Rearing of metazoans in the absence of microbes is truly an extension of the pure culture concept.

Sterile Plants

Early Investigations

Plant physiologists of the nineteenth century learned to grow plants in the absence of microorganisms before the establishment of the pure culture concept by Koch. Healthy plant and animal tissues were found to be free from bacteria. Sterile plant tissues, seeds in pods or fruit, and embryos could be obtained by aseptic procedure designed to keep surface bacteria from the desired material. The development of techniques for rearing bacteria and plants in pure culture were the foundation and stimulus for germfree research with plant and animal tissues, fungi, and protozoa.

The apparatus used in the early isolation of biological systems was apparently copied from tools of the gas chemists and Laplace and Lavoisier, who in 1770 studied exchange of respiratory gases in animals. Indeed, some of the first work was performed by men who had collected and separated the gases of the atmosphere in bell jars. Studies on the role of atmospheric nitrogen in plant nutrition served as impetus for the refinement and further development of the apparatus. Finally, Pasteur's comment on Duclaux's work with sterile peas presented the concept that animals might be reared in the complete absence of microorganisms. Thus, in both philosophy and technology work with plants directly preceded germfree animal research.

Nitrogen Fixation

> Sow the golden wheat,
> Whence earlier you took away legumes.
> —VERGIL

Joseph Priestley (1796) noted a decrease in gaseous nitrogen when plants were grown in an inverted bell jar. When De Saussure (1838) could not repeat the work, the first great controversy of agricultural research was begun! The apparatus, techniques, and concepts developed during that half century of controversy over nitrogen fixation laid the ground work for experiments with germfree animals. In 1855, Boussingault found more nitrogen in plant products than he had added in a nitrogen balance study on farms. In the greenhouse he found 20% more nitrogen in *Trifolium* grown in burnt soil than was present in the seeds. He concluded that plants take

EARLY DATA OF BOUSSINGAULT (1838)

N_2 in produce	707.2 lb.
N_2 in manure	487.6 lb.
Excess N_2	219.6 lb.

nitrogen from the atmosphere. When Liebig criticized his experiments on the basis that he had neglected to account for nitrogen added in previous years, Boussingault repeated the experiment using aseptic technique and found no increase in nitrogen in the plants. He concluded that his first experiments were in error.

In 1853, G. Ville reported that cress grown in sand gained 4 to 40 times more nitrogen than was in the seed. In 1855, a French commission repeated Ville's work but discontinued its efforts when ammonia was found in the water (see Ville, 1855). Wilson (1957) has reviewed this early work in a delightful manner.

After many years of tedious work, Boussingault (1855) found lupines gained nitrogen while oats, wheat, and cress gained negligible amounts. Since there was not a great gain, he attributed the gain to ammonia in the air and "organic corpuscles" on the roots. He used a 124 liter metal-framed glass cage with pots inside. The air with 2–3% CO_2 was washed by passing it through pumice stone saturated with sulfuric acid and then passed through water for a wash. This apparatus was like that of Balzam (1937), Fred *et al.* (1932), and Lakey (1945) almost 100 years later. In 1858, Boussingault found no nitrogen fixation in sterile soil, while good fixation was obtained when he used unsterile soil. Lawes *et al.* (1861) found that plants died when grown in sterile sand in a sterile enclosure. In 1862, M. Jodin grew plants in a nonsterile, closed container and found that nitrogen disappeared from the gas. By this time the only clear head was that of Louis Pasteur. He predicted that living microbes were fixing nitrogen for the plants; he was shown to be correct 15 years later.

The experiments of M. Berthelot with artificial lightning were most interesting. When he used a very low emf he still observed

DATA OF M. BERTHELOT (1877)

	Start–End
Moist paper:	0.010–0.045 gm N
Sugar on moist paper:	0.012–0.192 gm N

nitrogen fixation; and with no emf fixation was evident; but with sterile sand in his container little fixation occurred. When paper was soaked in sugar, nitrogen fixation was increased.

It was 1885 before Berthelot was really convinced that the soil can fix nitrogen. A 4 liter jug (Fig. 2.1) was sterilized at 100°C for

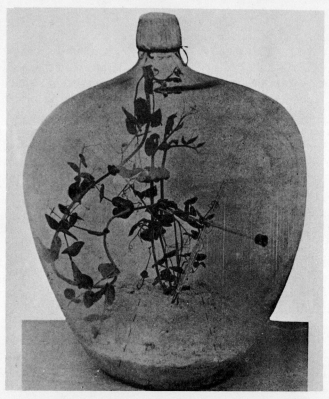

FIG. 2.1. Simplified germfree apparatus for plants. This type of apparatus was used for sterile plants by Hellriegel and Wilforth (1888).

2 hours and aerated with filtered air heated to 130°C. No nitrogen was fixed in such a jug, but when nonsterilized soil was added, nitrogen was fixed. Also in 1885, Duclaux reported experiments showing that peas would not grow under absolutely sterile conditions. His paper evoked Pasteur's comments that animal life would also be impossible without bacteria. Hellriegel and Wilforth (1888) noted that cultivated soil added to their sterile experiments allowed some plants to develop nodules. Only those plants which formed nodules survived and ac-

cumulated more N_2 than was formed in the seeds. They found the nodules to be full of bacteria. When this work was verified by Lawes and Gilbert (1891) the controversy ended. Work with sterile and monoinoculated plants continues in the study of nitrogen fixation reviewed by Wilson (1957). Recent work with nitrogen fixation is concerned with activity in cell-free extracts (Wilson and Burris, 1960). Botanists now use sterile plants for studies on physiology (Nickell, 1959), metabolism (Ryther, 1959), and tumor formation (M. Ward, 1960).

Algae Culture

One of the most active fields in plant physiology today uses pure cultures of algae in research. Mass culture of *Chlorella* is being explored for an economical protein source. The term "pure culture" has several meanings for workers in this field. The majority would agree with Orskov (1922) that a pure culture must consist of individuals which are known with certainty to be descended from one, and only one, cell. To the extent that there is disagreement regarding the term "pure culture" in this area this term becomes less useful in the over-all field of germfree research.

The techniques used to obtain a pure culture of algae are very similar to those used by bacteriologists. With some species pure culture is very difficult to obtain, whereas in others the pure culture is obtained quite easily. This apparently depends upon the type of mucous layer surrounding each cell. This active field began in 1890 when Beyerinck isolated *Chlorella* and *Scenedesmus* in bacteria-free cultures. Miquel (1892) isolated diatoms in pure cultures, and in 1894, Kossowitch isolated *Cystococcus* in bacteria-free culture. Chick (1903) was one of the few early workers to inoculate material into nutrient broth, such as bouillon, in routine bacteriological testing. Pringsheim began working with *Chlorella* in pure culture in 1912, and for over 30 years he maintained uninterrupted study of different algae. The use of ultraviolet light by Gerloff *et al.* (1950) and Allen's technique (1952) in which repeated transfers are made from the periphery of the fast spreading colony in order to obtain a colony free from bacteria have been used successfully by Kratz and Meyers (1955) in mineral and nitrogen nutritional studies of several blue-green algae. The classic techniques for the isolation of single celled microorganisms have been well reviewed by Hildebrand (1938). The groups of algae which are easily obtained are Chlorophyta, Euglenaphyta, and Phaeophyta. Diatoms and dinoflagellates can be studied quite satisfactorily with the same methods. Rhodophyta have been the neglected group of the algae according to Gerloff *et al.* (1950).

The early work in algae culture was reviewed by Richter (1911), and later work was reviewed by Bold (1942). More recent work was reviewed by Krauss (1958) who notes the increasing use of antibiotics in the isolation of algae and argues that many studies can be made in open culture in the presence of antibiotics or other chemicals. Tamiya (1957) reviews the mass culture work of algae as does the volume edited by Burlew (1953). As will be seen in the section on invertebrates, pure culture of *Chlorella* is sometimes used as food in dibiotic cultures of aquatic species.

Culture of Higher Plants

Knudson (1933) showed that given the proper pH, carbohydrate, and aseptic environment, the hosts of commensal plants such as orchids and heathers can be grown in the absence of the symbiont. White (1943) enumerated the methods useful in obtaining sterile plant seeds: plant seeds in fruit and pods are easily obtained in the germfree state by aseptic procedure; nuts and other hard fruits can be flamed; and chemical procedures must be used on grasses and other plant seeds. Bromine water, mercuric chloride, and calcium hypochlorite are used for the latter category. White also reviewed methods for rearing whole plants, parts of whole plants, and plant tissues in sterile culture. The bell jar apparatus used by him is most similar in principle to that used by Nuttall and Thierfelder (1895–1896). The more practical aspects of heat and chemical sterilization of seeds and soil were reviewed by Hartmann and Kester (1959). They listed several nutrient solutions for different plants and outlined methods needed for the aseptic culture of plants. Their discussion of disease-free clones for asexual propagation emphasizes the importance of virus-free stock. One novel method for obtaining virus-free plants is by aseptic culture of the growing tip. Since viruses sometimes move slowly through plant tissue, the growing tip may provide virus-free stock for the propagation of healthy plants.

Another link between the germfree plant work and that of animals occurred when the apparatus used by Hopkins *et al.* (1931) to study nitrogen fixation in plants was copied by B. E. Lakey (1945) for germfree chick work.

Germfree Culture of Tissues

As the first agricultural controversy over nitrogen fixation gradually diminished, another problem appeared which occupied almost four decades of slow development by plant and animal cell physiologists. That was the problem of the sterile cultivation of tissues and cells in the complete absence of microorganisms. Arnold (1887) had used an ingenious system to study leucocytes free of other living matter (he inserted porous material under the skin; when it was removed leucocytes had accumulated in it); and Ljunggren (1898) had already kept skin alive for weeks using aseptic fluid. Haberlandt (1902) suggested that interrelationships between cells and organisms might be carried out if studies with excised plant tissues could be accomplished. Haberlandt's suggestion was followed experimentally in the development of animal tissue culture methods. Jolly (1903) kept leucocytes in hanging drops for over 1 month. Harrison (1907) worked out an aseptic procedure for procuring nerve fibers from the living frog and keeping them on lymph clot for observation of axone formation by the cell alone. His student Burrows (1910) developed the plasma clot method to cultivate chick tissues. Burrows stated, "The success of the method depends on maintaining absolute asepsis. . . ." Methods for detecting the presence or absence of bacteria were well developed and well known from the classic work of Pasteur and Koch. Lewis and Lewis began studies on an artificial medium (nutrient agar and bouillon) in 1911. Carrel (1911) learned to maintain cells through serial transfer. He suggested (1912) that the first step in the use of cells in culture was to obtain pure strains. He then began his collaboration with Charles Lindbergh on the indefinite culture of chick heart fibroblasts (Carrel et al., 1938). Unfortunately the First World War effectively stopped advances in tissue culture for a decade before serious work with both animal and plant tissue culture began again; it has since continued at an ever accelerating pace.

Robbins (1922) found that autolyzed yeast and peptone increased the growth and survival of repeated subculture of sterile corn root tips. Nutritional inadequacy deterred the success with sterile plants, a pattern seen too frequently in the germfree animal work. One of those to whom W. J. Robbins had demonstrated his technique of repeated subculture of excised root tips was P. R. White, who noted as late as 1936 that no one had grown plant tissues in culture for an indefinite period. This situation changed dramatically in 1939. Gautheret reported the indefinite subculture of carrot root cambium; Norecourt reported the same thing; and, simultaneously, White reported the indefinite subculture of sterile plant callus in an artificial nutrient. This was a real milestone in botanical research. Sanford et al. (1948) pioneered in growing single cells in culture by providing adequate nurture. The reviews of White (1954), Paul (1959), and Wetmore (1959) on plant tissues complement the definitive work of Gautheret (1959). The effect of infection on the defense mechanisms of sterile excised orchid embryos has been studied by Gaumann et al. (1960). Most of the orchids tested were found to produce the mild, broad-spectrum antibiotic, orchinol, when infected with any of 19 mycorrhiza fungi which are symbiotic to them. This chemical defense of the orchid bulb allows a local infection but keeps the fungi from causing a general infection. When 24 saprophytic or semiparasitic soil fungi were inoculated into the orchids, no synthesis of orchinol was induced. Therefore Gaumann and Kern (1959) considered orchinol to be a plant antibody. Nickell (1953) used sterile plant tumors as a vehicle for the study of antibiotic action. Steeves et al. (1957) studied the nutritional needs of excised leaves grown in different media. Hildebrandt and Riker (1953) and M. Ward (1960) used callus tissue for in vitro studies in plant nutrition. Klein and Braun (1960) reviewed work with crown gall tumor induction in carrot discs and tomato plants using sterile extracts. Nickell (1956) devised a system for the continuous submerged cultivation of plant tissue as single cells under controlled aseptic conditions which permits manipulation of plant tissue as single celled homogeneous material. Steward et al. (1952) have used the roller-tube technique for the cultivation of plant tissues. Muir et al. (1958) grew plant tissue in culture with a variable speed shaker system similar to the systems used in microbial fermentation. Nickell (1959) grew substantial quantities of plant tissue in large volume carboy in submerged culture with forced aeration. The plant physiologists now have the techniques needed for studying plant cells and tissues effectively.

The methods of tissue culture of animal cells (Pomerat, 1951 and 1961) are used by a great number of able investigators; e.g., Eagle (1955) in nutrition, Wolff and Wolff (1961) in tumor transplants, Salzman in genetics (1961), and Moscona (1959) in cell interrelationships. However this field is as much in its infancy as is that of germfree plants and animals. Morgan (1958) reviews methods and nutritional requirements of animal tissue cells. Grace (1959) and Vago and Meynadier (1961) reported promising results with insect tissue culture. Several cultures can be maintained for the normal life span of the insect from which they are obtained. Murray and Kopeck (1953) have compiled a bibliography on tissue culture which is useful.

Cooper *et al.* (1959) report the growth of animal cells in continuous suspension culture. The power of microbial techniques has been transmitted to metazoan tissues. Germfree animals provide an ideal source of material for tissue and organ culture. This source is particularly useful for material from the intestinal mucosa. Ward (1961) reported the use of tissue from the gastrointestinal tract for the propagation of continuous cell lines.

Germfree Invertebrates

Pure Culture of Protozoa

While methods for obtaining sterile plant cells, tissues, and organs were being developed, techniques for rearing pure cultures of protozoa were being worked out. Lwoff (1923) obtained a protozoan free from bacteria almost a decade before others began work. The Herculean efforts of Glazer formed a practical basis for the separation of protozoa from bacteria and helped to define the nutritive problems which had to be solved for the axenic rearing of protozoa. The fruit of his seeds can be seen in the symposium on the "Growth of Protozoa," edited by Miner (1953) and "The Nutrition of Invertebrate Animals," by Kidder (1953). Glaser's review (1943) of sterile animal culture surveyed the early methods of aseptic technique with animal tissues and the value of having sterile cultures of protozoa and invertebrates. Migration upward of negative geotropic organisms results in sterile protozoa after 2–3 migrations in sterile water. The downward migration of positive geotropic organisms and the acceleration of this process by the addition of killed yeast cells gave success in two washings. Cleaning the encysted forms of some with 1.25–2.50% potassium dichromate solutions was successful. A V-tube with nutrient agar was used to cleanse many protozoans. A single passage of the protozoan through thickened media usually sufficed. Others have used centrifugation, repeated washing, micropipetting, and the addition of germicides. Antibiotics have been used extensively in recent years to obtain bacteria-free cultures of many protozoa (reviewed by Goldberg, 1959). Thompson (1958) has outlined a simple system for the continuous culture of axenic protozoa.

The nutritional requirements of protozoa, reviewed by Kidder (1953) and Hutner *et al.* (1953) are most varied. Some species have been relatively easy to rear on chemically defined diets (Seaman, 1952; Slater, 1952); others are strict parasites (and/or mutualites) to such an extent that workers have tried repeatedly and failed to rear them free from other living forms. Obviously, on the basis of information presently available, the latter cannot be reared completely germfree, and lack of adequate knowledge of nutritive requirements is again a major deterrent to progress in germfree research. The prodigious amount of work and the problems still remaining in the cultivation of *Endamoeba histolytica* (reviewed by Rees, 1955; and Meleney, 1957) is an example of slow progress in a difficult area. It is probable that the provision of better environments and one or more nutrients (or metabolites) to the parasite would make it independent of the host. Van Wagtendonk (1955) reviewed the axenic culture of ciliates.

Diamond (1960) has obtained two reptilian parasites, both *Endamoeba,* in the axenic state using crude material for diets. A review of the axenic work with one genus of protozoa, *Tetrahymena,* was presented by Corliss (1954). The well defined diets, the simple apparatus, and the ease of obtaining and maintaining large populations of these protozoa makes them extremely useful for studies in cytology, physiology, biochemistry, chemotherapy, morphogenesis, genetics, and cytogenetics. Johnson and Baker (1942) succeeded in maintaining bacteria-free cultures of paramecia. They obtained the sterile organisms by a combination of the migration-dilution technique of Claff (1940) and the washing technique of Parport (1928). They found that the bacteria needed for maximum growth rate could be replaced by fresh yeast juice. Later, Johnson (1952) found that hydrolyzed nucleic acid and mononucleotides would replace the heat-labile factor of yeast juice. This was confirmed by Miller and Johnson (1957), who found the nucleotides of guanine, cytosine, and uracil to be more active than the respective nucleic acids. These authors also reported the amino acid (1957) and fatty acid requirements (1960) of *Paramecium multimicronucleatum* before turning their talents to the culture of germfree metazoa, *sic* planaria. Paramecia also have been used in a variety of other studies, i.e., the identification of a steroid requirement in *P. aurelia* by Conner *et al.*

(1953). Kidder and Dewey (1951) have made extensive use of *Tetrahymena* for studies in biochemistry and nutrition. This is exemplified by their work with antimetabolites (Dewey and Kidder, 1960).

Pure Culture of Metazoa

Work with invertebrate metazoa has recently been summarized by Dougherty (1959) who reviewed the species which have been grown axenically, their natural habitat, the means by which they have been cultured, and the extent of axenic development. He emphasizes that, "those organisms sufficiently tamed for such cultivation are almost all easily accessible in nature." Marine invertebrates are the simplest of all living forms to obtain and rear axenically, as shown by the simple apparatus, procedures, and diets successfully used by early workers in the field. The eggs (easily sterilized with a germicide such as H_2O_2, chloramine-T, peracetic acid, and more recently antibiotics) are transferred to sterile bottles containing a wet nutrient mash in which the larvae hatch, feed, grow, and metamorphose. Complete life cycles of Diptera and other insects are readily studied following the methods of Glaser (1943), Trager (1947), and Stoll (1953a).

Phylum PLATYHELMINTHES

Class TURBELLARIA. Several species of planarians have been obtained in the germfree state by Johnson and Baker (1942), Miller *et al.* (1955), Zwillenberg (1956), and Miller and Johnson (1959). The latter workers have obtained both larvae and adults by repeated washing in sterile water followed by soaking in a mixed antibiotic solution. Antibiotic treatment with fungichromin used to obtain sterile *Dugesia orotocephala* caused a complete loss of pigment in this "black" planarian with no other visible changes (Johnson *et al.*, 1959). Problems of diet were considerable; few planaria would eat heat-sterilized liver, and it was not convenient to provide sterile fresh liver. Aseptically drawn blood, dried yeast, and egg yolk were found to be satisfactory for nutrition; however those individuals fed egg yolk did not survive. Mixtures of egg yolk and yeast or egg yolk and ethylene oxide sterilized liver allowed the survival of axenic worms, but growth was not comparable to that of conventionally reared controls. Johnson *et al.* are presently working on an "attractile" substance in fresh liver. Dougherty is attempting to rear some of the microturbellarians in xenic and axenic cultures.

Classes TREMATODA AND CESTODA. Of the several species of Trema-

TABLE 2.1

In Vitro Development of Parasitic Axenic Trematode and Cestoid Invertebrates[a]

Organism	Host	Nutrient Media	Development	Investigator
Trematoda				
Diplostomum flexicaudum	Larva: fish lens	Fish lens + Tyrode's solution.	Larval development (cercaria to metacercaria)	Ferguson (1943)
Diplostomum phoxini	Larva: snails and fish; Adult: birds	Chicken egg yolk + albumen	Maturation of larva (metacercaria eggs with abnormal shells)	Smyth (1959)
Posthodiplostomum minimum	Larva: snails; Adult: birds	Chick serum + yeast extract, etc.	Maturation of larva (metacercaria), with ovum and sperm production	Ferguson (1940)
Paragonimum westermani	Larva: snails, then crustacea; Adult: mammals	Chick embryo extract + cat erythrocytes.	Prolonged survival of advanced larva (metacercaria);	Yokogawa et al. (1955 and 1958)
Schistosoma mansoni	Larva: snails, Adult: mammals	(1) Amniotic fluid (2) Horse serum + 0.15% glucose (3) 50% Horse serum in salt solution + 1% erythrocytes	(1) Partial differentiation of immature adult (2) Maintenance of adult, with laying eggs (3) Near-maturation of advanced larval stage (schistosomula)	(1) Senft and Weller (1956) (2) Robinson (1956) (3) Cheever and Weller (1958)
Cestoda				
Ligula intestinalis	Larva: copepods, then fish; Adult: birds	Horse serum, etc.	Maturation (without growth) of plerocercoid, with reproduction	Smyth (1947, 1959)

Schistocephalus solidus	As above	Highly buffered horse serum	As preceding; eggs fertile	Smyth (1954, 1959)
Diphyllobothrium dendriticum	As above	Duck embryo extract + horse serum, etc.	Differentiation of plerocercoid fragments to gametogenesis	Smyth (1958, 1959)
Spirometra mansonoides	Larva: in copepods, then mice Adult: in mammals	Chick embryo extract + calf serum	Partial development from larval stages	Mueller (1958)
Taenia serialis	Mammals	Horse serum + NaCl	Limited development of larval stage	Coutelen (1929a)
Echinococcus granulosus	Mammals	Hydatid fluid + human ascitic fluid	As above	Coutelen (1927); Deve (1928)
E. multilocularis	Mammals	Human ascitic fluid + salt	As above	Raush and Jentoft (1957)

[a] Modified from Dougherty (1959).

toda obtained in the germfree state (Table 2.1), only one has been used in both the larval and adult stage. A greater variety of work and somewhat more success has been obtained with the cestodes. The two classes may be considered together since there are many similarities in methods, diet, and stages of development. The parasitic nature of most of the members of these two groups presented difficulty in obtaining a suitable environment for their axenic culture. This was especially true in the development of the diets satisfactory for growth and differentiation. Generally, the problems here appeared to be more difficult than those with free-living nematodes. Larvae are often readily available by aseptic removal from the intermediate hosts (Smyth, 1959).

A complete life cycle of a single species in either class has yet to be obtained in axenic culture. The diets used generally include serum of the adult host for each parasite, and there has been little progress in obtaining chemically defined diets. Since many larvae occur in sterile environments, this stage is most frequently used in axenic research. The different stages of development of cestode and trematode larvae give several precise criteria of success according to Smyth (1959) who points out that much of the work with adult parasites has used only the criterion of survival as a measure of success. Other criteria which should be used are histological condition, maturity, behavioral patterns, and infertility. Smyth's system of growing tapeworms in cellulose tubing was a great technical advance (1954).

Phylum Aschelminthes

Nathan and Laderman (1959) have obtained one rotifer, *Brachionus variabilis*, in axenic culture and have maintained it several days. Eggs were sterilized by exposure overnight to a mixture of penicillin, streptomycin, chlortetracycline, and actidione in the proportions of 1,000 units, 100 units, 50 units, and 0.1 mg per ml respectively. They also studied *B. variabilis* in dibiotic culture with *Chlorella*. Dougherty and Solberg (see Dougherty, 1959) reported they have obtained growth in this species when grown axenically. Later work indicated that a slow growing bacterial contaminant had been overlooked. More recently, Dougherty et al. (1960c), have reared this species in tribiotic culture: *B. variabilis* with *Chlorella pyrenoidosa* and an unnamed bacterial species. They maintained *Lecane inermis* tribiotically in malted milk and filtered pond water, with *E. coli* and another gram-negative, rod-shaped bacillus. A late communication from this trio (1960d) indicates a greater success; they can maintain *L. inermis* in dibiotic culture with an unidentified bdelloid in the absence of all other organisms. These workers also were able to grow *Philodina acerticornis* in dibiotic culture with *E. coli*. These rotifers are bacteriophagous; attempts to rear them without living bacteria met with limited success. Dougherty is presently attempting to grow *P. gregaria,* a species from the Antarctic continent, in dibiotic culture. This species is highly resistant to desiccation and repeated freezing and thawing.

The class Nematoda has been studied extensively during the past two decades. A modification of Dougherty's summary of this class is presented in Table 2.2. Nicholas and McEntegart (1957) presented improved methods for the procurement of bacteriologically sterile eggs from members of this class. Success with *Caenorhabditis briggsae* by Dougherty *et al.* (1959), Nicholas *et al.* (1959), Dougherty and Calhoun (1948b), and Dougherty and Hansen (1956a,b,c) indicates that terrestrial nematodes are easily rendered axenic and easily maintained with diets which contain natural material and extracts. They could not rear species of this class on chemically defined media (a *holidic* diet). Hence, they speculate that the requirement for an unidentified growth factor (named Factor Rb) may be characteristic of the group. Interesting studies were begun on the source and role of DNA using triturated thymidine in the diet of these organisms (Nonnenmacher, 1961). These workers are actively attempting to cultivate a large number of marine nematodes. Nicholas (1956) was able to confirm the work of Zimmerman (1921) by rearing the aquatic nematode *Turbatrix aceti* (the vinegar eel), in axenic state. He used diets similar to those proven successful with the terrestrial Rhabditida.

Axenic cultivation of insect parasitic nematodes was accomplished by Glaser (1940) with sterile kidney as an effective stock diet. Stoll (1959) reported that *Neoaplectana glaseri* was carried 14 years (219 generations) *in vitro*. Studies on the nutritive requirement indicated a possible similarity of the growth factor required for this organism with the Rb factor of Dougherty (1951b). Several free living stages of *Bacterophogous strongyles* have been maintained axenically in media containing natural juices (serum, embryo extract, liver extract, or tissue homogenate). Several synthetic media were tried for the growth of *Nippostrongylus muris* without success; the larvae survived but would not grow. The addition of embryo homogenate serum allowed

TABLE 2.2

AXENIC DEVELOPMENT IN THE CLASS NEMATODA[a]

Organism	Habitat	Nutriment	Development	Investigator
Rhabditis anomala	Terrestrial (saprophagous)	"Liver medium," etc.[b] Chick embryo extract + C.D.[b]	Many generations Several generations	Nicholas *et al.* (1959)
R. pellio	Terrestrial	Raw liver extract	As above	Dougherty and Calhoun (1948)
		Chick embryo extract + C.D.	As above	Dougherty (1953c,d)
R. axei	Terrestrial	Chick embryo extract + autoclaved liver extract	Egg to adult, no second generation	Nicholas *et al.* (1959)
Caenorhabditis briggsae	Terrestrial	"Liver medium"; chick embryo extract + autoclaved extract, etc.; liver protein fraction + chick embryo extract + C.D.	Many generations	Dougherty *et al.* (1956a,b,c); Nicholas *et al.* (1959)
		Chemically defined diet	Slow maturation and limited reproduction	Dougherty and Hansen (1956; Dougherty *et al.* (1959)
C. elegans	Terrestrial	"Liver medium" Chick embryo extract, etc.	Many generations (1 yr.) Several generations	Nicholas *et al.* (1959) Nicholas *et al.* (1959)
Neoaplectana glaseri	Parasitic (insects)	Raw liver extracts + liver infusion broth	7 years	Stoll (1953b, 1959)
		Casein hydrolyzate	"Development" of third stage (dauer) larva	Stoll (1948)
N. chresima	Parasitic (insects)	Autoclaved beef kidney or liver, etc.	As above	Glaser *et al.* (1942)

Organism	Type	Medium/diet[b]	Result	Reference
Strongyloides ratti	Parasitic (mammals)	Chick embryo extract + various supplements	Egg to filariform (third) larval stage	Weinstein and Jones (1957a)
Ancylostoma caninum *A. duodenale*	Parasitic (mammals)	Chick embryo extract; rat liver extract	Egg to filariform (third) larval stage	Weinstein (1953)
A. braziliense	Parasitic (carnivores)	Rabbit kidney extract, etc.	As above	Lawrence (1948)
Necator americanus	Parasitic (man)	Chick embryo extract + various supplementations	Egg to third larval stage	Weinstein (1954); Weinstein and Jones (1959)
Haemonchus contortus	Parasitic (ruminants)	Liver extracts + yeast, etc.	Third larval stage to end of fourth larval stage	Glaser and Stoll (1940)
Vippostrongylus muris	Parasitic (rodents)	Chick embryo extract + various supplementations	Egg to adult (yield variable), but no reproduction	Weinstein and Jones (1959)
Heligmosomum skrjabini	Parasitic (rodents)	Chick embryo extract + Sigma liver or rat serum	Egg to near maturation	Jones and Weinstein (1957)
Ascaris lumbricoides	Parasitic (pigs)	Yeast extract, peptone, etc.	Limited growth from egg	Pitts and Ball (1955)
Dirofilaria immitis	Parasitic (larva: in mosquitoes; adult: in dogs)	Dog serum + C.D.	Maintenance of larval stage (microfilaria)	Earl (1959)
		Tissue culture medium 199	Maintenance of adult stage (filaria)	Earl (1959)
Wuchereria bancrofti	Parasitic (larva: in mosquitoes; adult: in man)	Human serum + glucose + saline	Limited development from larval stage (microfilaria)	Coutelen (1929b)
Eustrongylides ignotus	Parasitic (larva: in fish; adult: in birds)	Broth + glucose, etc.	Prolonged survival larval stage	Von Brand and Simpson (1945)

[a] Modified from Dougherty (1959).
[b] C.D. = Chemical diet; etc. indicates a variety of other materials were added.

development in about one-half of the worms; however, reproduction was not obtained. Similar results were obtained with the human hookworm *Necator americanus* (Weinstein, 1954; Weinstein and Jones, 1959). Limited success was obtained when these workers attempted to rear the parasitic nematodes *Strongyloides ratti, Ancylostoma caninum, Ancylostoma duodenale,* and *Heligmosomum skrjabini.* Sterile eggs would hatch but the larvae would not mature properly. Similarly, *Ancylostoma braziliense* and *Haemonchus contortus* had rebuffed the pioneering efforts of Glaser and Stoll (1940) and Lawrence (1948) respectively.

Vertebrate parasites from the orders Spirurida and Enoplida have also been recalcitrant to all attempts to rear them. Earl (1959) maintained the larvae and microfilariae of *Dirofilaria immitis* for a short time with a chemically defined medium. They could be maintained several weeks when dog serum was added to the medium. His review of his own work and that of others indicated that success with rearing filariae through several generations with chemically defined media should not be expected in the near future.

Nutritional knowledge deficiency clearly limits the usefulness of this phylum for other experimental work.

Phylum ANNELIDA

Dougherty and Solberg (1960) reported successful cultivation of the annelid *Enchytraeus fragmentosus* (Class Oligochaeta), in dibiotic conditions with *Escherichia coli,* and have recently succeeded in growing it in germfree culture (Dougherty and Solberg, 1961).

Phylum MOLLUSCA

Chernin (1957, 1959) obtained sterile snails, *Australorbis glabratus* from germicide treated eggs. Limited growth was obtained with a diet of dried brewer's yeast and formalin-killed *Escherichia coli.* Since conventional snails have been reared through several generations with a syntype diet used for laboratory mammals (Luckey, 1960), rapid progress may be expected in germfree snail nutrition. E. H. Michelson obtained embryos from the uterus of a large ovoviviparous snail (*Vipporus japonicus*) by microsurgery. This technique, reported by Chernin (1959), promises to be one way of avoiding the heavy use of drugs in the procurement of axenic snails.

Phylum ARTHROPODA

Class CRUSTACEA. The only crustacean to be reared axenically is *Artemia salina*, the brine shrimp (Provasoli and Shiraishi, 1959).

Class INSECTA. "Necessity, rather than mere academic interest, has therefore made the axenic culture of invertebrate metazoa a goal for biologists" (House, 1959). Insect larvae were obtained and grown axenically by Guyenot and Delcourt as early as 1911. Küster (1915a) reported that Guyenot started in 1907 and Bogdanow began working with sterile fly larvae in 1898. A milestone in progress was reached in 1946 when Schultz *et al.* reared *Drosophila melanogaster* axenically on a chemically defined medium. A decade later many workers learned to rear other insects in sterile culture using chemically defined diets. The compounds and elements required were remarkably similar to those used for microbial and mammalian species. More important, no major differences were found in the qualitative nutrient requirements for plant parasitic, animal parasitic, or nonparasitic insects.

Review of attempts to rear axenic insects confirms the view that one of the major problems is diet. Very few species have been reared axenically through reproduction. Dougherty (1959) has done real service in reviewing the axenic work as reflected in Table 2.3. The successes recorded are pitifully small when compared to either the abundance or the importance of this class of invertebrates. As noted by Fraenkel, nearly all of the insects used in the laboratory are either insects that feed on dry foods such as flour or grain or the larvae of mosquitoes and flies. This leaves real opportunity for pioneering work in this field. House (1962) has recently reviewed this field.

Bogdanow (1906, 1908) reared germfree fly larvae in order to study the ability of the maggots to form fat from a "fat free" diet (*sic* blood) without any possibility that the maggots were consuming fat already produced by action of microorganisms. Bacteriologically sterile eggs were obtained by treating clean eggs (which were usually sterile without treatment) from fresh meat with 5% $HgCl_2$ solution for 1.5 minutes in a glass wool spindle. The eggs were then rinsed with sterile water. Bagdanow found sterile meat was not a good food for the larvae unless he added sterile trypsin, or bacteria with proteolytic activity. *Bacillus pseudanthracis* greatly improved the growth of the flies, while unidentified cocci were without effect.

Wollman (1911) repeated the work of Bogdanow using similar

TABLE 2.3

AXENIC GROWTH AND DEVELOPMENT IN THE CLASS INSECTA[a]

Organism	Nutriment	Development	Investigator
Order Coleoptera			
Anthonomus grandis	Soybean protein + corn oil + dried yeast + cellulose + sodium alginate + C.D.[b]	Egg to adult	Vanderzant and Davich (1958)
Order Diptera			
Culex pipiens molestus	Various media casein hydrolyzate + C.D.	Egg to imago	Lichtenstein (1948)
Culex pipiens pipiens	Alcohol-sterilized yeast	Egg to imago	Buddington (1941)
Aedes aegypti	Liver extract + heated yeast (larva); defibrinated blood (adult)	Several generations	Trager, in Glaser (1943)
	RNA[b] + C.D. + casein	Egg to imago	Singh and Brown (1957); Trager (1948)
Culiseta incidens	Casein, dried yeast, etc.[b]	Egg to imago	Frost et al. (1936)
Calliphora vomitora	Meat; etc.	Egg to imago	Bogdanow (1908); Wollman (1911, 1922)
C. vicina	Vegetable oils + RNA + C.D.	Egg to pupa	Sedee (1952, 1954)
Lucilia caesar	Meat	Egg to imago	Wollman (1911, 1922)
Phaenicia sericata	Various mixtures	Egg to imago	Michelbacher et al. (1932); Hobson (1935a,b)
Phaenicia cuprina	Casein + yeast + agar, etc.	Egg to fully developed larva	Lennox (1939)
Chrysomya rufifacies	As preceding	Egg to fully developed larva	Lennox (1939)

Organism	Diet[b]	Result	Reference
Phormia regina	(1) casein + agar + C.D.	Egg to adult, without reproduction	Brust and Fraenkel (1953); Cheldelin and Newburgh (1959)
	(2) RNA + agar + C.D.	Egg to adult	House (1959)
Pseudosarcophaga affinis	RNA + agar + C.D.	Egg to adult	House (1959)
Kellymyia kellyi	RNA + agar + C.D.	Several generations	Glaser (1943)
Musca domestica	Heated swine liver + yeast, etc.	Egg to adult, with reproduction	House (1959)
	Casein + agar + RNA + C.D.		House and Barlow (1958); Brust and Fraenkel (1958)
Hylemya antiqua	RNA + agar + C.D.	Egg to adult	Friend et al. (1959)
H. cilicrura	RNA + agar + C.D.	Egg to imago	Friend et al. (1959)
H. brassicae	RNA + agar + C.D.	Slow, limited growth	Friend et al. (1959)
Drosophila melanogaster	Casein + agar + RNA + C.D.	Seven generations	Sang (1956, 1957, 1959)
	RNA + agar + C.D.	Egg to adult	Schultz et al. (1946); Hinton et al. (1951)
	C.D. + agar	Several generations	Hinton (1959)
Order Lepidoptera			
Pectinophora gossypiella	Corn oil + agar + C.D.	2 generations	Vanderzant (1957); Vanderzant et al. (1958)
Galleria mellonella	Petroleum-extracted yeast + Pablum + cholesterol	Larval growth	Waterhouse (1959)
Achroia grisella	As preceding	Larval growth	Waterhouse (1959)
Pyrausta nubitalis	Casein leaf-factor concentrate, etc.	Egg to advanced larva	Beck (1960)
Chilo suppressalis	Dried brewer's yeast + dried rice plant powder + cellulose + C.D. + agar	Egg to pupa	Ishii and Hirano (1955)

[a] Modified from Dougherty (1959).

[b] C.D. = Chemical diet; RNA = ribonucleic acid; and *etc.* = a mixture of several other things.

methods. Wollman used either 1–4% $HgCl_2$ or 10% H_2O_2 as disinfectant. The germfree flies at first grew more slowly than contaminated control flies, but later they grew at a faster rate, and no substantial differences were found after 8 days. Wollman added single species of bacteria to the maggots. *Escherichia coli, B. proteus,* and *Micrococcus pyogenes,* var. *aureus* were stimulatory; *Bacillus putrificus* was deleterious. These experiments were continued by Guyenot (1913c). He obtained reproduction for the first time in "germfree animals" in May, 1911. He found that yeast improved his potato diet and sterilized baker's yeast alone was an adequate diet. Two generations appeared within 1 month yielding 10,000 flies (*Drosophila ampolophilla*). Loeb and Northrop (1916) confirmed the work of Guyenot using yeast to feed sterile *Drosophila.* They reared 12 successive generations of bacteria-free flies. Wollman (1919, 1922) found that germfree flies would live longer than conventional flies. About the same time Bacot and Harden (1922) showed the need for "vitamin B" in *Drosophila. Drosophila* nutrition with axenic adults for egg production has been studied by Sang and King (1961).

Baer (1931), Buchman and Blair (1932), and others used sterile blowfly larvae in the treatment of suppurative conditions. No attempts were made to obtain a complete life cycle in germfree conditions. The larvae of the black blowfly, *Phormia regina* (Meig.), were reared under germfree conditions by Brust and Fraenkel (1958). The qualitative requirements of B vitamins by this organism were similar to that of the white rat. *Phaenicia regina* has recently been reared to adulthood on a chemically defined diet in axenic state and has been used to study the production of proteases (Cheldelin and Newburg, 1959). Several groups are presently studying the nutritive requirements and interrelationships in this organism.

Trager (1935) borrowed the medium of autoclaved liver extract and autoclaved yeast from Glaser (who had found it suitable for rearing paramecia in germfree state) and was able to rear the yellow fever mosquito, *Aedes aegypti,* through many generations in the axenic state. A sterol was required and nucleic acids stimulated pupation. Similar requirements were found by Brust and Fraenkel (1958) for larvae of the housefly, *Musca domestica* L. A synthetic diet containing folic acid supported growth at a slow rate.

An interesting confirmation of the positive role of microorganisms in insects comes from studies on the onion maggot, *Hylemya antiqua* (Friend *et al.,* 1959). Larvae reared axenically grew at a slower rate than did contaminated larvae on a great variety of diets. When grown in dibiotic culture with a bacillus, the larvae did not root at random through the liquid diet but fed mostly in the areas where bacterial colonies had become established. These workers did not study this "bacterial attractant or nutrient," but they have succeeded in growing axenic larvae on a chemically defined diet. Coincidentally, axenic onion maggots cannot live on sterilized onions. Fraenkel (1959) is convinced that intestinal microorganisms are not important in the nutrition of most insects studied.

One of the interesting studies to come from the insect work follows the lead of Friedmann and Kern (1956), who had determined that the wax-eating honey guide could not digest wax when the organisms in the intestinal tract were repressed. However, Waterhouse (1959) fed wax to sterile moths and noted that they could digest fatty alcohols, acids, and esters in the absence of the bacterial flora. Although symbiotism is important to some insects (Koch, 1954), Fraenkel (1959) noted that the requirement of many insects for 8 or 9 B vitamins precluded any great contribution by the intestinal microorganisms to the nutrition of their host.

Special nutrients, as nucleic acids, are required by a variety of insects; other nutrients, such as carnitine, are found to be the special requirement of a single genus, Tenebrio (Fraenkel, 1959). Hinton (1959) has shown interrelationships between environment, inheritance, and nutrition in axenic Drosophila. He concluded that the genetic control of metabolism in metazoan organisms is complicated by multiple genes, modifiers, and other variables. Brookes (1956) and House and Barlow (1958) found that Musca domestica L. required the usual B vitamins for growth.

H. L. House (1959) gave a clear presentation of the status of axenic rearing of insects and some of the problems involved.

As early as 1910 Delcourt and Guyenot explored the possibility of rearing larvae of Drosophila melanogaster Meig. (= D. ampelophila Loew) on a more or less precisely defined synthetic medium, and grew them aseptically. Techniques were developed to rear uncontaminated maggots for surgical use and were widely used about 25 years ago. Techniques continued to be improved by various workers, and in 1946 Schultz et al. for the first time reared a multicellular organism, D. melanogaster, axenically on a chemically defined medium of pure amino acids, vitamins, salts, and other substances. This was done subsequently with other insects, including the Asiatic rice borer Chilo suppressalis (Wlk.) (= C. simplex Butl.), the onion maggot Hylemya antiqua (Meig.), and the pink bollworm Pectinophora gossypiella (Saund.), the larvae of which feed on specific plants; *Phormia regina* (Meig.), and *Calliphora vicina* Desv. ($= C.$ *erythrocephala* (Meig.), larvae of which cause myiasis in animals and birds; and *Pseudosarcophaga affinis* (Fall.), an endoparasite of the prepupae of the spruce budworm *Choristoneura fumiferana* (Clem). The real significance of these accomplishments is evidence that parasitic insects can be reared axenically on chemically defined diets composed of nutrients in simple ionic and molecular forms. Reviews on insect nutrition show, moreover, that phytophagous insects and those that attack animals have nutritional requirements that are very similar to those of other kinds of insects.

House noted that the dietary requirements for even the parasitic forms were qualitatively similar to those determined for mammals. Minor differences in qualitative requirements were important. Equally important in the successes obtained was a clear understanding of the chemical and physical character of the environment: the proper pH, osmotic pressure, consistency of medium, physiological stimuli and, as Sang (1959) would add, the extent of crowding. Dr. House has worked continuously on germfree insects since 1946. He and his collaborators, Dr. J. S. Barlow and Dr. J. F. Bronskill, summarized their methods in a personal communication:

With the viviparous dipteran, *Agria* ($= Pseudosarcophaga$) *affinis* (Fall.), the larvae used on experimental diets are dissected from the gravid female submerged in weak formalin, then transferred to an aseptic (germicidal light) chamber where the formalin is pipetted off, and the larvae are transferred to sterile test tubes containing food medium. With insects that lay eggs, such as *Musca domestica* L., the eggs are washed in soapy water, rinsed in sterile water, transferred to the aseptic chamber and washed with weak formalin or other germicide, rinsed in distilled sterile water and put into sterile test tubes containing food medium. Antibiotics have been fed to insects to sterilize the gut, but they have exhibited harmful effects.

The insects are reared individually on chemically defined diets. Any that appear contaminated, judging from microbial growth or breakdown of the medium, are discarded. Originally the contents of each rearing tube were plated on four kinds of bacteriological media to detect aerobic and anaerobic bacteria, yeasts, and molds. This is no longer done as the food media seem to show the presence of contamination just as well as the above tests did. The bacteriologist at our institute has made complete checks of our larvae, including tissue sections, from time to time and found no evidence of microorganisms present in our insects or experimental diets. Our stock cultures from which gravid females, or eggs, are obtained are not kept free of contamination. Test insects on experimental diets are only handled germfree until larval growth is complete and they are ready to pupate. Though some may pupate (and even produce flies) under aseptic conditions, asepsis is usually broken just before pupation when the larvae are transferred to clean sawdust.

An idea of the simplicity of apparatus used by House and associates is given in Fig. 2.2.

Although nutritional problems of Arthropoda are usually paramount, some insects present special problems in the procurement of sterile material. Intracellular symbionts, particularly in ovarian tissue, have plagued workers who attempt to rear sterile cockroaches (Brooks

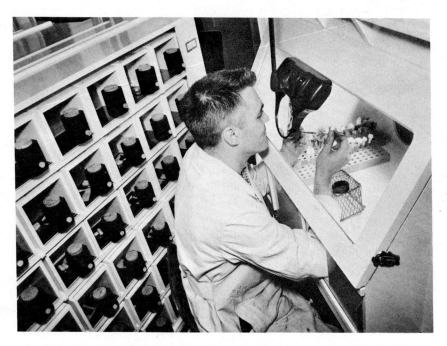

Fig. 2.2. Simplified apparatus for germfree insects. Dr. H. L. House manipulating larva of *Agria affinis* under germfree conditions for nutritional research. Photograph courtesy of Canada Department of Agriculture.

and Richards, 1955). The term symbionts is appropriate because the insects will not grow or survive when the "bodies" are removed. The cockroach, *Blattella germanica* (L.), has been reared (House, 1949a,b) under germfree conditions on a chemically defined diet. The presence of an intracellular parasite in the ovaries of these insects has been suggested, but it has not been shown unequivocally. Waterhouse and McKellar (1961) found that chitinase is released into the digestive tract of the American cockroach, *Periplaneta americana*, in the absence of microorganisms. Continued work by Waterhouse and Corne and the recent migration to Canberra of Nichols from Liverpool and Smyth from Dublin should accelerate significant work in the rearing and use of germfree invertebrates at the Australian National University.

Germfree Vertebrates

Development of Concepts, Apparatus, Methods, and Diets

The first experiments in germfree animal research so profoundly affected subsequent work that they are presented in detail. Subsequent chapters will present the methods used, nutrition, and characteristics of germfree vertebrates. Nuttall and Thierfelder pointed the way for others to follow; their many contributions in their few experiments left techniques that could be improved, but few fundamental innovations to be produced by those who followed. Technical developments, important to the first germfree animal trials were the use of cotton for air filtration by Schroeder and Dusch, Pasteur's finding that steam heat is more effective than dry heat in killing bacteria, the use of the bell jar and other enclosures to provide a sterile environment, improvements in the use of antiseptic solutions, the ability to work aseptically, the transfer of sterile material, and the systems provided by Koch and others for systematically detecting microorganisms. Parallel to these advances were the first studies on the nature of the intestinal flora and the work of Kijanizin (1894a,b, 1895) on the presentation of sterile food to animals.

The idea of rearing germfree animals was first expressed by Pasteur in 1885 during his contemplation of the work on nitrogen fixation with sterile and inoculated plants by Duclaux. Pasteur had presented the work of his student Duclaux to the French Academy of Science, after which he gave his own comments. The statement of Pasteur may seem oracular to the uninitiated. It is actually a clear statement of a proposition which was most reasonable to one who had been deeply embroiled in the controversy over spontaneous generation (in which the key was the complete destruction of all microbes within one environment) and who had helped develop the concepts of fermentation by microbial species. Pasteur knew the problems which beset those who would isolate, cultivate, and classify bacteria; he was the leader in developing the specific germ theory of infectious disease, and now the work of his student Duclaux (1885) with sterile plants reviewed the problems and technical progress which had accumulated so rapidly in the experimental development of all these areas. He addressed his remarks with the full understanding of a genius knowing that a new field of research could and should be opened. He knew that all of the essential techniques for work with germfree animals were available as proven tools in the repertoire of the new microbiology. He also knew that blood, tissues, and embryos *in utero* and in eggs were bacteriologically sterile. Pasteur's comments to the French Academy of Science are presented as the *leit motif* of germfree animal research.

Remarks on the Preceding Note of M. Duclaux

by M. Pasteur

French Academy of Science, 1885

In presenting this note of Duclaux, I take the liberty to offer an idea for an experiment which comes not only from the evidence which I give to the Academy in his name, but also from work, no less distinguished, which he has already done on the role of bacteria in digestion.

For several years during discussions with young scientists in my laboratory, I have spoken of an interest in feeding a young animal (rabbit, guinea pig, dog or chicken) from birth with pure nutritive material. By this expression I mean nutritive products which have been artificially and totally deprived of the common microorganisms.

Without affirming anything, I do not conceal the fact that if I had the time, I would undertake such a study, with the preconceived idea that under these conditions, life would be impossible.

If this work could be developed simply, one should be able to study digestion by the systematic addition to the pure food, one or another single microorganism or diverse microorganisms with well defined relationships.

A chicken egg could be used without serious difficulty for this type of experiment. Before the chick is hatched the exterior could be cleaned of all living organisms; then the chick would be placed in a cage without any kind of microorganisms. In this cage where pure air is given, the chick would also be supplied with sterile food (water, milk, and grains).

Whether the result would be positive and confirm my preconceived view, or whether it would be negative, in other words, that life would be easier and more active, it would be most interesting to perform the experiment.

Except for the local press, the only immediate reaction to Pasteur's statement was that of Nencki, the Swiss chemist who had first analyzed ptomaines a decade previously. In contrast to Pasteur's suppositions, Nencki (1886) argued that life should indeed be possible without bacteria; after all, did not the microbes of the intestinal tract produce toxins such as indole and skatole? He noted that the digestive

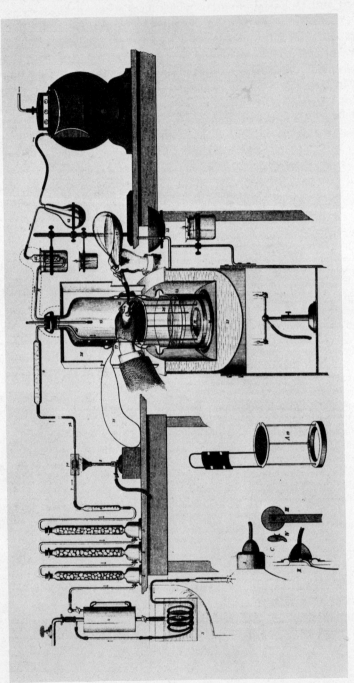

Fig. 2.3.

juices of animals with no bacteria could digest polysaccharides and fats. He hoped that, "we shall one day attain a digestion without irksome gas and stinking products." Nencki predicted that animals with no bacteria should be more healthy and live longer than contaminated animals. Schottelius (1899) believed, with Pasteur, that life without bacteria was not possible and pointed out the fact that digestive juice may be expected to have bacterial metabolic products (enzymes) according to the work of Buchner. This defined the argument supported so elegantly by the wit and knowledge of E. Metchnikoff on one side and balanced on the other side by the failures of Nuttall and Thierfelder, Schottelius, and Mme. O. Metchnikoff in their attempts to rear germfree animals. The experiment of Kijanizin (1895) may have unduly influenced the thinking of scholars at the turn of the century. Kijanizin placed conventional rabbits in a sterile metabolism

---

FIG. 2.3. Apparatus of Nuttall and Thierfelder (1896–1897) for germfree guinea pigs.

I and II. Detail of rubber retractable nipple and its attachment to the cage. The nipple is pushed through the bulb. III and IV protector to keep animal from eating the rubber.

1. Prefilter for air. 2. and 3. Water bath for temperature control of air supply. 4. Water bellows pump gives positive air pressure in the apparatus with 3–6 changes of air per hour. 5. Calcium chloride drying towers (concentrated sulfuric acid was used later). 6, 9, and 12. Cotton air filters. 7 and 8. Air sterilizer with burner under platinum coil (7a). The block was kept red hot. 10. Tube to carry air to the level of the guinea pig. 11. Air outlet in a hot fluid bath to prevent moisture condensing on the outlet filter (12). The insulating cover (dotted line) kept all of the outlet lines warm. 13. Pressure control bulb to ensure positive pressure within the germfree cage (the 1% $HgCl_2$ solution acts as a back pressure trap). The air flow is measured as it exits through the gas meter (14). 15. Bell jar with thermometer with a polished rim connected to the bottom cylinder (16) with heavy rubber band (total volume is 6 liters). 17. Slit connection of balloon (21) through glove (20) into germfree chamber. 18. Guinea pig. 19. Wire grid on stand holds animal above the waste chamber. The glove protector slides down to keep the animal away. 20. Glove attached to jar opening as detailed in II. 21. Balloon with cotton pads wrapped in tissue which are used as bedding. The pads are fed into the cage through the glove slit (17). 22. Sterile milk in flask. 23. Holding bath for the milk flask with temperature control. 24. Rubber band used to keep a tight seal between two polished rims of the bell jar and waste cylinder. 25. Oil layer over the water in the waste chamber is useful to reduce the humidity in the bell jar. 26. Thermometer. 27. Water bath used to maintain the animal at 25°C. 28. Glass walled box to help keep temperature constant.

cage and allowed only sterile air, water, and food to be given them. They gradually lost weight, showed a negative nitrogen balance, and died. Kijanizin concluded that death was due to decreased numbers of bacteria. This work was used as indirect evidence that decreasing the bacterial population was harmful to the host.

Germfree animal research began when Nuttall and Thierfelder (1895/96) tried to rear germfree guinea pigs in their laboratory at the University of Berlin. Their primary purpose was that of all investigators during the first two decades of germfree experimentation: to determine whether life is possible in the complete absence of microorganisms. They placed Cesarean-delivered guinea pigs into a sterile bell jar adapted for the purpose and fed them aseptically drawn and sterilized milk. The first animal was germfree, appeared to be healthy, and weighed as much as the control at 8 days, when it was sacrificed for examination. They concluded that the presence of bacteria in the intestinal tract is not necessary for the life of guinea pigs or other animals, or man, at least so long as the food is purely of animal origin. This was their answer to Pasteur's remark of 1885. Their second publication was based on several animals fed nutritious cakes of vegetable materials. The animals from their next three experiments were contaminated, but the two guinea pigs from the fourth and fifth experiments were carried 10 days and found to be germfree. The germfree animals did not gain as much weight as did the controls. They concluded that bacteria are needed for adequate digestion of vegetable foods. They gave up work with guinea pigs because it was "too complicated and uncertain" and tried experiments with chicks. Because the literature of the period indicated that chicks could not be obtained free of bacteria, they had not followed Pasteur's suggestion about chicks originally. In a preliminary experiment they examined the tissues of unhatched chicks and found them to be sterile. Two unsuccessful experiments with one contaminated germfree chick in each experiment discouraged them from further work. Although the work of these two pioneers in the field was limited it established the techniques which were modified by men who followed their path to success.

In the work of Nuttall and Thierfelder, one can see the major elements of germfree research as they exist today. These pioneers studied all situations carefully and usually came up with an acceptable answer. In order to obtain germfree guinea pigs they learned to determine time of parturition. They developed anesthetic procedures which would not too adversely affect the young. They worked out the surface sterilization of the abdomen, procedures of aseptic Cesarean operation for small animals, and aseptic transfer of the young from the uterus into a sterile environment. Sterilizing of the environment was not really different from that used by the plant physiologists, except for the complexity of the apparatus. Nuttall and Thierfelder had to determine the kind of food to be used and the sterilization of the food, of large quantities of air, and of other material. They worked out a system for the collection of excreta in order to study the metabolism of the animals. The manipulation of the animals by means of rubber gloves was an innovation which required the connection of rubber to other material. They apparently used antiseptic solutions to introduce other material—food, water, or utensils. Such a germicidal trap is still used. They sterilized milk and devised nipples for feeding newborn mammals. Their system for testing germfree animals was very similar to that used in germfree plants, but they should be given credit for a systematic test for sterility in germfree animals and for the first observations of germfree animals. They described differences between contaminated animals and germfree animals; i.e., the enlarged cecum of the guinea pig which plagues experimenters today.

Nuttall and Thierfelder believed that the evidence from their guinea pig studies indicated that bacteria are required for the digestion of natural products but not for homologous food. Schottelius, on the other hand, suggested that the weight increases they obtained in guinea pigs were primarily a filling of the gut and contended that decreased weight of the germfree guinea pig was good evidence that bacteria are needed for proper digestion in higher animals. He was careful to point out the difference between the questions, "Is there life without bacteria?" and "Are bacteria necessary for the life of higher animals and for the human?" He would answer both questions in the affirmative. On the other hand, O. Metchnikoff suggested that the germfree guinea pig experiments of Nuttall and Thierfelder *were successful.* She pointed to the fact that the animals lived for many days and *grew.* This controversy continued for the rest of their lives. The problems they attacked were far from easy. During the next six decades several groups unsuccessfully tried to rear healthy guinea pigs, but only recently has this species been reared through one complete generation in the germfree state by B. A. Teah in 1959.

Rearing Germfree Vertebrates

Pisces

Germfree fish have been obtained by Baker and Ferguson (1942) and by Shaw (1957), and were mentioned by Reyniers and Trexler (1943b). In all cases, the fish used have been of the small, viviparous species.

Baker and Ferguson (1942) used the small tropical platyfish, *Platypoecilus maculatus,* obtained from Mexican waters. It is 4 or 5 centimeters in length and readily available from commercial fish hatcheries. It bears about 20 young every month and is readily adaptable to many experimental problems. Pregnant females were immersed in alcohol for 3 minutes and then in tincture of iodine for 7 minutes. The tincture of iodine was removed by an alcohol bath and finally by an ether bath. This effectively sterilized the continuous epidermis which covers the scales of the fish and gave a dry sterile surface for the operation. Incision into the abdominal cavity allowed a sterile pipette to be introduced, and gentle suction produced a rupture of the ovary containing the embryos which were drawn into the pipette and placed in a dish containing sterile water. Such a procedure gave 10–15 young per female. The young were then distributed singly or in pairs into cotton-plugged bottles containing about a liter of water. Sterile food was introduced once or twice a month and the fish were observed to eat in normal fashion.

Bacteriological examination was made by placing whole fish or samples of the water in which they had lived into infusion broth and meat media incubated at room temperature and at 37° under anaerobic and aerobic conditions. Almost all fish were found to be free of microorganisms. Mold occasionally was found in some of the containers. In most cases when it occurred, microbial contamination had been seen by inspection of the aquarium, which showed mold or turbidity before the bacteriological culture test was run. The fish were maintained for as long as 4 months and grew considerably, although no reproduction was obtained. The authors believe that nutritional factors were the principal cause for the lack of continued growth and reproduction.

In the nutritional study they found that fish fed agar particles apparently died of starvation. The contents of the yolk sac were depleted, and their decline was gradual with weakness and progressive emaciation signaling death. The young fish showed almost no growth, since they remained only about 1 centimeter long until they died at 2–3 weeks. Some growth was seen when commercial fish food was given, and the survival time was 60–90 days. Growth was rapid during the first month but gradually decreased. When sterile nematodes were added to the commercial fish food, growth was somewhat better and the survival period was then 75–120 days. When the fish were fed the nematodes alone, *Neoaplectana glaseri*, the fish grew and survived as they had on the commercial fish food. When the nematode diet was supplemented with heat-killed algae or autoclaved housefly larvae, or when pond water was substituted for tap water, no real advantage was seen. Obviously, further work needs to be done before this species is acceptable as a normal tool for germfree research. Apparently, the major problem was nutritional and should not be insurmountable with our present knowledge of the effects of sterilization upon nutrients.

Shaw and Aronson (1954) found that the eggs of *Tilapia microcephala* could be sterilized by dipping them in 0.04% formaldehyde solution in water for 10 minutes. When these eggs were aseptically transferred to sterile water they hatched and developed into germfree fry. In a later communication, Shaw (1957) reported on 25 trials with 10 eggs in each group. Later, 8 of the 25 trials remained germfree. The eggs which were not germfree died during the experiment, indicating that certain bacteria were harmful contaminants for the fish. Although they were not fed, the germfree fry survived 2 or 3 weeks after hatching. They used a large quantity of their own yolk for their food. Eventually, these fry died of starvation after the yolk was absorbed. Some of the dead fish were kept as long as 4 months when they were then discarded. They did not disintegrate, and no microorganisms could be cultured from the dead fry when inoculations were made into nutrient broth, nutrient agar, and thioglycollate media.

Shaw suggests that the cichlid fish might be more appropriate for germfree experiments than the platyfish, since the platyfish appeared to require live food for their maintenance, and *T. microcephala* can regularly be raised on dry food which could be easily sterilized. It is noted that Shaw never worked out a system for feeding his germfree fish. Further advantages of this species are the larger number of fertile eggs which are available, the ability to raise many fish together with little care, and the reproduction at frequent intervals during the entire year. Thus far no one has reared germfree fish for an extended period.

Amphibia

Three investigators have attempted to rear amphibia. O. Metchnikoff and Wollman worked with the grass frog (*Rana temporaria*), and Moro worked with tadpoles of the toad (*Pellobates fuscus*). All three apparently had the same purpose—namely to determine whether life was possible without bacteria. In addition, O. Metchnikoff noted the desirability of working with vertebrates which would be easier to rear germfree than guinea pigs or chickens. The work of O. Metchnikoff (1901) was outlined by her husband, Eli, who sincerely hoped that she would obtain evidence that life was indeed possible without bacteria. Madame Metchnikoff removed the outer envelope of an egg containing a mature embryo of *Rana temporaria*, rinsed many times with sterile water, and placed in a sterile environment. When the embryo hatched it was fed bread which had been heated to 110°C in a sterile flask. When fed bread, both sterile and nonsterile tadpoles developed more slowly under experimental conditions than did tadpoles under normal conditions. At 80 days, by which time normal tadpoles are completely transformed, the sterile and nonsterile experimental tadpoles showed rudiments of the metamorphosis period. These differences may be due to space, aeration, and food. Therefore, she concluded it is much better to compare the sterile and nonsterile tadpoles under the same conditions. She started with 80 tadpoles; 31 of them died the first day; 42 were contaminated; and 7 remained sterile throughout the experiment. Of the 42 contaminated tadpoles, 7 lived for the 80 days, while of the 7 sterile tadpoles, 5 lived past the 65th day. This would tend to indicate as Wollman (1913) suggested that bacteria under these conditions make living conditions worse. The size and weight of the contaminated tadpoles was variable but, in general, they were larger than those of the sterile tadpoles. The largest germfree tadpole was equal in size and weight to that of the smallest contaminated tadpole.

In a 34-day experiment the 4 survivors of 8 germfree animals weighed an average of 0.025 gm and were 1.2 mm long in contrast to the controls (contaminated with bacteria from the intestine of a conventional frog) which averaged 0.076 gm and were 2.3 mm long. The germfree tadpoles showed no tendency toward limb formation and were less vigorous than the controls. All the controls metamorphosed; 2 of the 4 germfree animals survived being placed in a contaminated environment and developed normally. Wafers and egg white were the main food constituents used, with milk being added as a supplement.

Moro (1905) repeated the experiments of O. Metchnikoff using toad tadpoles with greater attention to details, such as maturing of the embryos, but with no greater success. His aeration system was more efficient. The eggs were collected in a 1% boric acid solution as a disinfectant. The outer membrane (containing many microorganisms) was removed and the eggs were washed in flowing water, the next jelly coating was removed, and the eggs placed in 0.3% boric acid.

Wollman (1913) used *Rana temporaria,* as had O. Metchnikoff. He sterilized the eggs at hatch with sodium perborate or hydrogen peroxide and with dilute "antiformine." The newly hatched tadpoles were kept about 1 week to test sterility and the sterile ones put in rearing bottles which had been cotton stoppered. He fed a paste of meat and bread. To test sterility, the material from the bottle was diluted with bouillon and incubated as a broth and with gelatin at 37°. Wollman also examined the intestinal contents of the tadpoles microscopically to show that they were sterile. In his first experiment in 1911, he reared only 1 sterile tadpole. It was well developed at 24 days. In his second experiment, he had 16 sterile tadpoles and 15 contaminated tadpoles. The contaminated tadpoles were reared in an open crystallizing dish which had its water changed every 2 days. In the third experiment, he had 29 sterile tadpoles and 30 contaminated tadpoles. The observation that all the contaminated tadpoles died the first day verified the findings of O. Metchnikoff that certain bacterial strains are harmful to tadpoles in confinement. Wollman noted that all the sterile tadpoles at the age of 1 month were as large as the largest contaminated tadpoles, and most of them had well developed legs by 30 days.

In 1912, Wollman ran another series of experiments. The data are given in Table 2.4. Results indicated that the sterile tadpoles grew at a rate equally fast and sometimes faster than the contaminated tadpoles, and again many contaminated tadpoles died when microorganisms were present. Generally, the development of the posterior legs of the conventional animals was faster than in the sterile tadpoles. Wollman concluded that this shows that a wide variety of animals are able to eat and develop normally without the help of microbes; he knew the results obtained with the guinea pigs of Nuttal and Thierfelder; he had just learned of the first germfree goat of Küster, and he knew his own results with sterile flies fed enzyme digested food and that Guyenot had concluded germfree flies reproduced better than contaminated flies. The pictures presented by Wollman illustrated that the tadpoles were not well developed, had not matured well, and were far from a complete metamorphosis even in the sterile condition. Since all contaminated animals died, no comparisons can

TABLE 2.4

GROWTH OF GERMFREE TADPOLES, *Rana temporaria*[a]

Experiment	Age	Germfree tadpoles (length in mm)	Contaminated tadpoles (length in mm)
1	1 month	26, 28, 29, 30	21, 27, 28
2	1 month	20, 21, 21, 26, 28 32[b], 40[b]	30, 32, 32, 35

[a] Data from the 1912 experiments of Wollman (1913). The length of 1 day old tadpoles was 13–16 mm.
[b] Posterior legs well formed.

be made. This series of experiments indicates that Amphibia have not developed properly in the absence of bacteria. Later experiments with nonsterile tadpoles (Luckey, 1961a) have shown that tadpoles grew and metamorphosed when fed a syntype diet, but as noted by the early investigators, the development was much faster in a balanced aquarium.

AVES

Several species of germfree birds have been reared including a variety of chickens, turkeys, and quail. It is apparent that other species such as ducks, geese, and pheasants could be easily obtained in sterile condition. The chicken has been the classical animal of germfree research. It was used in all major laboratories up to 1950 with the possible exception of those of Miyakawa, Glimstedt, and Gustafsson.

Nuttall and Thierfelder (1897) showed that the chick embryo was sterile while the surface of the egg shell was not. When their attempts to sterilize the surface failed they stopped germfree experimentation. Schottelius (1899) verified the fact that the inside of the egg can be sterile. He learned to sterilize the outside of the surface and obtained sterile chicks.

Obviously, the ease of obtaining new material makes the germfree chick well suited for germfree research. It is easily maintained; it learns to eat and drink by itself; it presents no foster mother problems and is independent as soon as it has hatched. It will eat a variety of feeds, and taste is not a major factor with this species. The species grows rapidly and occupies a much larger space within a few weeks; however, this may be a distinct advantage since large quantities of biological material are available. Heart punctures can be made very easily without anesthesia, and most tissues are large enough for biochemical analyses. The germfree chicken has been well studied because it is a suitable tool for nutrition studies, for biochemical studies, and for morphological, physiological, and serological examination. The strains of chickens used have the greatest drawback in their variability and size. Inbred strains of chickens are not as uniform as those of mice and rats. Thus, larger numbers of animals or greater differences must be obtained before the work reaches statistical significance.

Schottelius (1899) ran preliminary experiments on the bacteriological status of the interior and exterior of the egg and on means of sterilizing the egg surface. In order to correlate the weight of the newly hatched chick with the weight of the egg at setting, he also studied water loss in the hatching eggs and the weight of chicks given no water. He did this so that he would not have to weigh newly hatched chicks in a germfree environment. He next cleaned a large room in the new Institute of Hygiene at the University of Freiburg for the sole use of his experiments with germfree chicks. Near the center of this room he built a series of cubicles (see Fig. 2.4). Other details of his cubicles and his operation will be given later. The inside of the cubicle was kept sterile. The operator entered after donning a sterile gown and gloves and stepping in the antechamber. Very surprisingly, after all these elaborate precautions to keep the chicks germfree, Schottelius placed his contaminated control chicks in a container next to that of the sterile chicks in the same sterile cubicle. Later, he more wisely kept the contaminated chicks out of the cubicle area.

The germfree chicks of Schottelius (1899) fed millet, chopped eggs and shells, ate continuously, gained some weight (see Table 2.5) for 12 days, after which they became progressively weaker. The first experiment was stopped at 17 days when the chicks appeared moribund. Since growth was acceptable in conventional chicks reared in similar cages next to those of the germfree chicks and since they were fed in exactly the same way, Schottelius concluded that intestinal bacteria are essential for the adequate nutrition of the animal. He, therefore, became interested in what microbial species may be required in order to translate such results to practical human hygiene. In 1900, Schottelius began experiments designed to find such an

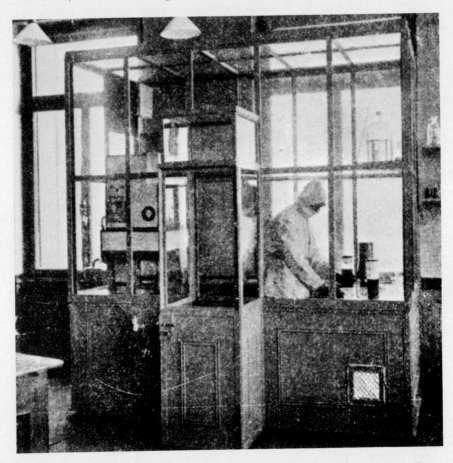

Fig. 2.4. Sterile room of Schottelius (1908a). Note the entry cubicle in the center, the air filter at the lower right, and the incubator inside the room to the left of the entry.

organism. In the first experiment, 4 germfree chicks were maintained until 2 of them became weakened at 8 days. Then, this master of the germfree technique slid a glass partition into place to divide the cage into two completely separate, identical, germfree cages, each containing 1 strong and 1 weak chick. Into one of the compartments he poured 20 gm of nutritive fluid inoculated with fresh excreta from conventional chicks. This fluid was poured over the food and floor and a few drops were added to the water. The weak germfree chick died at 10 days of age and the weak inoculated chick died at 15 days. The strong chick which remained germfree, continuously rushed to and fro along the middle glass wall as if trying to get to the other chick. On the 16th day of life this animal was visibly tired and on the 21st day it died. This germfree chick lost 10 gm or 23.5% of its body weight. The control chick weighed 52 gm at 3 weeks of age. This was 6 gm above the calculated hatch weight. In 1901 this experiment was repeated with 4 chicks, 2 of which were inoculated with a pure culture of *"Bacillus coli gallinarum."* One of the sterile chicks died on the 11th day and the other on the 12th. The monoinoculated chicks survived. Later, Schottelius (1908a) repeated these experiments using two separate cages because the sliding glass panel was too complicated. He concluded that he had shown conclusively that bacteria are needed for animals which are fed heterogeneous foods. He believed the growth of the milk-fed germfree guinea pigs of Nuttal and Thierfelder was not a true test and predicted that these animals would require bacteria if fed their usual plant food. He pointed out that his results conformed to those of Metchnikoff and those of the plant physiologists. He completely ignored the action of the bacteria on the food before the chicks ate it and of the nutrients (vitamins and protein) present in the 20 gm bouillon used as inoculum.

Later, Schottelius (1913) agreed that life was possible without bacteria ("since every bacillus shows it can live and can thrive without bacteria") as demonstrated by the absence of microorganisms in the intestinal tract of parasites and other organisms. The question to be considered was whether warm-blooded animals and human beings could live without bacteria. He observed that long range experimentation in germfree research is excessively expensive and cannot be oversimplified. The technical ability of Schottelius was superb, but unfortunately knowledge of nutrition at that time was not adequate for his efforts to bear fruit. His total number of sterile chicks was quite small for this decade of hard labor. How different this field would be if he had started 30 years later. Modern reviewers (see Reyniers *et al.*, 1949b) who note Schottelius' failure to obtain growth in germfree chicks cite his poor diets and the destruction of vitamins by heat sterilization as the suspected cause of his failure.

Eli Metchnikoff, as head of the Pasteur Institute, finally sent one

TABLE 2.5

GROWTH OF GERMFREE AND CONVENTIONAL CHICKS

Investigator	Year	Days	Number	Gain in grams per day	
				Germfree	Diet and cage control
Schottelius	1898	4–17	10	(0.3) −0.5 to 0.7	0.6
	1899	11	1	−1.4	0.8
	1899	13	1	−1.0	2.0
	1899	21	1	−0.5	1.5
	1899	25	1	−0.7	1.5
	1899	29	1	−0.5	0.5, 0.7
	1900	12	2	−1.3, −1.1	0.3
	1900	30	1	−0.5	0.6, 0.4
	1901	10	2	−0.1, −0.1	0.7
	1901	11	1	−0.1	0.6
	1901	18	1	−0.6	
	1908	16–23	7	No growth	Inoculated chicks grew
	1908	28	11	Poor growth	All inoculated
Cohendy	1907[a]	13	2	0.6, −0.7	0.4, 0.6, −0.5
	1908	20	1	3.0	2.0
	1908	15	2	2.0	1.0, 1.5, 2.3
	1909	33	1	1.3	1.9
	1910	6–40	4	Poor growth	—
	1911	35	2	0.5, 0.7	0.1, 0.5, 0.6, 1.0
	1911	12–22	3	Poor growth	—
	1911	45	2	0.2, 0.6	0.2, 0.2, 0.3, 0.4

				4.2, 8.5, 8.9, 9.6 All died, See text	5.8, 6.3, 7.4, 7.8 All died
Balzam	1937	59	4	4.2, 8.5, 8.9, 9.6	5.8, 6.3, 7.4, 7.8
	1937	10	4	All died	All died
	1937	68	7–1	See text	—
Reyniers	1938	6	2	2.3	3.8
	1938	10	2	0.7	—
	1938	11	3	5.3	6.4
	1938	12	2	2.8	4.3
	1938	15	1	5.3	—
	1938	18	1	7.2	6.8
	1939	4	2	0.0	4.0
	1939	5	1	−2.0	−0.6
	1939	8	2	2.0	—
	1939	10	2	3.6	—
	1939	11	1	3.3	1.8
	1939	17	1	3.9	6.4
	1939	21	4	1.2	—
	1940	5	3	3.4	5.2
	1940	10	1	5.1	6.0
	1940	12	4	3.8	—
	1940	23	5	4.3	7.0
Reyniers and J. Reback	1940	30	2	7.5	7.7
	1940	30	4	5.4	2.3
Reyniers and E. Foley	1940–42	34	16	3.6	—
	1940–42	22		4.4	5.6
	1940–42	28		5.1	

a Done at Freiburg with Schottelius.

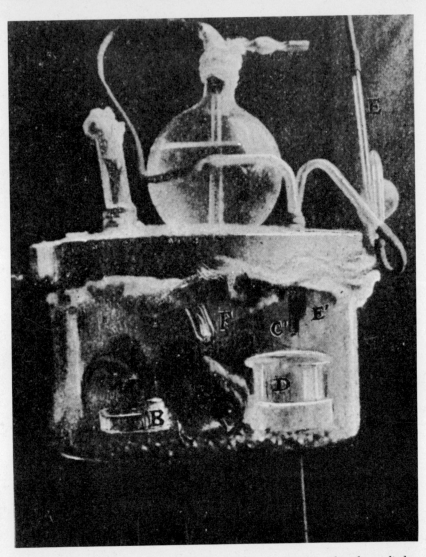

FIG. 2.5a. First germfree chick cage of Cohendy (1912a). This glass cylinder (15 × 28 cm) had the lid made by layers of cotton pressed between two wire screens with a metal rim made bacteria-tight by layers of cotton between the lid and the cylinder. Food was introduced into the shallow container (B) through the glass tube through the lid above it (the seal between this tube and the lid was a cotton filter). The other opening in the lid contains two tubes. One (C) leads from the water storage to the waterer (D) in the cage. The other (E) is connected to a vacuum pump which draws air through the cotton roof into the germfree cage. Sterile 20 day embryonated eggs were aseptically placed into the sterilized cage and the cage placed into an incubator having a glass door. The tube of broth (F) was intended for bacteriologic control; it remained unused.

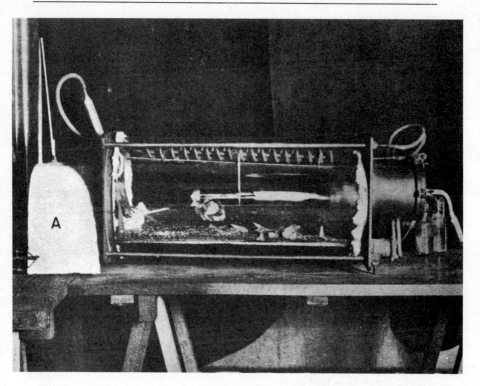

Fig. 2.5b. Second germfree chick stage of Cohendy (1912a). This glass cylinder (80 cm long and 35 cm in diameter) has a bronze plate bolted together and sealed to the ends of the cylinder with cotton and rubber gaskets. The left plate contains a small tube for the admission of cotton filtered air, and a large opening into a 25 cm copper brooder (A) attached. This opening has a woolen curtain which retains the heat of the brooder and has a slit in the center to allow easy passage of the chick into either chamber. The end of the brooder had a small door which was unscrewed to allow aseptic entry of sterilized eggs. The brooder is lined with asbestos to retain body heat and has a pierced nickel plate floor over a taut canvas cloth kept moist from the overflow of the water fount. A water cooled condenser is attached to the top of the plate on the right side of the cylinder. Moisture removed by this coil drains into the water fount. The plate on the right has 3 openings with metal stoppers gasketed with cotton. On the inside is a metal grill to protect them from the chicks and on the outside a screw cap is attached. The top opening contains a stopcock through which the air exits. This can be removed to allow tongs to be used inside the cage. The center opening is large enough that one can reach through with a hand. The small opening at the bottom serves to remove waste. These openings are used only under the protection of a rubber tent sterilized with mercury chloride spray.

of his outstanding young men, M. Cohendy, to learn germfree techniques from the acknowledged master Schottelius. Here, Cohendy learned how to obtain germfree chicks. The following year, 1908, he returned to the Pasteur Institute where he performed several experiments in a simple cage made from a glass cylinder (see Fig. 2.5a and b). The workings of this cage are described in the history section on cages. The daily variations of his diets are suggested in Table 2.6. It is

TABLE 2.6

DIETS OF COHENDY

Day	Diet
	First Experiment
1	None
2	Dry bread crumbs and egg yolk
3	As on day 2 plus a mixture of ground corn, potatoes, rye, barley, and lettuce
4–15	As on day 3 plus milk
5	
6	As on day 3 plus millet and flies
7–12	As on day 3 plus chopped egg and chickory
	Second Experiment
1–2	None
3	Whole crushed, (hard cooked) egg and sand
4–6	As on day 3 plus flour
7	As on days 4–6 plus rice, milk, and grains[a]
8–11	As on days 4–6 plus rice and milk
12–19	As on days 4–6 plus 8 flies
18–23	As on days 4–6 plus lettuce
24	As on day 3
	Other Experiments
1–11	As second experiment plus meat and fat

[a] A variety of grains were used: thistle, sorghum, white and red millet, mohar and flax seeds.

noteworthy that the chicks of Cohendy did grow (see Table 2.5), and that he was able to draw the memorable conclusion that life without microbes is possible for one vertebrate, the chick, which normally has a rich microbial flora. He found that germfree chicks resembled contaminated chicks as far as their gross morphology, development, and appearance was concerned. However, most germfree chicks exhibited an extraordinary appetite when food was available and they excreted copiously. He showed that germfree chicks have great resistance to hunger, cold, humidity, and thirst. When they were returned to conventional (polycontaminated) life they grew to adulthood. He also maintained chicks with a single organism and found that this could be harmful. For example, germfree chicks which became contaminated with *E. coli*, at 25 days weighed little more than half as much as conventional birds kept in a similar cage and fed sterile diets. The two monocontaminated chicks weighed 75 and 62 gm while the three conventional birds weighed 120, 102, and 95 gm respectively. Küster (1913a), critical of the conclusions of Cohendy, would have no comparisons made unless all conditions of the control group were exactly the same with the exception that it be inoculated. Küster gave Cohendy credit for important advances toward the solution of the question of germfree life but noted his work did not answer the question.

Twenty-five years after Cohendy's last germfree chick work, N. Balzam (1937, 1938) studied the effect of the intestinal microflora on the B-vitamin requirement of the chick. In his first experiment, 4 germfree chicks showed good growth and normal development for 59 days (see Table 2.5). Since the diet he used contained no vitamin C, he concluded that chicks do not get vitamin C via the intestinal microflora. His balance data are presented under "characteristics" (Chapter 5). In the second experiment, yeast was omitted from the diet to study the "vitamin B" requirement; all germfree and conventional chicks died within 6–10 days. Both groups showed typical beri-beri (thiamine deficiency) syndrome. Balzam suggested that the difference between these data and those of Schottelius could be explained by the wet food presented to the inoculated chicks of Schottelius which may have fermented after it was sterilized.

Balzam's third experiment was designed to give a quantitative estimate of the yeast required. Seven germfree chicks were fed the yeast-free diet. At 9 days the only survivor exhibited severe polyneuritis and the diet was supplemented with 10% yeast. The chick doubled its weight in 1 week. When the yeast content of the diet was lowered to 2.5%, the growth rate decreased to less than 3 gm/day. When the yeast was increased to 8% of the diet, the chick showed an immediate response to 15 gm gained each day. At 68 days it weighed 450 gm and was taken outside where it continued to gain 14 gm per day. Balzam interpreted his work as evidence that the intestinal microflora gave practically no protection against B-vitamin deficiency.

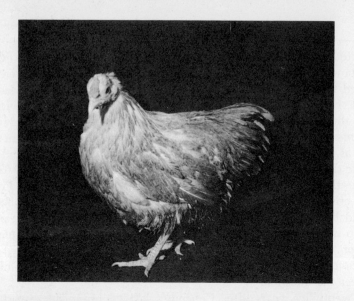

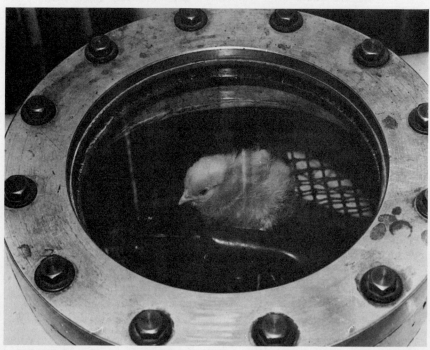

FIG. 2.6. First reproduction in germfree vertebrates. *Upper:* Germfree Wyandotte Bantam hen. *Lower:* Second generation white Wyandotte Bantam chick.

R. Naito (1937) developed his own method for rearing germfree chicks and Akazawa (1942) used germfree chicks to study the effect of staphylococci, *E. coli*, and an aerobic spore forming bacteria upon the chicks. A summary of the work of the students of Matsumura was given in 1948 by Tanami (1959) who continued these studies with guinea pigs. The major works are presented in the chronology.

Reyniers and associates (1949b) perfected the experiment with germfree chicks. The early work (Reyniers *et al.*, 1949b) with chicks fed commercial mash produced erratic growth responses (see Table 2.5) but in later work, diets were developed which gave consistently good results. Reyniers and Trexler (1943b) developed heavy-walled metal equipment which is strong enough to withstand steam pressure sterilization (see Chapter 3) and is adaptable for a variety of experimental uses. The group at the University of Notre Dame, Forbes *et al.* and Phillips and associates, the workers at Chiba University in Japan, and this author have contributed the major portion of information about germfree chicks which is presented in subsequent chapters. Germfree birds have been reared on both practical and synthetic type diets, and germfree white Wyandotte Bantams have been reared through egg production and to the second generation (Fig. 2.6a and b) by Reyniers *et al.* (1949d).

Although chicks have been the most used of the species in Aves, turkey and quail are also useful. No systematic data have appeared on turkey (Luckey *et al.*, 1960) or quail (Reyniers *et al.*, 1960) comparable to the quantity available on chickens. For this reason and for the reason that methods developed for rearing germfree chicks appear to be adapted easily and successfully in rearing other avian species, emphasis has been placed upon the chicken.

MAMMALIA

Guinea pigs. The guinea pig is another classic animal of germfree research. The first experiments with germfree animals were performed with guinea pigs and have been described. Guinea pigs were used by most investigators, because as stated by Nuttall and Thierfelder (1895–1896), "Of all the mammals concerned, it alone was useable" (without a prolonged suckling period). Most workers have been frustrated by the difficulties involved in raising and feeding germfree guinea pigs and by the enlarged cecum which prevented the study of normal development and reproduction for half a century. In spite of these difficulties, guinea pigs have been studied for various research problems, and the results have been major contributions to the annals of germfree research. The pieneering work of Nuttall and Thierfelder (1895–1896) with germfree guinea pigs was the introduction to germfree animal research and needs no repetition here.

The third period of the germfree work of Cohendy was devoted to the rearing germfree guinea pigs (Cohendy and Wollman, 1914). They maintained guinea pigs in the germfree state for 16–19 days and found that the germfree guinea pigs were similar to the controls. Both were underfed according to the standards of today. Eight years later, Cohendy and Wollman (1922) collaborated to study vitamin C deficiency and virus infection in germfree guinea pigs. They obtained scorbutic animals in one experiment, and in another experiment they successfully inoculated *Vibrio cholerae* into guinea pigs which harbored *Staphylococcus.*

Glimstedt (1932) was able to rear germfree guinea pigs for 2 months. He fed the animals from a catheter five times daily. The base diet used was milk with plasma added for protein and cream added for fat. The calorie/protein ratio was adjusted to correspond to that of guinea pig milk, and vitamins A, B, C, D, and E were added. Oatmeal was used in small quantities to improve the appetite. Guinea pigs fed this material became "hungry crazy" and bit everything possible. The second diet used consisted of 88% soy bean flour, 7% filter paper, and 5% McCulloms salts. The guinea pigs grew poorly (Fig. 2.7)— both germfree and control—but life was maintained. At last, emphasis could be taken from the question of "Is life possible without bacteria?". Glimstedt made extensive plans for studies on the lymphatic development, metabolism, reproduction, physiology, nutrition, biology, and medicine. A summary of his morphological study and his observations on the underdeveloped lymphatic system is given in Chapter 5. Reyniers (1932) attempted to rear germfree guinea pigs as living culture media to study microbial heredity and changes. In 2 years he obtained 6 germfree guinea pigs of which the 3 that survived the day of operation lived 4, 5, and 8 days respectively. No details of equipment, diet, or character of the animal was given. Reyniers and Trexler (1943b) and Reyniers (1946a) indicated that germfree guinea pigs developed normally for about 3 weeks, after which the growth rate decreased and death occurred at about 2 months. The animals were very active, appeared starved, and ate ravenously.

Thorbecke *et al.* (1959) confirmed the findings of Glimstedt on the underdeveloped lymphatic system, using guinea pigs which were in a much better state of health. Miyakawa (1959b) and his associates studied the effects of tuberculosis in the guinea pig. After many years of trial at the University of Notre Dame, Phillips and associates (1960) worked out diets which successfully maintained guinea pigs

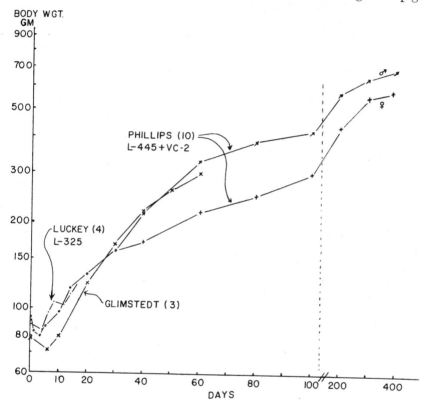

FIG. 2.7. Guinea pig growth. The number in parentheses gives the number of animals represented by the curve.

for the required period of time, and studied guinea pigs inoculated with a single protozoon or with a protozoon and a single bacterial species. The guinea pig has been brought to reproduction in the completion of a germfree life cycle by Teah (Fig. 2.8) at the University of Notre Dame and, more recently, by Phillips and Newton at the United States Public Health Service, National Institutes of Health. Many of these guinea pigs appeared to be in good condition, but the phenomenon of the enlarged cecum is ever present.

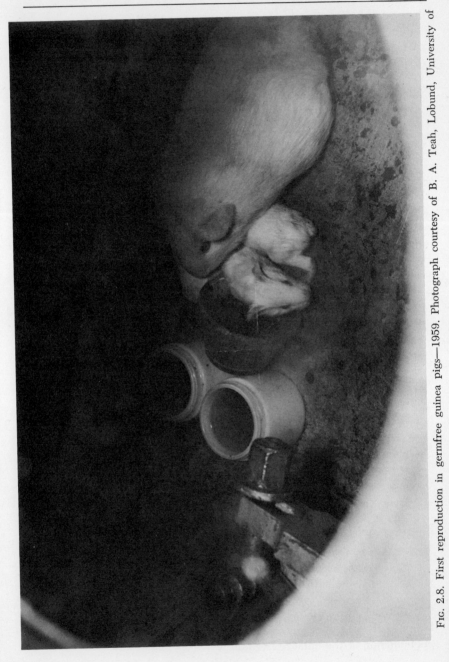

Fig. 2.8. First reproduction in germfree guinea pigs—1959. Photograph courtesy of B. A. Teah, Lobund, University of Notre Dame.

Rats. Germfree rats may be easily obtained in large numbers by a Cesarean operation of a dam prior to parturition. Unfortunately, at birth the animals are quite helpless. It is most difficult to hand-feed newborn rats and care for their every need until they can forage for themselves without recourse to letting them suckle their mother or a foster mother. Reyniers and Trexler (1943b) reported difficulty due to the small size and immature condition of rats at birth. Gustafsson (1946) weaned a few germfree rats which did not grow satisfactorily. All had enlarged ceca and reduced size of thymus and lymphatic organs. In 1947, he obtained growth of germfree rats that was equal to the growth of control rats fed via stomach tube. His diet was steam sterilized milk with added casein hydrolyzate, vitamins, and minerals. The growth of one germfree animal which grew well is given in Fig. 2.9. Gustafsson (1948) gave a full report of 23 experiments with a total of 76 germfree rats. These rats had voracious appetites and excreted unformed feces. The impressive difficulty of Gustafsson was the small size of the germfree cage. His subsequent work was done with a much larger apparatus (1959b).

In the early work of Reyniers *et al.* (1946) germfree rats could be weaned only occasionally (less than 3%) and the growth rate was poor (Fig. 2.9). Some of these were reared to maturity. In their experiments vitamin C minimized the bloating in hand-fed rats, increased the growth rate, and lowered the mortality.

In the first of two long-term experiments one animal was weaned and carried 298 days before it became contaminated with two species of bacteria. Since it was not sacrificed until 1 month later, the autopsy observations have little meaning (excessive fat in the abdomen and around the heart, ovaries, and uterus). The second experiment with 4 weaned germfree rats also became contaminated. These rats were free from bloating during the pre-weaning period and were continued as diflora rats with *Aerobacter aerogenes* and a gram-positive coccus. Each of 3 female rats gave birth during the 244 day experiment; 20 young were born and 14 were weaned. The legends given for the pictures and blood data of these rats are misleading since the rats were not germfree at the end of the experiment, as indicated by the dates, ages, text, and the high white blood cell counts recorded.

The problems and progress in the hand-rearing of germfree rats is presented in detail in the chapter on nutrition. The culminating effort of Pleasants (1959) resulted in diets, apparatus, and techniques which were adequate to wean 85% of the rats. The first colony of germfree

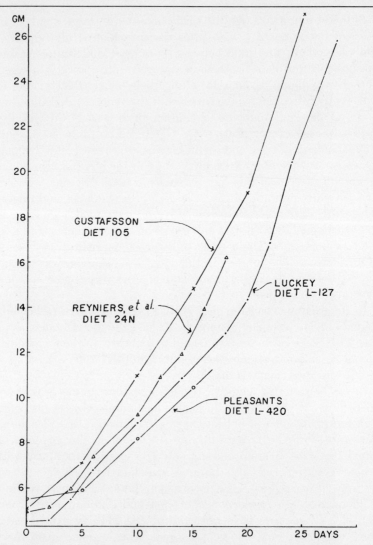

FIG. 2.9. Growth rate of hand-fed germfree rats (average of 10 rats in each group, excepting that of Gustafsson).

rats was started in 1950 (Fig. 2.10). Colonies are now in existence at the University of Notre Dame, The University of Lund, the National Institutes of Health, United States Public Health Service, and the Walter Reed Army Medical Center. Most germfree rats are plagued with enlarged ceca; however the size is not large enough to prevent growth and reproduction (12 generations of germfree rats are reported by Reyniers, 1959b) but it is an ever apparent problem and is being studied by Wostmann and Bruckner-Kardoss (1959). The germfree rat can be accepted as an experimental tool with certain reservations.

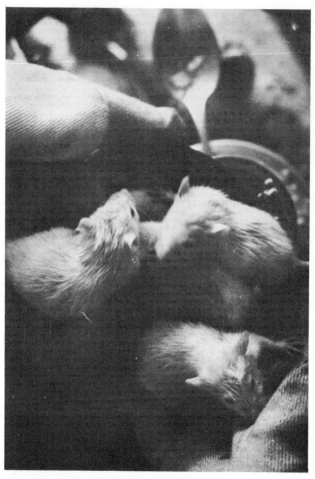

FIG. 2.10. First second generation germfree rats weaned. Note canvas gloves used to protect rubber gloves when handling animals or doing rough work.

Most people using the germfree rat today do not begin their own colonies but obtain stock material from one of the colonies listed above or the animal farms listed in the chronology.

Mice. Sporadic attempts to rear germfree mice have been made by

Reyniers and associates (1943b) throughout two decades, and until the germfree rat problem was solved the difficulties with mice were not surmounted. Shortly after it was learned how to raise germfree rats routinely, Pleasants (1959) tackled the problem of rearing germfree mice and succeeded very soon in obtaining colonies. Extensive studies on the germfree mouse have not been made. Growth of hand-fed germfree mice is given in Fig. 2.11. Several major problems remain to be solved before acceptable mice can be reared by hand: Swiss

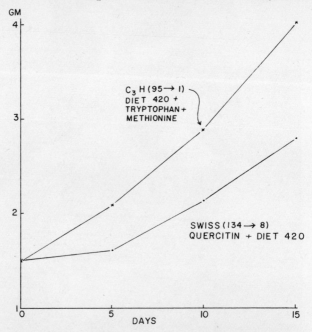

FIG. 2.11. Growth of hand-fed germfree mice (Pleasants, 1959). Numbers in parentheses indicate success (number at start → number weaned).

mice have cataracts, leg deformities, and rachitic rosary; C3H mice are more difficult to rear and very few were weaned. Since colonies of germfree mice were started, other strains of mice are available by means of foster suckling following a Cesarean operation. Eleven generations of germfree mice have been reared (Reyniers, 1959b), and as Trexler (1959a) has noted, the best picture of the germfree status is possible when the studies can be followed through many generations. A photograph of one of the 5 germfree mice autopsied for this presentation is given in Fig. 2.12.

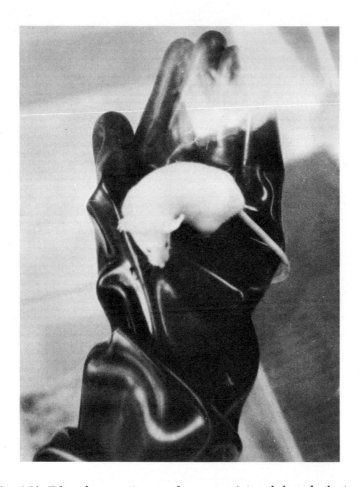

Fig. 2.12. Fifteenth generation germfree mouse (viewed through plastic cage wall).

Rabbits. Germfree rabbits have been reared at the University of Notre Dame by Luckey and Teah (unpublished) (Fig. 2.13) and by Pleasants (1959). The enlarged cecum problem was more serious in this species than in any other. The growth rate was good for hand-feeding (Fig. 2.14) and 23% of those obtained by Pleasants were weaned. Most of the rabbits which reached adult size died due to complications resulting from enlargement of the cecum. Consequently, the species has not been studied thoroughly. The general appearance

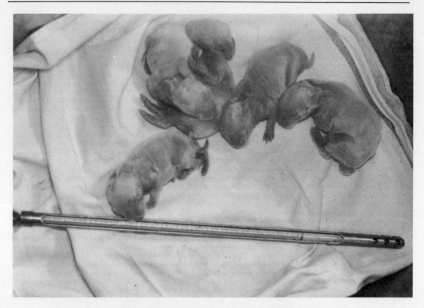

Fig. 2.13a. Newborn germfree rabbits.

and growth of this animal is quite comparable to that of a conventional animal. The rabbit is large enough at birth for it to be easily hand-fed, but it has not been brought to reproduction in the germfree cage. It should be noted that the conventional rabbit has been raised on synthetic diets and on sterilized synthetic-type diets through reproduction (Luckey, 1961a). Pleasants and Wostmann (1959) reported that maturity and reproduction in the germfree rabbit were thwarted owing to deaths caused by the enlarged cecum. Pleasants has recently (1961; personal communication) reared germfree rabbits which have reproduced.

Monkey. Germfree monkeys have been reared by Reyniers and associates (1943b). They found no major problems in obtaining germfree monkeys, and the growth rate was quite acceptable (Fig. 2.15). The development and general appearance of the germfree monkeys were comparable to that of conventional monkeys. The first monkey was contaminated at 31 days, the second survived several months. Both animals appeared to be healthy. At the present time no systematic study has been made of this species.

Dogs. The rearing of germfree dogs has been attempted by Schottelius (mentioned in 1902), Glimstedt (unpublished; mentioned by

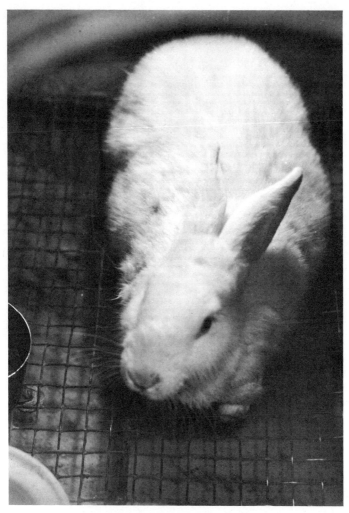

FIG. 2.13b. Mature germfree rabbit.

Gustafsson, 1946), and by the Notre Dame group (unpublished).
Thus far, all have found that they could obtain germfree dogs, but
the majority of germfree dogs still carry worms. Therefore, routine
production of germfree dogs must await the cleaning of dogs to rid
them of the worms. Such procedure is quite possible. The data obtained from germfree dogs are limited to those of pups (Phillips, 1960)
and what appears in Chapter 5 in this volume. It should be noted

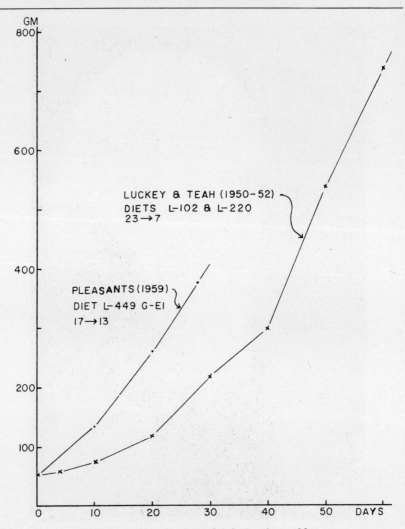

FIG. 2.14. Growth of hand-fed germfree rabbits.

that the nutritional problems of the dog have not appeared to be major ones, and conventional dogs have been reared to maturity on synthetic-type diets (Luckey, 1961a).

Ruminants. Küster began working as assistant to Schottelius. His view broadened until he became interested in more than providing data for the controversy regarding the possibility of life without bacteria. After leaving Schottelius, he began germfree research with goats in order to have enough material for serological, histological, physiological, and nutritional studies. He noted that goats are also good food utilizers, are easily raised on a bottle, and that the goat "possesses a great life energy." His pilot experiment (1911) showed that a young kid could be obtained germfree by Cesarean section. In

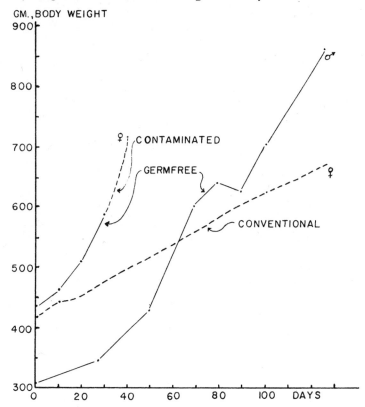

Fig. 2.15. Growth of germfree monkeys (Reyniers and Trexler, 1943b).

his second experiment (1912), the kid was delivered in a sterile tent and passed into a sterile box fitted for urine and feces collection. This animal died before eating, but it was found to be germfree. The germfree kid of the third experiment (1912) ate goats' and cows' milk and gained 2 lb in 12 days; it became contaminated on the 11th day. After moving to Dahlem, Küster performed the fourth operation. The kid obtained was reared germfree until a glove tear contaminated the chamber at 36 days. The condition of the animal, its food intake, and weight increment (Fig. 2.16) were comparable to that of conventional goats, and the utilization of sugar and fat was good. Küster's (1915a) laborious method for obtaining sterile milk exemplified the care and precautions required in germfree experiments. Milk was drawn asep-

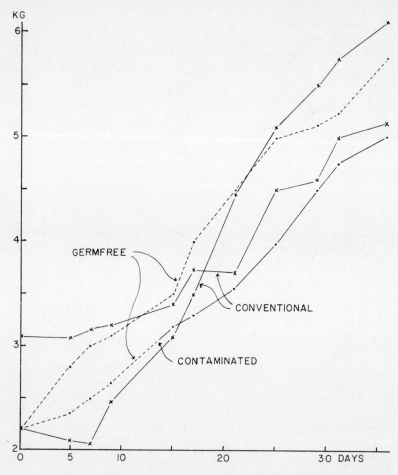

FIG. 2.16. Growth of germfree goats (Küster, 1913b).

tically from the cow through sterile cotton filter into a sterile bottle; this was heated for 15 minutes in a hot water bath on 5 successive days and the stopper pushed in without removing the paper cover. These bottles were watched for any sign of microbial action for at least 6 months. The milk used in the last experiment had been collected 12

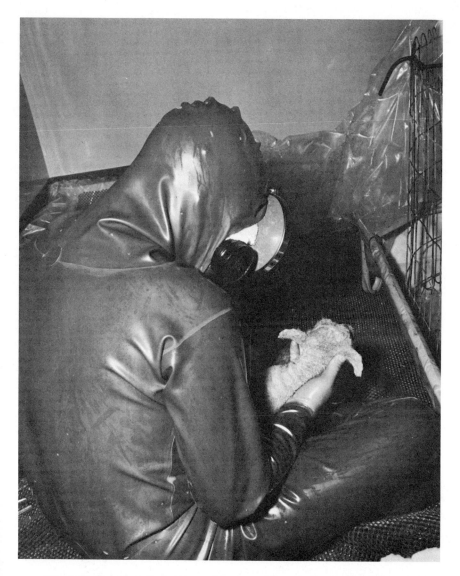

Fig. 2.17. Germfree lamb in germfree room. Photograph of author by R. Noll, University of Missouri.

or more months previously. Smith and Trexler (personal communication) have recently attempted to raise germfree goats. The first attempt apparently gave a monocontaminated goat. It is anticipated that Smith will continue this work at the University of Michigan.

Germfree lambs have been obtained by Luckey (1960) and by Smith and Trexler (1960) (see Fig. 2.17). The germfree lamb has the gross appearance and development of contaminated lambs, although no thorough study has yet been made of them. It is notable that the Notre Dame workers used sterilized milk for the lamb diet, while Luckey fed a synthetic-type diet which had proven to be successful with conventional lambs through 2 seasons of feeding.

Pigs. Germfree pigs have been obtained by Landy *et al.* (1961) at the University of Arkansas using the Cesarean operation and are expected to be used for surgical studies, since the pig is closely related to the human from a morphological viewpoint. They are fed fortified cow's milk without hand-feeding and grow at a rate as fast as that of conventional pigs. It should be mentioned that germfree pigs are actually obtained in operations for disease-free pigs, but they are not maintained in a sterile environment. These pigs are reared in the system which could be used for gnotobiotic animals (Young, 1959).

Summary

Throughout the written history of man the concept of infectious agents, such as miasma in the air, has been expressed. The concept of an invasive agent carried with it the concept of evasion and isolation which was one of the first and major methods for fighting infectious diseases. This is seen in the Bible and is stated throughout the history of microbiology even before van Leeuwenhoek discovered microbes as living organisms. With the advent of knowledge of the variety of microorganisms came the early studies on attempts to isolate one species from another. The pure culture concept of Koch and the methods developed by the early microbiologists was most useful in the separation of one species from another and led to the mechanical foundation for the establishment of pure cultures. Single cell isolation has taken many forms. The methods found to be useful for bacteria were directly applicable to protozoa, fungi, and other microorganisms as well as isolated tissues and cells of plants and animals.

The methods of germfree research were largely worked out by the plant physiologists and the microbiologists of the nineteenth century.

The plant physiologist borrowed apparatus and methods from the gas chemist who had learned to separate one gas from another. The work of Pasteur and others on spontaneous generation and the germ theory of disease gave excellent methods for the complete sterilization of enclosed systems and the detection of microorganisms. From the microbiologists the early botanists learned how to sterilize rearing chambers with heat and how to keep them sterile while sterile air was being introduced. The use of this technique in the nitrogen fixation controversy was a colorful prologue to germfree animal work. During the end of the controversy on nitrogen fixation, Duclaux reported his rearing of peas with and without bacteria. This report challenged the imagination of Pasteur enough for him to state that he would, if he had the time, like to undertake experiments with germfree animals— with the preconceived notion that life without bacteria would not be possible. Nencki's reply that bacteria are indeed harmful since they produce noxious compounds led to another controversy; namely, is animal life possible without bacteria? This problem was approached experimentally in 1897 by Nuttall and Thierfelder who used guinea pigs and chickens and very shortly thereafter by Schottelius with chickens. Success in rearing germfree plants, plant cells, and tissue cultures occurred simultaneously with the development of the rearing of animal tissues and cells free from other species. The next development was the rearing of metazoa free from bacteria. Work with the rearing of the species of aschelminthes, annelids, and insects in axenic culture has been reviewed. Since the early work with chicks was not successful, O. Metchnikoff and Moro turned to amphibians. Several attempts were made to rear sterile tadpoles. Germfree fish have been obtained, but never reared successfully. While germfree chicks were obtained by Schottelius (1898–1908), he lacked an adequate knowledge of nutrition to raise them successfully. In 1912, Cohendy reared germfree chickens by giving a wide variety of material as a diet. Cohendy showed that life and growth of vertebrates was possible without bacteria. Cohendy's work was verified by Balzam in 1937 who obtained acceptable growth in germfree chicks. Balzam also began a study of the effect of the intestinal microflora upon vitamin B production and utilization by the host. Reyniers and his associates undertook the study of germfree chickens through several decades, and germfree chickens were reared through reproduction with the diets of Luckey in 1949.

Rearing of germfree guinea pigs had been attempted unsuccessfully by Nuttall and Thierfelder in 1896 and was attempted again by Wollman and Cohendy during the second decade of this century. During the end of the third decade Glimstedt began to work with germfree guinea pigs. He was able to maintain them for 1–2 months and in 1936 gave the first full view of a germfree animal with all its morphological characteristics. Reyniers and associates made several attempts to raise germfree guinea pigs but it was not until the decade 1950–1960 that germfree guinea pigs were reared successfully by Phillips and Wolf and carried reproduction by Teah in 1959. Both Gustafsson and Reyniers and associates were able to rear germfree rats prior to 1950. Diets devised by Luckey led to the first reproduction in germfree mammals and in 1950–1960 germfree colonies of germfree rats were obtained. Following the success with germfree rats, germfree mice were reared by Pleasants in 1957, and colonies of germfree mice are now available for research. Luckey and Teah reared germfree rabbits in 1952, and in 1961 Pleasants obtained reproduction in spite of problems with the enlarged cecum. Küster, 1911–1913, reared germfree goats to 2 months of age and others have attempted to rear germfree lambs, pigs, and monkeys for short periods. Bacteria free dogs have been obtained but thus far no one has successfully reared germfree, worm-free pups. The success obtained with the major laboratory animals would encourage the view that others could be readily made available for germfree research.

CHAPTER 3

Germfree Animal Techniques

Cages

Theory

The philosophy of isolation as applied to the animal as a biological unit, the elimination of contamination and the theoretical needs of the instrumentation of the principle of isolation were considered by Reyniers (1943; 1959b,c) and Trexler (1960c). A germfree animal must be obtained and maintained in an environment separated from the ubiquitous microorganisms in and about us. Although examples have been presented in the first chapter where no mechanical barrier existed, a dependable mechanical barrier is essential for experimental work. In accordance with the philosophy that degrees of biological isolation exist, the isolation involved in germfree research is relative, not absolute. The animal has indirect contact with the experimenter through a viewing glass and rubber gloves or other mechanical pickup system; and the isolation of a germfree animal from living microorganisms does not necessarily involve isolation from biologically distinct products of microorganisms. Thus, several degrees of biological isolation (germfree, antigen-free, and virus-free) are of current interest. Fortunately, the requirements of the barrier are very similar for these several degrees of isolation. The barrier might be active physiologically as well as passive physical material; consider the tissues, cells and fluids of the uterus, or the egg shell and membranes which harbor the sterile embryo. Sometimes nonturbulent air flow or physical distance in a small tube separates one environment from another for effective microbial sterility. Pasteur used the latter method to show that air-borne agents did not penetrate into sterile flasks when air currents were excluded. The air of some germfree cages currently in use is exhausted through an open tube. The constant positive pressure inside and the outflow of dry air assure maintenance of sterility.

In consideration of the ideal germfree cage, it must be remembered that neither a complete physical barrier nor thorough sterilization of the chamber can prevent indigenous microorganisms from entering. An impermeable mechanical system can keep exogenous microorganisms from entering the cage, but a major break in the mechanical barrier must always accompany the introduction of the animal into the system. Physiological, serological, and immunological barriers are as important as physical barriers at this point. It would be most difficult to obtain germfree animals if a parasite were passed *in utero*. Gard (1959) found 100% incidence of an intracellular parasite in one strain of mice. Therefore, stock free from such contaminants must be used for germfree research.

The physical barrier might be as simple as a flask plugged with cotton. Much of the work with plants, tissue cultures, and invertebrates employed Erlenmeyer flasks. Or the barrier might be a most complex mechanical device, a room, or a building. The complexity and the size have little to do with the principles of operation; an intact mechanical barrier is needed to separate all living microorganisms from the animal being studied. It should be emphasized that control of the biological variable in an isolator is a refinement of enclosures used for other purposes. Other enclosed systems control physical factors such as barometric pressure, temperature, humidity, sound, airflow, light, and composition of gases; these are factors which can be exactly controlled in many types of enclosures. The difference between these systems and germfree cages is simply the modification of the mechanical unit to control the living forms present as another parameter under the control of the investigator. The systems considered in this chapter can be used for other gnotobiotic work by inoculating germfree animals with one or more known microorganisms.

Since a complex variety of germfree cages exist, an exemplar (Fig. 3.1) will illustrate the essential elements of the system. A germfree isolator, cage, or tank might have any or all of the elements given in the stereotype exemplar. The main physical barrier surrounding the animal may be comprised of metal, plastic, glass, or rubber. A glass port may be used for light, viewing, or photography. The air inlet and the air outlet usually are mechanical filters; sometimes both filtration and heat are used. In one small germfree unit (Fig. 3.2) the air outlet was simply a 0.5 meter tube. The air flow and the air pressure were controlled by the size of the orifice at the end of the tube. Both gravity and air flow prevented the entrance of microor-

ganisms as long as the tube remained dry. Another essential part of
the physical barrier is a rubber or germicidal gasket between one part
of the unit and another; i.e., the connection between the glass port
and the tank. Most germfree tanks have a means for manipulation:
gloves gasketed into the side of the tank; mechanical arms, as in the

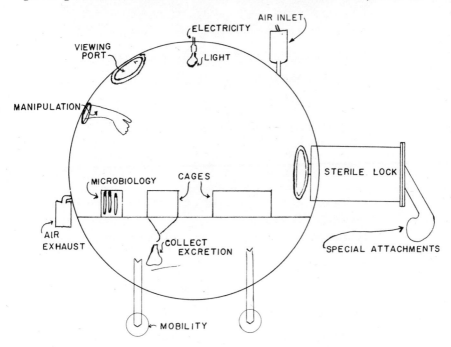

Fig. 3.1. Exemplar. The exemplar typifies the main parts of the germfree
rearing tank or isolator. The essential quality is that the barrier remain intact and
prohibit bacteria from entering.

tank of Miyakawa (1959c) (Fig. 3.3); or a man in a sterilized suit
(see Fig. 2.17) in a germfree room. The barrier usually has a means
for connecting one unit to another. In the exemplar this is done through
the sterile lock. Material is admitted through the outside door, sterilized, and taken into the tank through the inner door. The sterile
lock is sometimes a germicidal trap. Much of the adaptability of the
exemplar comes from ingenious use of the sterile lock. The outer door
may be glass to admit more light; it may have an opening for a
germicidal gas; it may have a special attachment for bringing eggs
through a germicidal trap; or it may be used to introduce cooling,

heating, or temperature control units to make an incubator out of the sterile lock. The tanks usually have a plug to bring electricity inside, but simple isolators eliminate this requirement. Since modern labora-

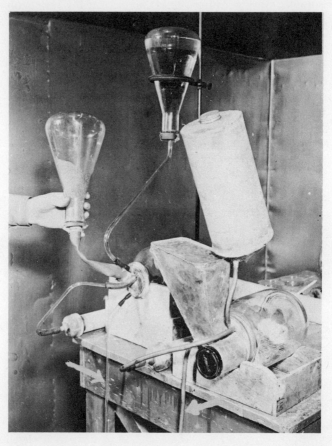

Fig. 3.2. Simplified germfree chick cage. These churns jars have specially adapted lids for feeding, watering, introduction of eggs, air supply, and exhaust. The free flow air exhaust is a tube about ⅔ of a meter long extended downward. (T. D. Luckey, 1956, *Ann. N. Y. Acad. Sci.* **78**, 130.)

tories require mobility, heavy tanks have wheels. Mobility of equipment is usually preferable to having long connections for sterilization. The tank must have a means of being sterilized; this is usually accomplished with steam in metal isolators, germicides in plastic isolators, and sometimes radiation in folded plastic isolators. The isolator usually contains a coarse screen floor or a floor with bedding; often it

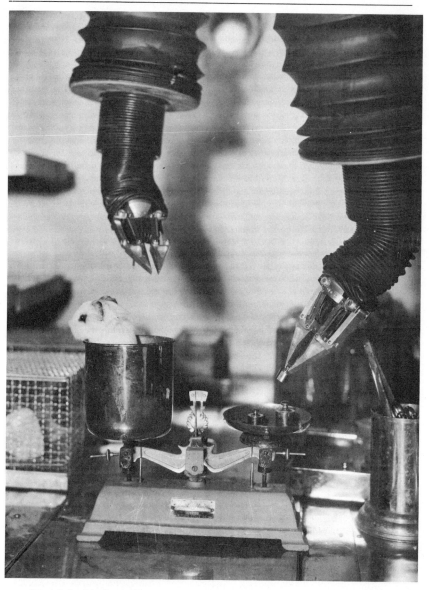

FIG. 3.3. Mechanical arms in germfree isolator. The tank of Miyakawa (1959c) has special adaptations for using mechanical arms in the rearing cage. The fingers are delicate enough to hold the guinea pigs, to feed and bathe them, and to take cultures. The Cesarean birth was performed in an attached Reyniers operating unit. (Photo courtesy: M. Miyakawa (1959) *Ann. N. Y. Acad. Sci.* **78,** 40.)

has a means for the collection of excreta. Within the isolator there are usually cages to contain the germfree animals; these animal cages must have a means of holding food and water supplies. Other parts of the tank can be used for storage. All germfree tanks have a means for gnotobiotic monitoring. A constant supply of sterile air, or oxygen, is required, and control of humidity, temperature, and air pressure are

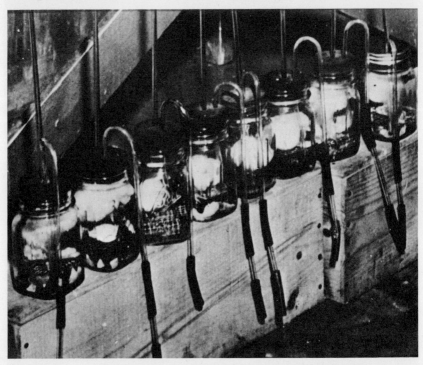

FIG. 3.4. Simple germfree container. Chicks were maintained in individual half-pint jars until sterility tests could be run on them. The germfree ones were then aseptically placed in a larger unit.

essential. Finally, most tanks have a large door to facilitate cleaning and maintenance.

Tanks are made to fit the purpose of the investigator. Small cages are made for short term work and special cages are made for transportation. Simple jar systems (Fig. 3.4) have been used by Schottelius (1908a) and Luckey (1956a) to test for sterility; and a glass jar with a rubber glove was designed by Reyniers *et al.* (1959a). Probably the ultimate in simplicity for a germfree container is that used by Gustafsson (1959a). Germfree rats were simply placed in a canning

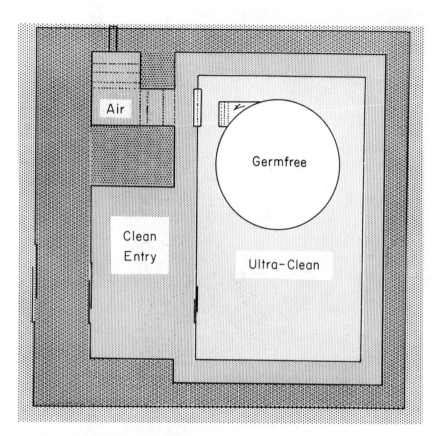

Fig. 3.5. Diagram of germfree room. This illustrates the versatility of the principles of isolation. This isolator is a simply designed area made with conventional labor and materials. The germfree tank in the room gives maximum security against contamination. The room itself has been used as an isolator. (T. D. Luckey, 1956, *Ann. N. Y. Acad. Sci.* **78**, 134.)

jar and taken from the sterile cage through the germicidal trap into another sterile cage. The air within the jar is adequate for several minutes. The other simplified germfree isolator is the plastic envelope.

Most germfree cages are large enough to hold 5 to 50 small laboratory animals. However, large cages have been made, germfree rooms have been found useful (Luckey, 1960), and suites of germfree rooms such as that of de Somer and Eyssen (1962) and germfree buildings are within the realm of engineering possibilities.

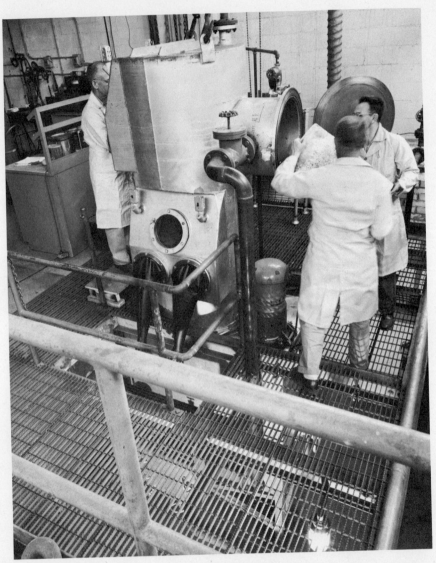

FIG. 3.6. Use of isolator for commercial chemical reactions. Here an atmosphere different from air is needed. No oxygen can be admitted to this particular reaction. Note the similarity in structure, concept, and practice between this apparatus and a germfree isolator. (Photograph by courtesy of Creamer-Trowbridge Co., Providence, Rhode Island.)

The ideal germfree system has a series of barriers between the germfree animal and the outside world. Such a system in which a germfree tank is placed within an ultra-clean room is shown in Fig. 3.5 (Luckey, 1956a). The ultra-clean room itself was microbe free for repeated experiments without being recleaned. This minimized chances of contamination from leaks in the tank. Constant positive pressure within the isolator (inaugurated by Nuttal and Thierfelder, 1896b) and means for repair of leaks are essential for routine operation.

Although germfree applications will be emphasized in this presentation, the cages and concepts presented are generally applicable to use with inoculated animals. A parallel development has occurred in equipment for work with virulent infectious agents and chemicals in controlled environment (Horsfall and Bauer, 1940; G. B. Phillips *et al.*, 1955; Walton, 1958; and Gremillion, 1960) as illustrated in Fig. 3.6.

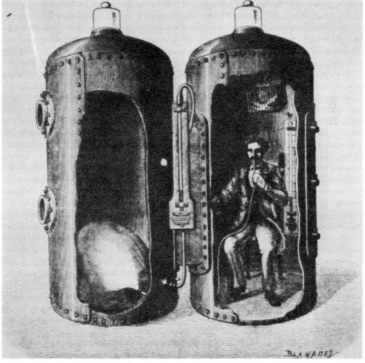

FIG. 3.7. Altitude chamber of Paul Bert. This drawing of 1878 illustrates the parallel development of gas chambers and germfree isolators; the barrier must be gas tight in both cases.

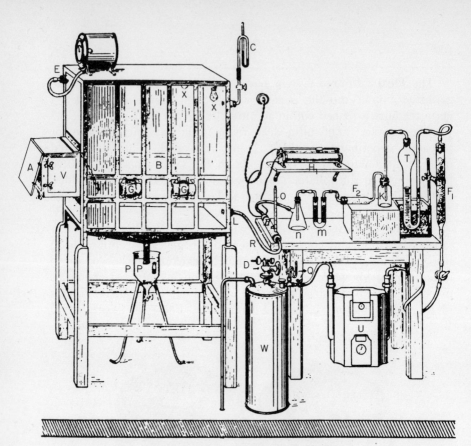

Fig. 3.8. Küster apparatus for rearing germfree goats. Note the use of gloves gasketed into the outside barrier of the isolator. Note also the use of metabolism cages to reduce moisture. This is the first isolator to incorporate a sterile "tunnel" into it (Küster, 1915c); although Cohendy had a similar area in his cylinder.

A. Outer door to the ante chamber.
B. Glass windows of sterile chamber. The bottom of this chamber is a funnel to reduce the moisture of the cage.
C. Manometer to indicate positive pressure inside.
D. Safety valve on the air supply.
E. Air outlet.
F. Sterile cotton filters in the air supply.
G. Rubber gloves gasketed onto the cage; they were rolled up when not in use.
H. Electric heater and rheostat for sterile air.

J. Door between ante chamber and sterile chamber.
K. Vessel to catch droplets of sulfuric acid from T.
L. Entry for sterile air.
M. Drying tube.
N. Dust trap to protect the electric heater.
O. Thermometer in the sterile air line.
P. Paraffin oil sealed the funnel and collected excrement from the sterile chamber. Urine underneath the oil could be obtained through the stopcock at the bottom.

Historical Development

The development of isolation systems and the presentation of cages of historical interest which are not in use at the present time were given in Chapter 2. The first isolation systems were the simple flasks (Fig. 2.1) and bell jars (Fig. 2.3) used by the early chemists for the collection of gases. This type of cage was used by the plant physiologists during the controversy on nitrogen fixation. Thus, it was quite natural that Nuttal and Thierfelder would modify the bell jar for their first germfree animal experiment. The modified bell jar has been used also by Cohendy (1912a), Balzam (1938), Reyniers and Trexler (1943b), and B. Lakey, E. McCoy, P. Wilson, and the author (see Lakey, 1945) at the University of Wisconsin. Bell jars are not as convenient as they appear to be for this purpose; the germicide tends to get splashed into the animal compartment and the high humidity is difficult to control. The connections required and the excessive humidity of the bell jar suggested the closing of the open end. The two ends of the cylinder of Cohendy (1912a) (Fig. 2.5b) and the lids of the churn jars of Luckey (1959c) (Fig. 3.2) have adaptations for feed, water and air supplies, and eggs. Such apparatus worked very well and could be sterilized in an autoclave. This simple cage was modified into more sturdy boxes: the storage cages of Reyniers (1943), the early cage of Gustafsson (1948), or the box cage of Luckey (1959c). All of these cages had limited use and needed further development (H. T. Miller and Luckey, 1962).

Gas isolation systems assumed the shape of a cylinder; one of the earliest was the altitude chamber of Paul Bert in 1878 (Fig. 3.7). When these were used under water, diving bell and submarine techniques developed. The modified cylinders were made airtight to withstand a pressure differential and thus were microbe impenetrable. The parallel development of the Papain digester, the Koch sterilizer, and the Arnold pressure sterilizer (see Bulloch, 1938) led to the modern steam pressure cylinder used for sterilization. Progress in these areas was reflected in the concepts, design and operation of the

---

Q. Manometer on the air supply line.
R. Air supply line.
S. Prefilter on incoming air (not shown) and positive pressure pump beneath the floor.

T. Sulfuric acid drying tower for air.
U. Flow meter.
V. Ante chamber.
W. Air storage chamber.
X. Electric lights.

Reyniers and Chiba germfree apparatus used today.

The early plant physiologists also used a sterile box with sterile air, sterile sand, and sterile seeds to study nitrogen fixation. This was developed by Küster (1915c) into an acceptable animal cage (Fig. 3.8) with the important innovations of arm-length gloves, a sterile lock, and a germicidal entry. This apparatus was the prototype of that used by Glimstedt (1936a) and in the early work of Reyniers (1943). Reyniers strengthened his square wooden unit with steel girders in an effort to make it withstand steam pressure for sterilization.

Modern Isolators

The simple jar and storage cage have been modified into a compact rearing box for germfree chickens* (Fig. 3.9), by H. T. Miller and Luckey (1962). It is a 24 gauge stainless steel box with a ¼ inch Pyrex plate glass top for viewing. It is sterilized within an autoclave with the top slightly ajar to readily admit steam. Following sterilization, sterile food is aseptically placed in the food hopper and sterile water administered through a ⅜ inch i.d. copper tubing and rubber tubing. Prefiltered air must pass three thicknesses of filter down number 50 before entering the germfree cage. The air outlet is the glass wool gasket between the glass and the stainless steel surface. Eggs are introduced through a germicidal bath into the bottom of the cage. This cage proved to be useful for short-term experiments with germfree chicks (Miller, 1962).

The modern version of the thin walled metal tank which is sterilized inside an autoclave is the light weight stainless steel tank† designed by Gustafsson (1959a). Since the pressure is the same on the inside and the outside during sterilization, the thin walled apparatus may have a large glass window and may be made in a variety of shapes (Fig. 3.10). The tank is lighted by fluorescent bulbs above the glass window. The window rests on a soft rubber gasket which forms the inside of a groove filled with germicide after autoclaving. A variety of animal cages can be used inside the tank. Water and food storage compartments are incorporated into the ends of the cage. The rubber glove has a heavy upper sleeve, 1.5 mm in thickness, fastened to the tank wall. Heavy duty surgical gloves are attached to the upper sleeve with a special clamp and secured with rubber

* Available from A. S. Aloe, Scientific Division, St. Louis, Missouri.

† Available from Separator, Lund, Sweden, and A. B. Rudelins and Boklund, Stockholm, Sweden.

cement to make a good seal. The surgical gloves can be changed during an experiment or between experiments, while the sleeves can be used repeatedly. Air sterilization in the Gustafsson cage is accomplished by a combination of incinerator and filters. Preheated air passes through filters of glass wool, asbestos, and Carborundum maintained at 300°C. The air reaches 200°C for a short time before it is

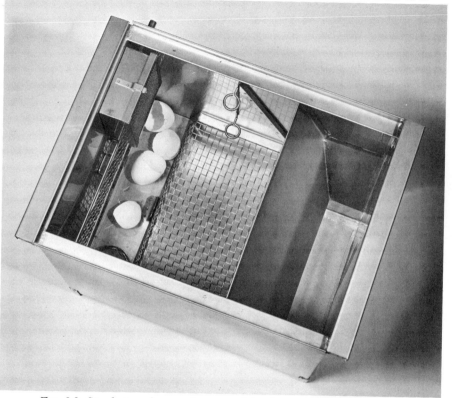

FIG. 3.9. Simple germfree rearing cage of Luckey and Miller. This cage provides germfree birds with minimum expense and effort. (Photo courtesy of A. S. Aloe and Company, St. Louis, Missouri.)

cooled by heat exchange and taken to the interior of the cage. The exit air is sterilized by the same procedure. Sterilization of the exhaust air is essential when pathogenic organisms are being used inside the isolator.

Heavy metal tanks* which can withstand steam pressure steriliza-

* Available from Reyniers and Son, Chicago 13, Illinois.

tion (Reyniers and Trexler, 1943b) have been modified for a variety
of uses (Reyniers, 1959a). The standard Reyniers isolator (Fig. 3.11)
is a metal cylinder, usually 12 gauge stainless steel, about 150 cm long,
and 72 cm in diameter. Attached by sturdy construction are the end

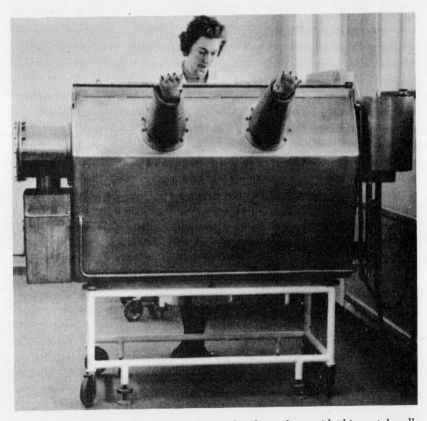

Fig. 3.10. The Gustafsson germfree tank. This isolator with thin metal walls
is sterilized inside an autoclave. The top is a large glass plate which makes viewing the interior very easy. Note the germicidal trap at the left which is a permanent part of most of these cages. (Photo courtesy: B. Gustaffson, 1959, *Ann.
N. Y. Acad. Sci.* **78**, 19.)

closures, one or more viewing and light ports, a supply lock, rubber
gloves, air filters, steam opening, drain, electricity inlet, and wheels.
The diameter and the length may be increased to make an examination unit or a surgical tank in which operators work from either side.
The surgical isolator (Fig. 3.12) has a compartment under the opera-

tion stage into which a pregnant animal may be placed for the Cesarean operation. The operating board may be moved upward until the abdominal surface makes extensive contact with the plastic sheet

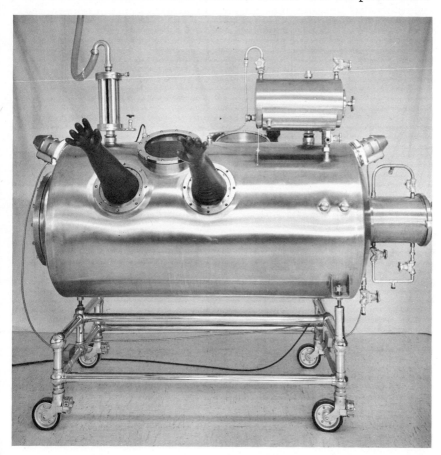

Fig. 3.11. Reyniers germfree isolator. This isolator has been a standard unit for many years. Note the sterile lock, the arm-length gloves, the air filter and exhaust above, and the viewing port. (Photo courtesy: Reyniers and Son, Chicago, Illinois.)

which is gasketed across the opening of the operation stage. A variety of units may be assembled through either lock-to-lock or end-to-end connections (Fig. 3.13). These self-contained units* can be used

* Available from Fisher Scientific Co., Pittsburgh, Pennsylvania.

in any room which has an electric outlet, and they contain a battery operated emergency system. If a shape other than cylindrical should be desired, heavier metal must be used in the walls* in order to withstand the pressure and vacuum (Fig. 3.14). Vacuum imposes the greater strain: one old cylindrical cage of light metal imploded while

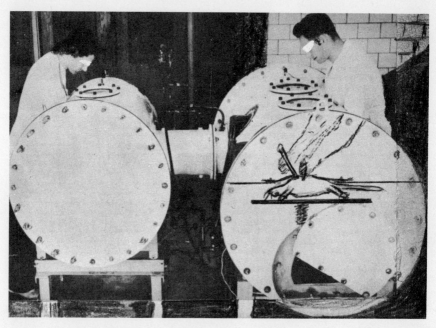

FIG. 3.12. Modified photo of the Reyniers operating cage. The operating cage, *right*, is actually divided into two complete compartments. The two compartments are separated by a plastic film. The operator cuts through the plastic and through the abdominal wall of the mother to extirpate the uterus. The young are then taken from the uterus in the operating cage and passed through the sterile lock into the rearing cage; then the inner door of the rearing cage is shut.

none have exploded to the author's knowledge. A comparison of isolator sizes and uses is given in Table 3.1. Each unit can be seen to resemble the exemplar in many respects and each has its individual characteristics and advantages. Review of the work at Chiba University (Tanami, 1959) indicates these workers started with improved heavy wall tanks developed by Naito (1936) and later used the designs of Reyniers *et al.* (1946) and Gustafsson (1948).

* Produced by S. Blickman, Inc., Weehawken, New Jersey.

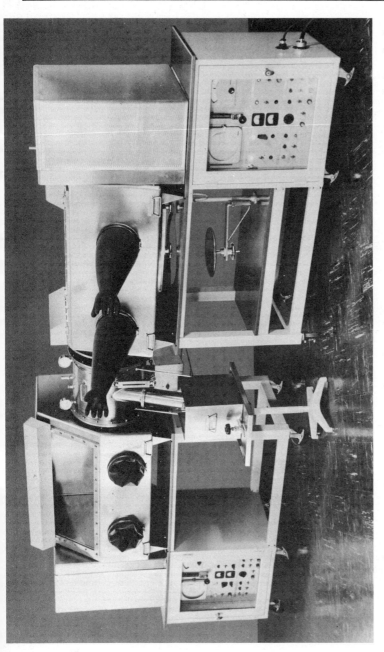

Fig. 3.13. The self-contained units of Fisher, Kewaunee, and Horton. Note the germicidal entry attached to the large sterile lock connecting the two units. The unit on the right is an operating cage, the one on the left is a rearing cage. The panel at the end of each cage contains all the instrumentation needed to sterilize and to operate the cage. Much of the lower part of the units are used for an emergency battery operated unit. (Photo courtesy: Fisher Scientific Co., Pittsburgh, Pennsylvania.)

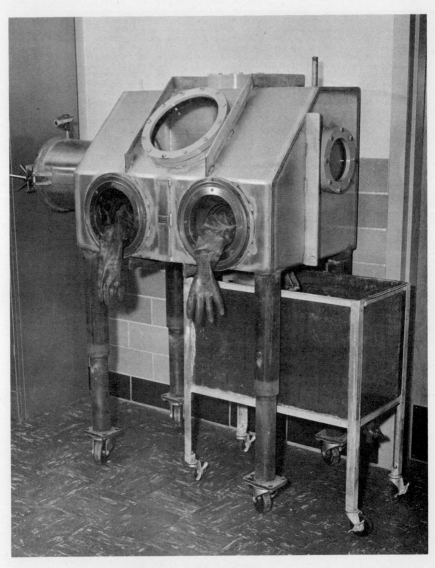

FIG. 3.14. Luckey-Blickman isolator. Heavy stainless steel isolators can be made in a variety of shapes and still withstand the pressures of steam sterilization. Note that this isolator has both a large germicide trap and a sterile lock. (Photo courtesy: S. Blickman, Inc., Weehawken, New Jersey.)

TABLE 3.1
MODERN ISOLATORS

Identity	Structure	Approximate floor space (cm²)[a]	Sterilization Cage	Sterilization Air	Germicide trap	Visibility	Advantages	Disadvantages
Reyniers #100 #200 #300 #400	Heavy steel	5,900	Steam, direct	Filtration	±	Fair	No large autoclave needed	Needs special laboratory
Reyniers, Ex.	Heavy steel	7,100	Steam, direct	Filtration	±	Fair	Versatility	Not adaptable to many laboratories
Miyakawa	Heavy steel	28,000	Steam, direct	Filtration plus heat	+?	Good	Isotopes	Cumbersome
Sito	Heavy steel	7,000	Steam, direct	Filtration	−?	Fair	—	—
Luckey-Blickman	Heavy steel	6,000	Steam, direct	Filtration	+	Fair	Versatility	—
Fisher-Horton-Kewaunee	Heavy steel	6,400	Steam, direct	Filtration plus heat	±	Good	Self-contained	Cost
Gustafsson	Light steel	5,000	Autoclave	Filtration plus heat	+	Good	Easy animal transfer	Slow glove exit; plate glass
Hickey-NIH	Light steel	7,500	Autoclave	Filtration	+	Good	Versatility	Slow glove exit; plate glass
Luckey-Miller	Light steel	900	Autoclave	Filtration	+	Good	Simplicity	No manipulation
Phillips, A. W.	Rigid plastic[b]	13,800	Chemical	Filtration	±	Good	Size is good for poultry and rabbits	Not easily moved
Trexler	Soft plastic	6,500[b]	Chemical	Filtration	±	Good	Adaptability	Susceptible to puncture
Levenson	Soft plastic	9,000[b]	Chemical	Filtration	±	Good	Adaptability	Susceptible to puncture
Envelope	Soft plastic	1,000[b]	Chemical	Filtration	−	Good	Adaptability	Susceptible to puncture
Luckey	Plastic coated room	102,000	Chemical	Filtration UV, precipatron	+[c]	Fair	Large numbers of animals	A single contamination is costly
Trexler	Plastic coated room	—	Chemical	Filtration	±	Fair	Large numbers of animals	A single contamination is costly
de Somer-Eyssen	Steel	—	Chemical	Filtration plus heat	+	Good	4 rooms	A single contamination is costly and very complicated

[a] From Hickey (1960) and author's estimates.
[b] Easily varied to fit the needs of each experiment.
[c] Germicide treated material is routinely taken into the room.

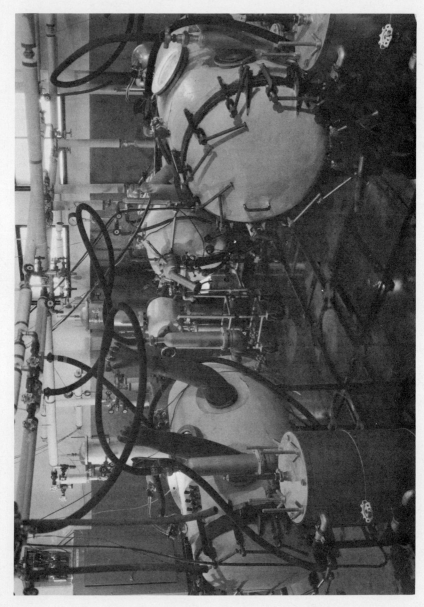

FIG. 3.15. Nakahara isolator. Germfree isolators used at Chiba University, resembled those of Reyniers but were apparently developed separately. (Photo courtesy: J. Tanami, Chiba University, Japan.)

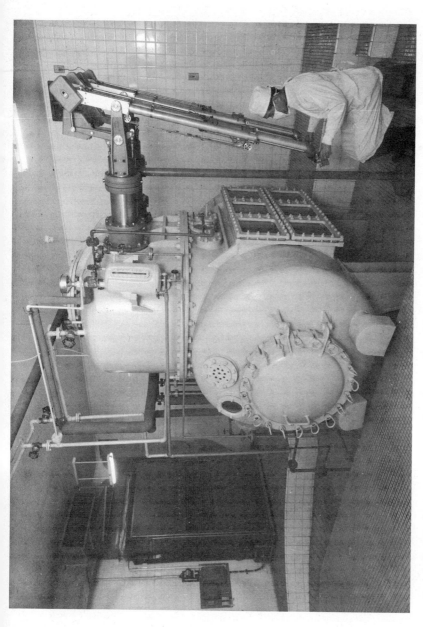

Fig. 3.16. Miyakawa remote control isolator. This elaborate cage is serviced by a large room full of equipment, yet its capacity is apparently small, approximately 8 guinea pigs. (Photo courtesy: M. Miyakawa, 1959, *Ann. N. Y. Acad. Sci.* **78**, 39.)

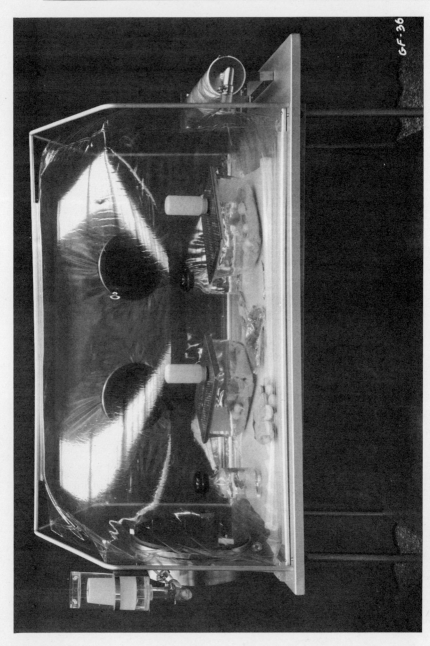

Fig. 3.17. Trexler plastic isolator. Note the simplified air sterilizer on the right and the free-flow exhaust at the upper left. The metal ring on the left allows this cage to be connected to standard metal cages. The simplicity, visibility, and adaptability of the plastic cages make them most acceptable. (Photo courtesy: American Sterilizer Company, Erie, Penn-

The apparatus developed by the Japanese workers at Chiba University (Nakahara, 1959) was a steel isolator (Fig. 3.15) which resembled those already described, although it was developed independently. The large unit at Nagoya University (Miyakawa, 1959c) (Fig. 3.16) was adapted to a Reyniers surgical unit for the Cesarean section. Following the operation the animals were brought into a large sterile chamber which has mechanical pickup arms similar to those used in chemical dry boxes. This is the only cage described in this section which is not available commercially. It is considered as a current model because it is the only germfree cage which can be used for highly active radio tracer work involving sterile animals. Except for this advantage it appears to be cumbersome and too expensive for adoption on a routine basis. As can be seen in the comparison, Table 3.1, this elaborate apparatus has very limited capacity. The mechanical arms are satisfactory for routine procedures such as picking up a guinea pig, testing it microbiologically, feeding it, bathing it, but the fingers are not delicate enough to do a variety of surgical operations. The cage apparently has functioned adequately to give this group material for studies on lymphatic development and wound healing in guinea pigs.

G. B. Phillips *et al.* (1955) showed that inexpensive plastic hoods could be made for bacteriological use. They presented the basic design and the concept of using plastic cages sterilized with germicidal spray. Refinements of the isolator* (Fig. 3.17) have been worked out by Trexler (1959b) who has shown their versatility, adaptability, and dependability. The susceptibility of the cages to puncture needs constant consideration; but with proper use of the cages, the rubber gloves remain the weak point. The food is packaged in a plastic bag and sterilized separately before being passed through the germicidal lock of the plastic tank. The plastic tanks are sterilized (Trexler and Reynolds, 1957) by spraying 2% peracetic acid with 0.1% surfactant (as Na alkyl aryl sulfonate), introducing formaldehyde or ethylene oxide, or by radiation of the isolator before it is inflated. While some plastics (i.e., Mylar† or Kel-F‡) can be sterilized with heat, germicides function adequately. Attachments can be made to the cage directly using a knife and glue. One of the forms used is a doughnut

* Available from The American Sterilizer Co., Erie Pennsylvania and from Germ Free Supply Division, Standard Safety Equipment Co., Palatine, Illinois.
† E. I. Du Pont de Nemours and Co., Inc., Wilmington, Delaware.
‡ The Visking Corporation, Terre Haute, Indiana.

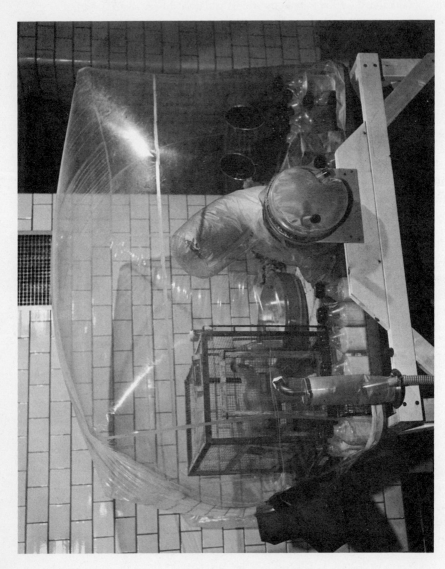

Fig. 3.18. Large plastic isolator. Plastic isolators are easily modified to fit the needs of the investigator: "they are built around an experiment." In this one the operator rises in a half-suit into the interior of the cage. This allows him to reach a greater sterile area. Note the germfree lamb in the cage in front of

shape with the operator in the center (Fig. 3.18) where he can reach
a greater number of rat cages inside the isolator. A flat-bottomed
bubble was developed for surgery (Figs. 3.19a and b) in which the
bottom of the bubble is placed over a surgery patient for sterile operation (Levenson, 1961; Landy *et al.*, 1961). The variety of plastic
(usually 12 mil polyvinyl) isolators includes small envelopes surrounding an animal-holding cage about 30 cm^3 and bubble chambers
which could be made the size of the room. The small isolators are
useful when a wide variety of microorganisms are to be used in
dibiotic experiments. Each of these units has one or more essential
attachments such as air inlet and air exhaust. The air outlet designed
by Trexler (see Reyniers *et al.*, 1960c) is efficient for large volumes
of air (Fig. 3.20). It is novel in that it relies on no filtration or sterilization of the exhaust air. When the air pressure becomes low, the
outlet air bubbles through a liquid germicide. Reverse air passage is
stopped by a column of liquid germicide. Lev (1962) developed a
simple plastic unit from nylon tube of 194 cm diameter. This material
("Portex," from Portland Plastics Ltd., Hythe, Kent) can be autoclaved for 30 minutes.

The advantages of the plastic isolator include economy and visibility; experiments are more easily observed, particularly by a group,
than they are in metal cages; photography is simpler; and the light
on all units in one room may be controlled by the room light. Separate
lighting for individual cages may be accomplished with black plastic.
The steel cages are not as well suited to the rearing of large animals
as the plastic isolators. A major advantage of the plastic over the
steel cage is the maintenance problem. Steel cages normally require
a complete maintenance shop; plastic cages with steel accessories
need little or no professional maintenance. Repair of the plastic, or
modifications such as the insertion of accessories, can be made using
glue, heat, or electronic "sewing machine,"* or the gasket system used
for metal cages. Trexler and Reynolds (1957) described the insertion
of a plastic sterile lock to take in or remove material from plastic
cages, while cages currently produced often have a metal ring
attached. This allows connection of a sterile lock, a metal cage, or
other attachments.

Hard plastic cages were developed by A. W. Phillips *et al.* (1960)
and they have some of the same advantages of soft plastic. These are
easily assembled without special equipment, easily repaired and

* Vertrod Impulse Sealer, Vertrod Corp., Brooklyn, New York.

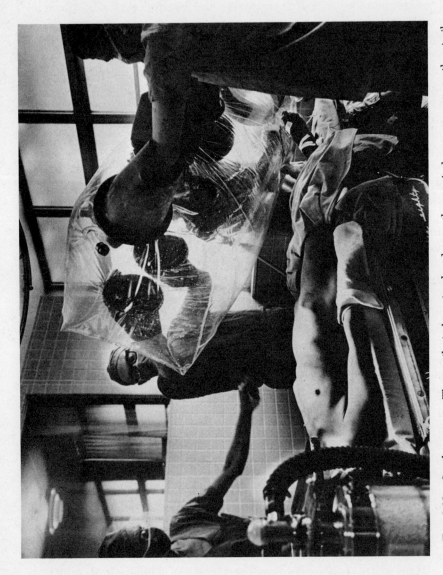

FIG. 3.19a. Sterile surgery. The sterile isolator is placed over the surgical area as soon as the sterile adhesive (sprayed on the patient by the assistant on the left) is semidry. This adhesive makes an airtight seal between the isolator and the skin.

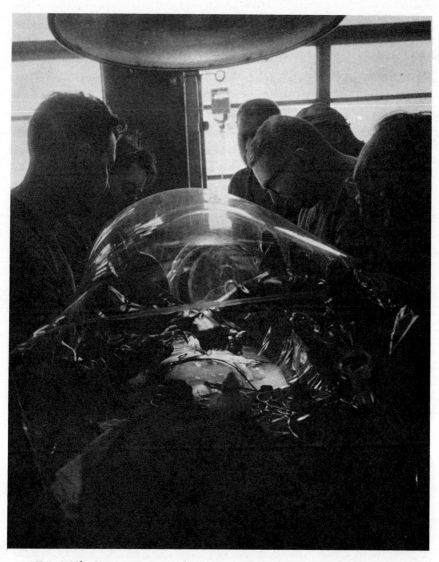

FIG. 3.19b. Surgeon J. J. Landy (wearing dark glasses) and assistant proceed
with cholecystectomy with little possibility of infection from the operating room.
(Photographs by courtesy of Dr. J. J. Landy, University of Miami Medical
School; they were provided by International Medical Press, Inc., New York City.)

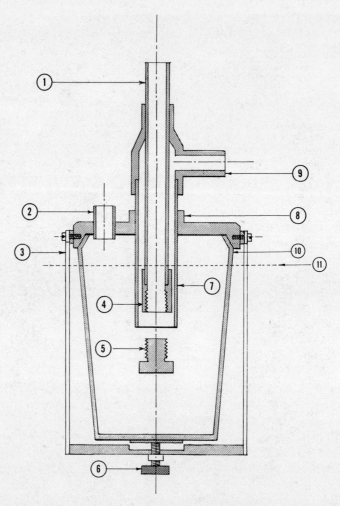

FIG. 3.20. Diagram of the Trexler-Reyniers exhaust air system. The air enters the center tube (1) from the germfree isolator and pushes the germicide out of the tube (7) allowing it to escape at point (9) without passing through a germicide or a filter. The opening at (2) allows the germicidal level to fluctuate without building up appreciable pressure. The plug (5) is used to close the system during steam sterilization. The dotted line (11) indicates the germicide level (2% Lysol and 15% glycerol in water) in the container. The use of the other parts is self-evident. (Photo from Reyniers *et al.*, 1960, *Lobund Repts.* 3, 18.)

modified, are sterilized with germicide, and offer visibility to the operator. Since the cage may be modified in the laboratory, the use of plastic allows greater freedom in design for special occasions. The Plexiglas cages of Phillips are rather large—1.7 meters in length, 1 meter in width, and 0.7 meters in height. The wall is almost 1 cm thick. Phillips used a germicidal bath for the introduction of sterile food.

Hickey (1960) compared the use of the Reyniers steel pressure chamber, the Gustafsson light steel chambers and the soft plastic isolators of Trexler. In addition the workers at the United States Public Health Service devised rigid plastic isolators and modified chemical dry boxes into germfree chambers. Hickey suggested that the viewing ports of Reyniers chamber require supplemental lighting, while control of the illumination in the plastic chambers was difficult except on a room wide basis.

Tanks similar to the germfree isolator are sometimes needed for carefully controlled experiments. These control tanks may be germfree isolators or simulated devices. The closer they are to the actual size, shape, and operation of the germfree cage, the better the control. As mentioned elsewhere, the best control is the germfree animal with the experimental animal being a gnotobiotic animal which has been inoculated with known forms of bacteria and maintained in an isolator under the same physical conditions as germfree animals.

Reyniers (1959a) described several germfree colony systems. Apparently the only one tested was a large tank 2.5 meters in diameter and 5 meters long (Fig. 3.21). It was entered by a man in a plastic diving suit. Details of the cage were given in the patent of Reyniers (1950). The operation was similar to that of the small tank: it was steam sterilized, the air was filtered through a mechanical filter, food and water were brought in through a standard isolator attached to the end, and a germicidal trap provided entry for the operator. The main difference was the sterilization of the suit of the operator. The suit was washed with detergent germicide before the operator entered a germicidal bath, 2% formaldehyde, in which he stayed for 30 minutes before he could enter the germfree tank. Since this unit was most difficult to operate and was susceptible to mechanical failures (see Trexler and Reynolds, 1957), details of its operation are not presented here. The large tank was more dramatic but less effective than a germfree room.

The germfree room of Schottelius (1908a) was built within a large

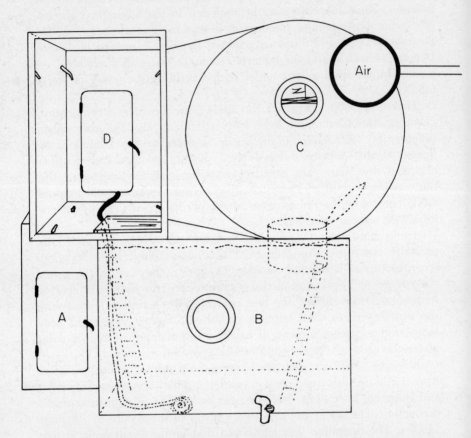

Fig. 3.21. Diagram of a large germfree tank. This germfree tank was 2.5 meters in diameter and 5 meters long. It was entered through door (A) where an exchange of clothes was made. The operator in an insulation suit then went from compartment (A'), directly behind (A), up a ladder into compartment (D) behind the door (D). A two-piece plastic suit was heat welded together around the waist of the operator. The operator came through the door (D) into the germicidal shower bath chamber. Following this cleansing bath he descended the ladder into the big tank (B) of formaldehyde. Note that the air hose originates from an opening in this tank; but notice also, in the center bottom, the quick exhaust for the tank in case of an emergency. The entry into the Leuven suite is similar.

laboratory which had everything removed and was thoroughly cleaned during the operation of the inner room. The entrance to the sterile room (Fig. 2.4) was a double door cubicle. Floor, ceiling, and side walls up to waist height were iron; the rest consisted of double glass plates sealed into the iron supporting unit. Two small boxes with cotton filters were sealed into the partition for ventilation without forced air. After donning sterile gown, pantaloons, and boots, one entered the entry chamber, closed the outside door, and entered the inner chamber through a second glass door. The inner chamber was 2.5 meters high, 2.5 meters wide, and 1.4 meters deep, a volume of almost 9 cubic meters. At one side of the inner chamber, the incubator rested upon a plate glass table. Another glass plate was an operating table; upon this rested the chick cage, which was made of glass and metal. The brooder was at constant temperature in an incubator with a liquid heat exchanger (5% Lysol solution pumped from the outer room). The eggs and chicks were maintained on asbestos. One thermometer was hung from the ceiling of the brooder room and another was placed with its bulb touching the floor of the brooder chamber. These thermometers contained red alcohol in order that they could be read easily from the outside with field glasses. A 10% Lysol solution was used to wash the entire partition; following this formaldehyde vapor was introduced (4 gm per cubic meter) for 48 hours. The suit was made in two parts, the bottom half completely covered the shoes; the top jacket was buckled over canvas pants with a belt. The sleeves were tightly closed with rubber gloves overlapping them for about 6 cm, and sterile rubber shoes were pulled on the feet. Rubber gloves and shoes were sterilized with mercuric chloride and the entry chamber contained a foot bath solution of 0.5% mercuric chloride. Entrance to the inner room was made once to begin the experiment, a second time to remove the unhatched eggs and egg shells, and finally at the end of the experiment. Enough food and water were provided to last the duration of the experiment. Full credit must be given for the painstaking care given to each detail by Schottelius. His experiments were successful from the viewpoint of microbial sterility.

Trexler (1960d) described a sterile room which had apparently not been used for germfree research. The room was of standard construction with the walls and ceiling of asbestos flexboard having a polyester resin impregnated glass cloth. The cement floor was coated with a plastic paint. Cages and equipment entered the room through a double door steam sterilizer. The air was admitted through a glass wool filter and the air outlet trap was similar to that used on other isolators. Trexler also experimented with plastic bubble rooms which could be sterilized with peracetic acid. No evidence is presented that the rooms have functioned for any extended period.

The germfree room built into the medical center at the University of Missouri (Luckey, 1956a) is diagrammed in Fig. 3.5. A conventionally built room with a hard, smooth, plastic coated interior surface was used. All crevices and joints were closed with caulking

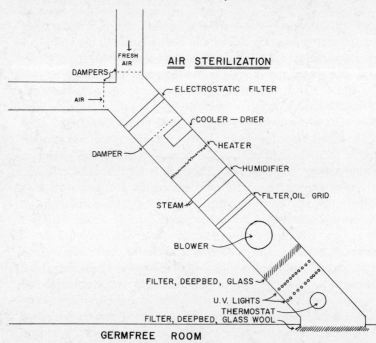

FIG. 3.22. Air sterilization. Diagram of the treatment of large quantities of air before it entered the germfree room. The precipatron was used only at the beginning of the work.

compound and painted with a plastic alkyl resin to give a complete seal. The room was $3 \times 3 \times 2.5$ meters. The air was brought into the room through a multiple sterilizing system (Fig. 3.22). In addition, a No. 50 glass down* filter 2.5 cm thick was sterilized with dry heat and gasketed over the end of the air line from the inside of the room. The air outlet filter was a single large Cambridge low pressure filter.†

* American Air Filter Co., Louisville, Kentucky.
† Cambridge Filter Co., Syracuse, New York.

Heat and humidity of the air line were automatically controlled. The inner door consisted of a double rubber or plastic dam with each flap overlapping the full width of, and 15 cm below the door. The air supply and pressure were great enough that a strong current of sterile air outward allowed no microorganisms into the room. On the floor of the room was a plastic sheet containing 5% diaprene chloride or 2% peracetic acid solution. The room was shown to be sterile and was used for as many as three successive experiments over a period of 2 months without being resterilized. The germicidal floor gave the room a self-sterilizing feature.

A large sterile area such as a room is most effectively used by a man in a sterile suit. Protective or isolation clothing has been known since the 17th century when weird outfits were worn by the physicians during plagues. These costumes covered the body completely, but were undoubtedly less effective than the physicians desired. Modern suits have been made of a variety of materials and designed according to the same principles as those used for isolators; all microbes must be kept from the animals. Again there has been parallel development with pharmaceutical and chemical industries which have needed to protect man from noxious or infective agents and harmful chemicals. This is a rapidly developing field with many advances in underwater and space suits proving applicable to the needs of gnotobiotic research.

Common denominators in the needs of different groups have accelerated progress. Plastics and rubber-covered cloth are the most used materials for sterile suits. Usually air is supplied through a plastic tube containing air inlet tube, air return tube, and communication line with the gases being forced through the hose. This practice is undesirable since positive pressure on the suit or hose invites contamination through pin-point leaks. Some plastics were useful for experimental design since they can easily be sprayed on a model of the desired size. The author used a rubber diving suit with success; entry was made through an opening in the middle of the suit which was subsequently closed with a germicide in a small plastic bag (Fig. 3.23). Connections between the mask and the head piece were gasketed with sterile gauze. The overlaps made with the surgical gloves over the rubber arms were sealed with a germicide. The suit was sterilized by a sponge bath of either 0.2% peracetic acid or 5% diaprene chloride. The operator entered the germfree room while still wet with germicide. In this particular suit no air hose was needed: a chemical mask was fitted with a double layer of 1 inch filter down number 50

placed in the exchange compartments. When the man breathed contaminated air in the entry room, an extra covering of sterile filter
down was placed over the mask. This system gave greater mobility

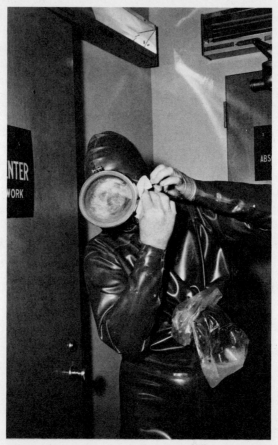

FIG. 3.23. Suit used in the sterile room. Note the umbilicus through which
the operator enters into and exits from the suit has a small bag of germicide over
the tied end. Sterile gauze is used as a gasket material between parts of the
rubber suit and the face mask. Freedom of movement is much improved by
elimination of the air hose.

and reduced the possibility of chance contamination when compared
with those suits having positive pressure air lines.

For hospital use, sterile areas and sterile suits are being developed
so that patients unable to fight infectious diseases (e.g., following

operation, sickness, or extensive radiation therapy) can be placed in sterile isolators to protect them from bacterial infection after a treatment. It is noted that in sterile surgery the interior of the patient is connected to a sterile compartment into which instruments are placed and surgeons' arms are inserted. Since direct connection is cut into the usually sterile interior of the patient from the sterile operation compartment, *no* extraneous microorganisms are admitted. Some of the incubators for premature infants are effective isolators. It is anticipated that patients harboring highly virulent organisms will be placed in disposable plastic isolators to prevent the spread of infection into other areas of the hospital.

Germfree Building

Since a man can be freed from an external supply of air by adequate filters in a helmet, by compressed air system, or by the use of compressed oxygen with CO_2 fixing agents, it is anticipated that buildings with several sterile rooms will be used in the future. A simple sterile building was proposed by the author at the University of Wisconsin seminar in 1945. A four-room sterile area at the University of Louvain (P. de Somer and H. Eyssen, personal communication, 1961) is the prototype for future developments (Fig. 3.24). As sterile techniques become better perfected the sterile building will provide colonies of sterile animals inexpensively. The present methods used in the operation of gnotobiotic colonies would require little change to adapt to large-scale germfree experimentation. The increased growth rate in germfree chickens might make it economically advantageous to market germfree poultry products.

Accessories

Sterile Transfer System

In any apparatus expected to operate for more than 3–4 weeks a sterile lock or germicidal trap is essential for adding more diet, water, and other supplies. The sterile lock or steam tunnel, as introduced by Küster (1913b), is simply a small two-door steamclave, the door at one end opens to the outside and the door at the other end opens into the germfree cage. It may be a steam jacketed sterile lock or a single wall lock; the former is more versatile than the latter. The sterile lock is often built permanently on the isolator; it may be 25–50 cm in diameter, 30–50 cm long, and built of 12 gauge metal or thicker.

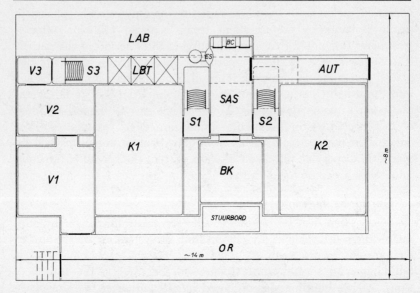

FIG. 3.24A. Germfree suite floor plan. This suite of germfree rooms being tested by Dr. P. de Somer, Dr. H. Eyssen, and Dr. M. Dedobbeleem, Department of Virology, Rega Institute, University of Louvain, promises to provide ample space for colonies and large-scale experiments. (See also facing page.) (Floor plan provided through the courtesy of Drs. M. Dedobbeleem, P. de Somer, and H. Eyssen, University of Louvain.)

V1 = Dressing room
V2 = Sterilization of the suite
V3 = Entry to bath
S3 = Bath (this liquid entry connects V3 to S1 and S2)
LBT = Bubble test for leaks in the suite
S1 = Entry to germfree room 1 or to SAS-room
S2 = Entry to germfree room 2 or to SAS-room
K1 = Germfree room 1
K2 = Germfree room 2
BK = Germfree room 3
SAS-room = Access to S1, S2, BK
           Access to germicidal trap, ES
           Access to inner door of autoclave, AUT
           Access to BC
AUT = Autoclave
ES = Germicidal trap
BC = 15 small hatching units
Lab = Laboratory
Stuurbord = Control panel
OR = Observation and control room

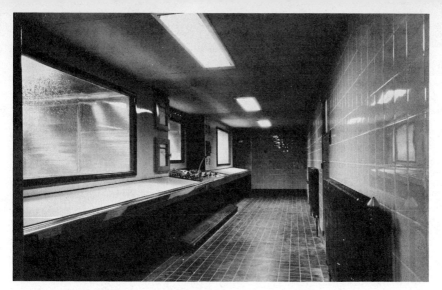

Fig. 3.24B. Observation and control deck of germfree suite. (Photograph courtesy of Dr. P. de Somer, Dr. H. Eyssen, and Dr. M. Dedobbeleem.)

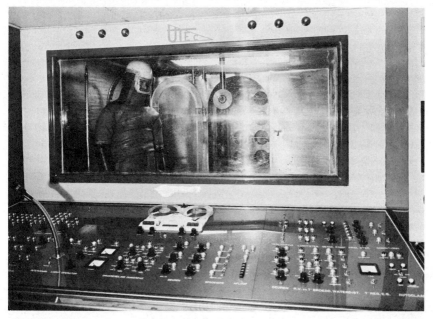

Fig. 3.24C. Control panel and central rooms. View through the small room (BK) and through the open double doors into room SAS having hatching units (BC) at the rear. The hose attached to the man's suite contains air inlet, air outlet, and communication lines. The pipe from the center of the ceiling carries germicide to the rotor which has dispersed liquid to sterilize the room (note remaining droplets on walls and window). The control panel gives a hint of the complex electronic and mechanical systems which occupy the basement. (Photograph courtesy of Dr. P. de Somer, Dr. H. Eyssen, and Dr. M. Dedobbeleem.)

The permanently attached lock may be equipped with an outer door having a sleeve for germicidal entry. Installation of a variety of outside doors gives versatility to the sterile lock. The outer door or the lock may have a freezing unit or a steam proportioning unit* for temperature control. This provides a good incubator for eggs. A liquid filtration system may be built into it. The sterile lock connecting two units together gives a system of germfree cages. Reyniers (1959a) illustrated several systems: particularly versatile for this purpose were the examination germfree units which were slightly larger than the rearing units and had more than one sterile lock. Since both ends of an examining unit could be removed, the ends could be provided with extra sterile locks. One of these could be used for incubation, one for sterilization, and one for freezing; or the two ends could be connected to the open end of the rearing unit to give one long versatile cage. The sterile lock could be attached directly to plastic cages, transportation cages, or storage cages. Both steam and germicidal sprays have been used to sterilize the interior and contents of the sterile lock. A vacuum may also be established in the sterile lock to concentrate fluids or to increase the rates of filtration. However, the use of pressure is preferable to vacuum for filtration. Reyniers and Sacksteder (1960a,b) reported other attachments which include the use of pressure filters for liquid filtration into a germfree isolator and a modified vacuum cleaner built into the outer door of the sterile lock.

Some isolators have a germicidal trap and no sterile lock; some have both. In cages where a germicidal trap is not part of the entrance system most germfree units will have occasion to use germicidal entries. An example is given by Reyniers et al. (1960a) in which the outer door of the sterile lock was replaced with a door containing a special tube (Fig. 3.25). This was sterilized as a part of the sterile lock; the end was submerged into a germicidal solution and the small door opened for entry of sterile eggs or small packages. Usually 2% mercuric chloride solution was the germicide. Material to be taken in was thoroughly cleansed and left in the germicide 5 minutes before being brought into the cage via a remote control device (small chain, wire, or string attached to an open net or nylon bag). The Gustafsson unit (Fig. 3.10) had a large germicidal trap in place of a sterile lock. The advantage of the larger trap as a component of the cage is that larger packages, as animals in jars, can be easily removed or trans-

* Minneapolis Honeywell Regulator Co., Philadelphia, Pennsylvania.

ferred. Quaternary ammonium compounds such as Septin* at 0.2% concentration are used as the germicide by Gustafsson (1948).

A third method for the introduction of material into soft plastic isolators may best be described as a *Cesarean entry*. The material is sterilized in a plastic container. The container is tightly glued to the isolator which immobilizes surface microorganisms. Then the barrier is cut with a red hot cautery, which kills any microorganisms near the opening, and the sterile material is transferred into the isolator.

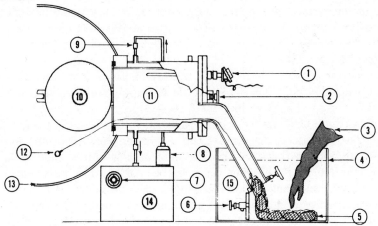

FIG. 3.25. Germicidal trap attachment to the sterile lock. Sterile eggs (5) are being taken into the cage (13) through the sterile lock (11) and the germicidal trap (15). The door (10) to the sterile lock will be closed and the eggs incubated in the sterile lock. The thermometer (1) will record the temperature while the steam proporting unit (14) will maintain the desired temperature for incubation. Note the ring (12) on a small chain which allows the operator in the germfree isolator to pull the eggs in a net to the desired position. Other items are: (2) handle to open and close the outside door of the sterile lock; (3) glove; (4) level of germicide; (6) door to the tube; (7) heat regulator; (8) heat-sensitive valve; and (9) steam inlet. (Photograph from Reyniers *et al.*, 1960, *Lobund Repts.* 3, 18.)

A fourth method was used successfully by the author to take material into the sterile room. Germicide treated packages of presterilized material were taken in through the tentflap door with the outward movement of sterile air providing ample protection. The operator entered several times daily following germicide sponging of the suit.

* 100% Septin from Pharmacia, Uppsala.

Transfer Cages and Holding Cages

A wide variety of transfer cages have been designed ranging from the simple glass jar which Gustafsson (1959a) used, to an elaborate transfer cage which can transport germfree animals for hundreds of miles. Most were sturdily built isolators with the means for attaching them to a sterile isolator to introduce a germfree animal. The transfer cage might have either a free flow filter or a forced air filter. The latter relied upon a battery driven motor to push air through a sterilizing system. These transfer units were normally sterilized in an autoclave before being attached to the sterile unit. Shipments of germfree animals have been made by land, sea, and air with no major difficulty.

Holding cages include a wide variety of cages, from the glass jar of Luckey (1952) which had a sterile air supply and exhaust attached and no means for providing food and water, to more complex units such as those of Reyniers *et al.* (1949b) in which the rigid walled unit had a special door, air supply, and a viewing port. The unit should be adaptable to the sterile lock system of a germfree cage. One of the simplest of the holding cages is the plastic envelope which had sealed into one end an air filter and could be attached to either a plastic cage or a sterile lock. The germfree animal and the food are placed in it from the germfree tank and the end sealed with heat, electronic sealer, or glue. The advantage of these sample cages was that a variety of experiments might be run with animals under different conditions, i.e., different microorganisms might be injected into germfree animals in order to make a variety of monoflora studies.

Cages

A variety of animal cages is needed inside the germfree tank, depending upon the experiment to be performed or the function of the isolator. To protect the gloves all cages must be fabricated with no sharp corners or edges. In experiments in which two groups are being compared within the germfree cage everything should be equal. For the antibiotic experiments two identical cages were made and placed in opposite ends of the germfree tank and a small light was placed over each group of chicks (Fig. 3.26). The size of feeders and waterers were equal and they were placed in the same part of the cage to eliminate variables as much as possible. The chicks were obtained from the same clutch of eggs and treated in the same manner. The only difference was the presence of antibiotics in the food of those on one side.

Sometimes a breeding cage is needed and sometimes a small cage for hand-feeding of mice or rats is needed. Often a metabolism cage is desirable; metabolism cages were actually a component part of Küster's (1914) cage and were the main cage used by Glimstedt

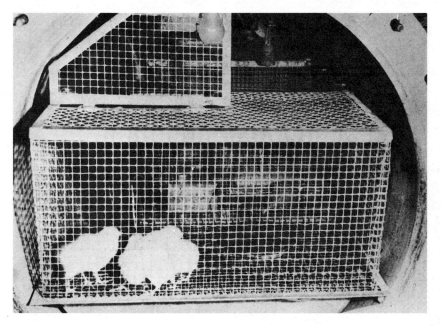

Fig. 3.26. Interior of germfree cage. Two groups of chicks are housed in identical cages with a light over each. (T. D. Luckey, 1959, *Ann. N. Y. Acad. Sci.* **78**, 133.)

(1936a). One advantage of these cages is the elimination of urine as a source of moisture. Animals should be confined in germfree cages in order that they may be easily cared for and caught; and they must be denied the opportunity to chew on the gloves. Even Nuttal and Thierfelder's (1896a) first germfree cage for guinea pigs had a glove protector device in it. And Küster (1915a) found that germfree goats would chew on the gloves if he forgot to put the glove protector over the opening. Rabbits are large enough and easily handled so cages are not always used for them. In this case a simple glove protector must be pulled over the glove port after each entry is made.

Since space within an isolator is limited, except in germfree rooms and large plastic cages, there is a tendency to overcrowd germfree animals. The animals need the same space whether they are germfree or not. Rats, hamsters, and young chicks each need 80 cm^2 floor space. Guinea pigs need twice this, and mice one-fourth as much as that needed for rats. Older chickens need 1000–1500 cm^2 depending upon the strain (size). Growth may be inhibited if too little space is permitted.

Gloves

As the weakest link in the system, the gloves receive the most care and attention. Neoprene shoulder length gloves* are usually 76 cm long and must have a good rim for attachment to a 22 cm diameter glove port. They are often pleated to give better ventilation and stretching. The rim acts as a rolled gasket built into the glove which is bolted to the cage via a ring clamp. Careful observation of the palm, fingers, and the fold next to the rim will allow animals to be transferred before gloves deteriorate. There should be a system worked out for patching gloves because pin-point holes and sometimes large holes can be discovered and patched without contamination if emergency preparations are adequate. The patch is made with rubber cement. Germicidal powder (boric acid) lubricates and helps to keep the gloves from accumulating a large quantity of viable bacteria. If a hole is discovered, a germicide should be used both on the inside of the glove surface and on the outside. Küster (1914) filled the glove with mercuric chloride, and quaternary N-compounds have been used. Dilute peracetic acid may be used since the oxidizing action would not be harmful for one or two washings. The rubber gloves should be protected from the worker by thin cotton gloves being put on the hands before insertion into the rubber gloves. This makes insertion easier and considerably decreases the amount of body oils which accumulate in the fingers and palm of the glove. The gloves must be protected from mechanical abrasion inside the cage by the use of canvas gloves during any and all heavy work: the opening of the inner door in which a heavy wrench must be used, the opening of water cans, and even in the handling of interior cages and animals. The inevitable problem with gloves is their aging due to oxidation; this is one reason why electrostatic filters are seldom used in germfree research. Even with neoprene gloves, the oxidation

* Pioneer Rubber Co., Willard, Ohio.

process is always a specter at work. However, good neoprene gloves could be used for many months and as many as 4–6 sterilizations are permissible.

Some cages such as the Fisher-Kewaunee-Horton isolater have glove ports so designed that new gloves can be inserted during the course of the operation. Also the lower part of the gloves of Gustafsson could be exchanged during the course of an experiment. This feature served as an adequate safeguard against the wear and tear on the hand part of the glove. However, equally vulnerable is that part of the glove around the glove port which is in contact with the metal and gets creased and stretched frequently. Since the gloves are vulnerable to excessive wear, animals should be transferred from one cage to another every few months in order that gloves may be replaced before they become aged or torn.

Electricity

An interior source of alternating electric current is essential for some germfree cages. The voltage should be standard for the locality. Electricity is needed outside for light and heat and is needed within the cage to operate such electrical facilities as cautery, homogenizer, etc. It is needed on the Fisher-Horton cage for the complete operation since many things are electrically activated. A simple electric plug having two lines is placed in the cage through a connector.

Steam and Air

The steam lines used for sterilization of germfree cages should have the condensation trap near the connecting unit and a metal screen to prevent small particles from entering the sterile tanks. Steam pressure of 17 psi is usually used for sterilization. Steam under pressure is also useful in cleaning cages. Pressure gauges and a recorder for the temperature of the steam as it leaves the sterile cage are useful. As mentioned previously, this is not as reliable a temperature guide as a thermocouple placed inside the cage but both are generally used.

Most cages have some device for temperature and humidity control. The temperature is normally maintained at 20–23°C. For young chicks the temperature should be maintained at 33–35°C the first week. It may be dropped 3° each week until ambient temperature is reached. The temperature rise during sterilization has been discussed. Humidity control is not easy to maintain since the animals give off much water in their excreta and spill water when drinking. The best humidity control is apparently a good source of sterile dry air. If the air line has a relative humidity of 10–20% and if the air flow were adequate, no problem with humidity is normally encountered. The air flow should be approximately 0.5 to 2 cfm, depending upon the size of the cage and the number of animals present. Less than 0.02 cfm per mouse, 0.05 cfm per rat, guinea pig, or small chick, or 0.2 cfm per large chicken or rabbit is inadequate. Small electric blowers for individual cages are used in some laboratories, others use central air supply. The air flow in the sterile rooms is much greater and can approach 20 cfm as entrances are made into the room.

Miscellaneous Items

Other potential sources of leaks are the rubber or neoprene gaskets used to seal glove ports, doors, electric plug, light ports, and viewing ports to the cage. As the rubber becomes worn it may cause leaks or not fit the doors properly, or the gaskets may become hard to seal properly. Horowitz *et al.* (1960) reports that Teflon gaskets are much superior to neoprene for this purpose. The Fisher-Kewaunee-Horton isolator uses heat-resistant, molded, silicon-rubber gaskets. Gaskets are frequently made in the cage-prep room from sheets of rubber, neoprene, or silicone-rubber 1–5 mm thick.

Provision must be made for observation of the animals by some means or another; there is little problem in the plastic cages where it is difficult to control light entering individual cages. Observation in the cages with the small viewing ports is not easy for more than one operator. A television system has been suggested for viewing the cages as well as details of operation, sterilization, temperatures, etc. This might be feasible for large-scale operations.

Isolators usually have a small balance for weighing the animals and for feeding and watering equipment. The sides and sometimes the space under the floor is used for storage and waste. A thermometer is part of the permanent equipment and bacteriological testing material is always needed. A simple system for admitting water is to use small cans with a solder seal which can be steam sterilized under pressure during the sterilization of either the cage or the sterile lock. A few small surgical tools for autopsy and a closed container for waste and the transportation of material or animals out of the cage are useful. A small cotton plug should be inserted into the exhaust air filter from the inside of any isolator which houses birds. This small plug should be changed every day as it collects the lint and dust from the feathers. If this surface were not kept clean, the residue would clog the exhaust system. The free flow exhaust (Fig. 3.20) thus has a special advantage for germfree fowl.

Minor items in the tanks include a small punch for opening water, milk, or vegetable cans, a wrench for opening the inner door of the sterile lock, an extra light bulb if an interior light were used, towels and gauze in order to keep the interior clean, extra bedding if the animals were on bedding, and a receptacle for waste and excreta. A syringe is often needed for anesthesia or drawing blood. If a large germicidal trap is available, glass jars may be kept in the cage to transfer animals from one cage to another. With an electric plug sealed into the unit a variety of electrical devices can be used inside the germfree cage. One of the most important of these is the electric cautery for operations. Other accessories are water pipes from the outside for maintaining a constant temperature incubator within the unit (introduced by Schottelius). This system was used for another purpose by Cohendy: he circulated cold water into the top of the small cylinder to condense water from the air for his chickens.

Mobility is desirable for germfree isolators. The soft plastic units are light enough to be placed on tables while the metal units are usually fabricated with ball bearing wheels or can be transferred on rolling racks to or from the sterilization panel. A special autoclave is needed for the Gustafsson units.

Sterilization

Methods and Use

While sterilization might be defined as the act of killing all living cells, the term has a slightly different nuance in germfree and possibly other operations. Apparently theoretical demands and laboratory testing procedures for bactericidal efficiency are more vigorous than those required for successful gnotobiotics. Possibly neither take into adequate consideration the multiplicity of vectors acting to reduce microbial numbers in a germfree experiment. Viable microorganisms may even be present in the germfree environment, but they remain inactive. Consider that spores trapped in grease may survive steam sterilization; yet it is most unlikely that the viable spores might be released to participate in any way in the experiment. Horton and Hickey (1961) sporadically found microorganisms in laboratory testing of radiation-sterilized diets; but no experiments were contaminated from the use of those diets. Whenever germicides are used for sterilization, there is always a good possibility that some spores have become inactivated rather than killed. Although the animals may test microbiologically sterile, neutralization of the germicide might reveal viable organisms. Mercuric chloride treated eggs could be shown to harbor viable spores on the egg shells if the germicide were neutralized; this does not occur in practice where there is enough germicide present to kill the microorganisms any time enough moisture is present to activate spores. From the practical viewpoint, germicides have been used effectively and they will be more widely used as more plastic isolators are used. Despite their theoretical handicap (see Davis, 1951) germicides are simple to use and routinely allow germfree experimentation. The use of various agents of sterilization in gnotobiotic techniques will be summarized; a more complete presentation of the use of germicidal agents may be found in Reddish (1954) and G. S. Wilson and Miles (1955).

Electromagnetic waves of the visible spectrum, or longer wavelengths, have bactericidal properties. Some ultraviolet (UV) rays with wavelengths between 2500 and 3000 Å are highly bactericidal. Ultraviolet lamps are useful as aids in cleaning air or space for germfree or gnotobiotic work. When used, they should be cleaned each week by wiping with alcohol or similar solvent, because UV rays penetrate dust and grease so poorly. They are rarely used as the sole means of sterilization. X-rays could be used for sterilization, but the use of X-ray machines for this purpose is unusual. The loss of energy in production of the X-ray is so great that the capacity of such machines is low; therefore, the time required for complete sterilization of any reasonable quantity of material makes this method impractical. A combination of β- and γ-rays from spent fuel sources was used by the author for the sterilization of material. Since the container stops most of the β-rays, a mixture of γ-radiation energies is involved. The higher energy rays are the most effective for penetration, but apparently the killing power of some of the lower energy γ-rays is equally good. A cobalt source with well defined γ-radiation was used in one laboratory. An electron beam with energies equivalent to that of γ-rays was used to sterilize diets with a Van de Graaf accelerator by Luckey et al. (1955); Phillips et al. (1959); Hickey (1960); and Horton and Hickey (1961). Generally 2 million rads was the minimum used for sterilization. Repeated tests with viable spores showed that 2 million rads minimum is effective for routine use (Miller, 1962). However, more has been used; Luckey *et al.* (1955) used 2.8 million rads minimum and Phillips *et al.* (1959) used 4–5 million rads. The bags were flattened to a thickness of 1 cm for electron beam sterilization and were kept to a proper thickness to correspond to the flux of the γ-ray source. Most of the diet received 10–100% greater quantity than the minimum due to the mechanics of radiation sterilization. Diet was packaged in double or triple plastic bags for radiation sterilization. The outer cover (if there were three covers) was removed before germicidal bath treatment. The radiation-sterilized diet was passed through the germicidal trap and a plastic bag removed. The sterile diet was then in a clean plastic bag ready for use. Another use which could be made of the high energy electromagnetic waves is the sterilization of plastic for use in germfree work. A plastic tent, cage, or isolator could be folded and passed under electron beam machine or in any environment with high γ-flux. This action not only sterilizes the material but makes it more resistant to heat and somewhat tougher; this explains the premium on radiation treated plastics. It is foreseen that the air around the nuclear reactors will be used as a source of clean, if not sterile, air for future germfree work. Such air might be useful in hospital recovery or surgery rooms.

Electricity as such has not been used in germfree or gnotobiotic work to accomplish complete sterilization. However, precipitrons (electrically charged filters) were used in air lines to help clean out all particles. The charge imparted to the particle prevented it from passing through the charged filter. This is an accessory similar to ultraviolet light since a precipitron is not generally used to sterilize air by itself. Electrostatic filters have the disadvantage that the production of ozone and related compounds are most detrimental to rubber. Since the rubber gloves of a germfree isolator are the weakest part of the whole system, electrostatic filters have not been popular in germfree research.

Ultrasonic waves undoubtedly could kill microorganisms but it is most difficult to kill *all* bacteria in a reasonable area. Undoubtedly, this is the main reason why ultrasonic waves have not been used in germfree work.

Dry heat of 140 to 200°C is most useful in presterilizing material for germfree cages: 140°C must be maintained for 3–4 hours for destruction of all viable spores; 160°C for 2 hours is acceptable, and 180°C for 1 hour is adequate for material with the usual low bacterial density. Therefore, operating materials, tubes, gloves, and bedding are wrapped in double sheets of paper and placed in a dry oven at 180°C for 1–1.5 hours. Apparently a temperature of 200°C for 30 minutes is adequate and 400°C will kill spores within 1 minute. The cage of Gustafsson used an air sterilization unit heated to 300°C. The main problem with using dry heat for a short period of time for an air system is that of raising the temperature of all particles in the air above 300°C for an adequate period of time. Depending upon the quantity of air flow, the amount of moisture present, the microbial population kind and number, and the amount of protein around the organisms, different resistances may be found. The real advantage of dry heat is that it can penetrate where water vapor could not, i.e., through a gasket, or into grease, or between two closely connected hard surfaces. Therefore dry heat is a most useful means for sterilizing material in gnotobiotics.

Intermittent heat sterilization of dry material, particularly food or seeds, has been used. It was most effective for liquids which would encourage the vegetation of spores. Boiling in water or other solutions has not proven to be as effective as might be desired. Although intermittent boiling could kill all the bacteria in an enclosed system, it was not used extensively.

Steam under pressure is the most reliable and useful means of killing all microorganisms. If air pockets remain in the material being sterilized, as in a finely powdered diet which was packed too thick, then the heat provided is essentially dry and is much less efficient than saturated steam. In practice, steam pressure of 17 lb per square inch or a minimum temperature of 123°C was used for 20 minutes or longer to sterilize most things. It is important to maintain the temperature at the stated level for the desired period of time. This is particularly important with large volumes in which heat penetration may take many minutes.

Sterilization by filtration was used for heat labile compounds; although bacteria-free filtrates could be obtained routinely, it was understood that these were not necessarily virus free. Of a variety of filters available, those most often used were Seitz filters, fritted glass filters, and membrane filters. All of these can be effective when used properly. The easiest to use, the membrane filter, is also the easiest to misuse. It is adequate for solutions which are not viscous. Pressure filtration should be used rather than vacuum unless the material can be tested following filtration. The use of vacuum in an isolator invites contamination.

Although a great variety of chemical compounds kill bacteria, very few of them are effective germicides. Acids and alkali are not practical and are no more effective than many inorganic and organic salts. Synthetic detergents, dyes, soaps, alcohol, ethers, phenols, and substituted phenols can all be used to kill bacteria, but few efficiently kill *all* spores. Some cresols are useful. Extremely active alkylating compounds, as ethylene oxide, ethylene amine, or beta proprio lactone, are effective, but quite toxic. The most promising compounds are strong oxidizing agents or those which decompose into oxidizing agents. Chlorine, iodine, hydrogen peroxide, and even concentrated sulfuric, nitric, or hydrochloric acids are germicidal compounds. In some respects peracetic acid surpasses hydrogen peroxide as an ideal germicide—it is readily soluble in water, easily stored, effective in dilute solutions, fast acting, volatile, germicidal in the vapor phase, highly sporicidal, readily inactivated, and it decomposes into innocuous compounds after releasing nascent oxygen. Unfortunately, *both* peracetic acid and hydrogen peroxide are highly corrosive to metals and concentrated solutions react explosively with organic material. The vapor of peracetic acid does not react as rapidly as the solution, i.e., all spores are killed within 30 seconds after contact with a 2% solution while it takes about 15 minutes to kill all spores with the vapor. Its effectiveness in an aerosol depends much upon the presence of moisture. Reyniers (1958) used 2% peracetic acid shower followed by a bath in 2% formaldehyde for 15–30 minutes to sterilize the suit of the operator of the large tank. Küster (1915c) used a hydrogen peroxide spray in the operating tent during an operation. Nascent oxygen from hydrogen peroxide is one of the best germicides. Küster also used a germicidal dye, vitralin, which he felt was most important to the maintenance of asepsis.

Mercuric chloride, alcohol, and ether were used by Nuttall and Thierfelder (1897) to sterilize glass surfaces and the abdomen of the guinea pig. They also used 0.1% mercuric chloride in 5% HCl to sterilize egg surfaces. Schottelius (1899) used 0.5% mercuric chloride solution as a foot bath in the antechamber of the room and for sterilizing egg surfaces. The eggs were then washed with sodium chloride to remove the mercury and dried with sterile cotton. It is interesting that he tried 10% mercuric chloride, which did not sterilize the eggs.

Cohendy (1912a) used the same solution and method for sterilizing eggs as had his teacher, Schottelius. Balzam (1937) immersed eggs for 2 minutes in 1% solution of mercuric chloride at 40°, following which they were brushed vigorously with an egg brush. Reyniers *et al.* (1949b) gave data for the sterility and hatchability of eggs treated with many germicides and different concentrations of mercuric chloride. After these studies and after the repeated use of different concentrations of germicides, the standard procedure of sterilizing egg surfaces with 2% mercuric chloride at 40°C for 5 minutes was adopted. Küster used 1% mercuric chloride solution to dip connections before use. Glimstedt (1932) dipped his cotton air filters in 1% mercuric chloride, then dried them. Thus, if they became wet, the germicide would be activated and kill vegetative bacteria.

The activity of mercuric chloride is in direct proportion to the amount of mercuric ion which enters the cell to react with sulfhydryl groups of proteins to denature enzymes. It is well known that this could be reversed by small sulfhydryl molecules, such as cysteine and thioglycolates. While mercuric ions are highly toxic to vegetative cells, they do not kill all spores. For this reason, egg shells are normally removed from a germicide cage after the chicks have hatched. If mercuric chloride on these eggs shells were neutralized, bacterial growth might result. Miller (1962) inoculated egg shells with spore-forming organisms, sterilized them with mercuric chloride, and fed small bits to germfree chicks. The chicks did not become contaminated despite the fact that when the mercuric chloride on those shells was neutralized, bacterial growth was obtained *in vitro*. Mercuric chloride is acceptable in spite of this, due to its absorption in the egg shell; any action which would normally allow spores to vegetate would reactivate the mercuric ions.

Alcohol and ether were used by Nuttall and Thierfelder for the sterilization of apparatus. Other workers have used alcohol and ether primarily to cleanse surfaces. Schottelius (1899) also used alcohol and ether to wash all surfaces of his cubicle and 10% Lysol solution for parts of the door frame and solid edges of the brooder. Following this, the cubicle was sterilized with 4 gm of formaldehyde vapor for 48 hours preceding the experiment. This was found to be quite satisfactory for sterilizing the area. If the humidity is high enough, this method of sterilization should be effective within 12 hours. Reviews on the action of germicides (see Reddish, 1954) indicate that formaldehyde gas is most active by virtue of dissolving in the water film on surfaces. The gas has good penetration power and the solution formed is both germicidal and sporicidal.

Küster (1915c) used 2% Lysol wash followed by sterilization with formaldehyde gas for his rearing tank. His sterile lock operated under pressure by heating water inside of the lock; he also heated formaldehyde solution in the lock. Balzam (1938) sterilized his apparatus by heating 10% formaldehyde at 40°C for 3 days. He then ventilated through a carbon filter to rid the apparatus of the gas. The apparatus of Glimstedt (1937) was sterilized at 50°C with 33% formaldehyde vapor after everything inside was presterilized at 110°C for 1 hour. Ammonia gas was used to neutralize the formaldehyde after 24 hours.

Sodium lauryl sulfate* (0.1% solution) was used to cleanse eggs prior to sterilization by Reyniers *et al.* (1949c) and Miller (1962). Although its bacteriostatic properties are mild, its cleansing action will greatly reduce the number of bacteria which must be killed or inactivated to give sterile chicks. Quaternary ammonium compounds have never been well accepted as sterilizing agents; however, diaprene chloride† was found to be effective in germfree experiments. Miller (1962) found that the material would sterilize eggs and the eggs had a good hatchability if adequate air flow was provided, while Luckey (1960) used it to wash the walls of the sterile room, as a germicidal solution for the floor and the surfaces of the rubber suit before entering the sterile room. Niss (1945) used 1 to 1000 Roccal‡ solution, a 10% solution of high molecular alkyl dimethyl benzyl ammonium chloride. The eggs were submerged in this solution at 40°C for 5 minutes. Bacteriological tests indicated that surfaces were sterile and sterile chicks were obtained.

Ethylene oxide, the simple cyclic ether, is one of the most potent germicides known. The compound is very volatile and toxic to man. The gas is extremely penetrating and most reactive at low humidity. It is also flammable and can be explosive; for this reason it is often diluted with Freon or carbon dioxide. These gaseous mixtures have 5 to 19% ethylene oxide in them. In the use of tanks with mixed gases it is well to remember that layering might occur; therefore, a full charge must be used if carbon dioxide is the diluent. Special autoclaves are made for sterilization with ethylene oxide. As might be

* Dreft, manufactured by Procter and Gamble, Cincinnati, Ohio.
† An effective quaternary nitrogen germicide, from Rohm and Haas, Philadelphia, Pennsylvania.
‡ Roccal from Winthrop Chemical Corporation, New York.

expected vacuum should be exerted to dispel air and the gas introduced under pressure to give maximum penetration. Heat increases
the bactericidal power of the gas. Large bags of bedding or 100 lb of
pelleted feed can be sterilized readily. A vacuum and adequate aeration are necessary to clear all the ethylene oxide from the food. As
mentioned in the discussion of diet sterilization, many changes occur
with this alkylating agent but diets can be properly sterilized with it.

Gustafsson (1959a,b) used tincture of iodine diluted 1 to 10 with
water to sterilize the abdominal surfaces of the mother rat for the
Cesarean operation. This was left for 10 minutes prior to the operation. Gustafsson (1948) also used Merthiolate, 1 to 1000, as a germicide around the window of this apparatus. Gustafsson has used a
variety of different fluids for the germicidal trap, but the best was
tincture of iodine diluted 1 to 200 with water. Unfortunately, the
fumes are disagreeable to both workers and animals and it is too
volatile for prolonged effectiveness. He has also used 1 to 1000
aqueous solution of cetyl pyridium chloride which has a high bactericidal activity, but its power diminishes with time. Hexylresorcinol
was used in a gasket powder to help inactivate any microorganisms
present where steam does not penetrate.

Cage Sterilization

An historical view of the early methods used for the sterilization
of the cage in which germfree animals were to be placed is presented
in Table 3.2. All workers used steam. Nuttall and Thierfelder (1897),
Schottelius (1908a), and Küster (1915a) used free flowing steam for
the major part of their apparatus. Cohendy (1912a) steam sterilized
his apparatus in a boiling pot of Koch at 99°C for 4 hours on two
separate occasions. All of these workers used steam under pressure to
sterilize utensils and material. Most workers used a germicidal compound for some part of the apparatus or as a cumulative germicide
before or after the steam. Steam and formaldehyde were used together
at 70°C for 2 days by Glimstedt (1936a). Sterile ammonia was used
to neutralize the formaldehyde: hexamethylenetetramine was formed
which gradually volatilized. Since sterile air was passed through the
cage for several days, cage sterilization and aeration took almost 2
weeks. Most workers employed an aseptic step; however, Reyniers
et al. (1943b) and Gustafsson (1948) performed operations in which
no aseptic step was involved. Schottelius (1908a) used a complete

TABLE 3.2

CAGE STERILIZATION BEFORE 1950

Investigator	Type	Agent	Pressure (lb/in.^{2})	Time (hr)	Temp. (°C)	Germastat	Aseptic step	Suit	Room treatment
Nuttall and Thierfelder	Bell jar	Steam and dry heat	0–1	?	100	Yes	Yes	Gloves	None
Schottelius	Roomette, metal hood	Steam and HCHO	0–1	1	100	10% Lysol HCHO (4gm/m^3)	Yes	Complete	Aseptic
Cohendy	Cylinder	Steam	15	$\frac{1}{2}$–8	99–120	?	Yes	No	Clean
Küster	Roomette	Steam and HCHO	0–1	?	100	Lysol and H$_2$O$_2$	Yes	Yes	Clean
Balzam	Metal cages	Steam and HCHO	30	—	121?	HCHO	Yes	Gloves attach	Clean
Glimstedt	Metal box	Steam and HCHO	0–5	1	50–110	"Tunnel" HCHO or Steam?	Yes	Gloves attach	—
Luckey et al.	Churn jar	Steam	17	$\frac{1}{2}$	126	No	No	No	None
Gustafsson	Inverted metal box	Steam	15	$\frac{3}{4}$	120	1:1000	Yes	Gloves	Clean
Reyniers et al.	Large cylinder	Steam	17	$\frac{1}{2}$	122	No	No	Gloves	None

sterile suit of canvas cloth. Schottelius was the only one who practiced
real asepsis in the room surrounding the sterile cage.

The germfree work today follows that of the early workers.
Gustafsson (1948, 1959b) used a tank which was sterilized inside an
autoclave. Hickey (1960) streamlined the sterilization of such light
metal cages as follows: air was removed by a 20 inch mercury vacuum
before the steam pressure was raised to 17 psi (pounds per square
inch). The pressure was relieved and a second vacuum drawn which
allowed the liter of water on the floor to boil. This vapor helped to
drive all air from the isolator through the partially open germicidal
trap; then full steam pressure was reapplied to the autoclave. Thermo-
regulators in dry diet inside the cage were used to maintain a temperature of 120°C for 30 minutes. Sterile air was admitted to the
isolator while it was still in the autoclave via a temporary filter. This
air maintained a positive pressure inside the isolator and the air
bubbled out through the germicidal trap until the incinerator on the
permanent air supply was heated to 300°C. The air was then introduced through the permanent sterilizer.

Details of sterilizing the heavy wall isolators and the sterile lock
were presented by Teah (1960). The tank was pretested under
pressure for 24 hours to see if it were air tight. Steam was allowed to
flow freely through the entire unit for 10 minutes to remove trapped
air. After maintaining a 26–28 inch mercury vacuum for approximately 7 minutes, free flowing steam was again admitted to the chamber for 10 minutes in order to exhaust all air. A fiber glass insulating
blanket was placed around the cage to reduce heat loss and to ensure
sterilization of the tank wall. Steam pressure at 17 psi, approximately
123°C, was maintained for 30 minutes to sterilize the tank. This
procedure also sterilized the glass wool filter. Air pressure was regu-
lated through a gas cock in the cover of the glove ports to keep the
gloves fully extended without distension into the interior of the cage.
This prevented the gloves from resting on the bottom of the tank. In
this manner excessive heat from the metal was avoided. Contact with
the bottom might prevent steam from reaching that part of the tank.
In some laboratories a vacuum was established following sterilization;
this was not only unnecessary, but it invited contamination through
pin-point leaks. Presterilized air was run through the tank to cool it
and to dry it to the desired humidity. The glove port covers were
removed and the isolator was ready to use.

Chemical sterilization of plastic cages was accomplished by washing all surfaces with 2% peracetic acid and 0.1% surfactant, then the peracetic acid was vaporized with continuous fogging for a period of 20–30 minutes. The saturated vapor was allowed to remain in the cage for 30 minutes; following this, sterile air was admitted for a period of 24–73 hours, depending upon the air flow, to drive out all residual vapor. Such procedure is more than adequate; shorter times have accomplished sterilization. Room sterilization was performed much as that for plastic cage sterilization. The walls were cleaned very carefully with a germicide and the room fogged 10 minutes one or two times, followed by aeration with sterile air.

Sterile Lock

The inner door of the sterile lock must remain open during the initial tank sterilization in order that the gasket surfaces become sterilized. During operation, the outer door is kept closed to reduce the microbial content of the lock. The operation of the sterile lock is very similar to that used for an autoclave or those germfree tanks which can withstand pressure. As mentioned previously much of the material to be placed in the sterile lock would be presterilized. The sterile lock can be used for gas, chemical, or steam sterilization. A single wall lock should have an insulation blanket around it during steam sterilization in order that the walls can be heated to the proper temperature. In order to take material into a germfree cage or to hook two germfree cages together, the inner door of the sterile lock must be properly closed. The outer door may then be opened and any material placed in the sterile lock may be taken from the germfree cage. The lock is cleaned with detergent solution and a germicidal compound is sprayed on the gasket surfaces of the doors. The sterile lock is packed using the principles of packing an autoclave in which materials rest on a wire screen and are not packed so tightly together that steam may not penetrate. If many small packages are being sterilized a metal perforated carrier may be used as a convenience for putting small packages into the germfree cage. The outer door is closed and a vacuum of 20 inches of mercury is created in the lock and held for 10 minutes to test for leaks using a pressure gauge. If no leak is indicated, pressure may be used to test for leaks employing the soap bubble technique or a Freon leak detector. Then free flowing steam is admitted until a temperature of 100°C is registered in both the jacket and the interior of the sterile lock; then steam pressure is admitted until thermocouples record 121°C for 25 minutes. At the end of the 25 minutes the steam supply is cut from the inner chamber while it is allowed to remain in the jacket, and sterile air is admitted to the sterile lock through a special filter available at the sterilization station. The heat in the jacket is cut off and the sterile lock allowed to cool. After the cooling, the inner door may be opened and the contents taken into the isolator. Heat to the animals is reduced during this sterilization by directing a stream of cold water on the germfree cage around the area of the sterile lock. However, considerable heat does irradiate into the germfree cage and into the room. Therefore any room in which a large number of sterilizations is to take place should have special ventilation. Sometimes the whole cage is packed full of diet, bedding, or other material, sterilized and tested for bacterial sterility before being passed into other germfree cages. Generally this requires more work and space than is warranted.

Before the outer door of the sterile lock is opened the inner door must be tightly closed and a vacuum pulled on the sterile lock to be sure that the inner door is properly closed. In order to take eggs or other heat labile materials in, the germicidal entry should be attached before the sterilization. At the end of the sterilization period the germicide should be added to the reservoir which would make a complete seal with the sleeve. Then the door at the end of the germicidal sleeve could be opened into the solution and pre-sterilized material taken in through the germicidal lock.

Chemical sterilization of the sterile locks is accomplished by (1) simply placing a small quantity of ethylene oxide, or other volatile germicide, in the lock and allowing it to vaporize at room temperature, (2) by bleeding in a spray of chemical; peracetic acid or ethylene oxide or its diluted mixtures, or (3) simply fogging the lock to drive the air out and to get thorough saturation of the area before shutting the door to the lock. Only the outside of the package needs to be sterilized. However, ethylene oxide sterilization of material can be accomplished in the food clave without presterilization. This sterilization is enhanced if the sterile lock has a jacket into which steam can be introduced to raise the temperature. However, the increased efficiency in sterilization does increase the heat of the cage, therefore, some of the advantage over steam is lost.

Horowitz et al. (1960) pointed out that the increase in heat load of the room was very pronounced during the steam sterilization of several isolators or sterile locks (see Fig. 3.27). Thus, when a number of tanks were sterilized during an 8-hour working day, the temperature

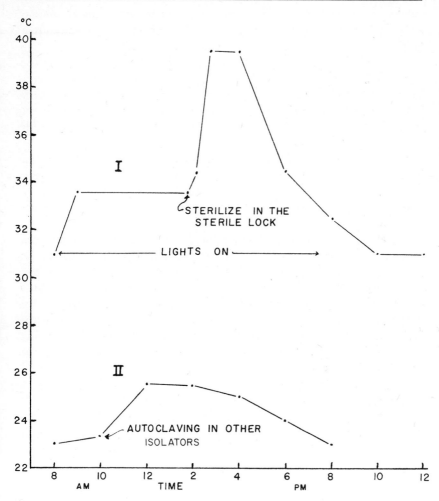

FIG. 3.27. Heat exchange. Temperature changes in the germfree isolator during steam sterilization of the sterile lock (I) and temperature changes in the isolator while other isolators are being sterilized in the same room (II). Taken from the data of Horowitz *et al.* (1959).

in the room rose 3–4°C above normal ambient temperatures (22–25°C). When this was added to the increased temperature from steam sterilization of the lock, the rats became quite uncomfortable. The temperature inside the cage should never go over 37°C for more than a few minutes. Another source of heat is the lights. Lights located outside of the germfree tank produce much less heating of the interior. Excessive heat may retard reproduction and has been known to kill valuable animals.

Air Sterilization

An historical view of air sterilization procedures prior to 1950 is given in Table 3.3. A prefilter takes out most particles. This allows the main filters to be used efficiently for a longer period of time. All investigators have used a prefilter for the air supply. Prefilters of Nuttall and Thierfelder (1897) were small tubes filled with cotton placed at the beginning of the air inlet and could be replaced as the cotton became filled with dirt. Since some microorganisms can grow through wet filters, most investigators also have had some system for drying the air. Nuttal and Thierfelder used potassium chloride tubes, Küster (1914, 1915a) used sulfuric acid, while modern investigators use a cold trap in the air line. Cotton filters were the main system for filtration for most workers until A. W. Phillips (1941b) showed the feasibility of using glass wool for this purpose, and glass wool filters were introduced by Reyniers and Trexler (1943b). Following cotton filtration. Nuttall and Thierfelder passed the air through a small platinum spiral heated to a red heat with a Bunsen burner. The air was then passed through a third cotton filter before it entered the sterile cage. In their apparatus the outlet air was taken through a sterile filter and bubbled through a mercuric chloride bath. Schottelius (1902) used a much simpler system for sterilization of the air, no heat was involved and only cotton filtration was used. The large clean room was supplied with sterile air. Large sterile pipes were filled with cotton for nonforced ventilation of the sterile room. The simple cotton filters were sterilized with the rest of the apparatus (using formaldehyde gas). The air inlet of Cohendy (1912a) was filled with two cotton filters, and the air was bubbled through mercuric chloride. The cotton filters were sterilized with the apparatus in the autoclave before the experiments begin. Cohendy apparently used suction to pull the air through the apparatus. Küster (1915a) pumped air with constant positive pressure through cotton filters, then bubbled it through mercuric chloride and potassium hydroxide for drying and for further insurance that no bacteria were admitted. This part of the apparatus was sterilized with dry heat before the experiment started. His exhaust air was filtered through a cotton filter. The system of Balzam (1937b) was similar to that of Küster; it had a prefilter in front

TABLE 3.3
AIR STERILIZATION

Investigator	Heat	Temp. (°C)	Germicide	Prefilter	Filter	Filter sterilized
Nuttall and Thierfelder	Yes	Bunsen	Outlet	Yes	Cotton	Dry heat
Schottelius	No	—	No	Yes	Cotton	HCHO
Cohendy	No	—	$HgCl_2$ + KOH	Yes	Cotton	Steam
Küster	Yes	180	No	Yes	Cotton	Dry heat
Balzam	No	—	No	Yes	Cotton	Steam
Glimstedt	No	—	Quinasol[a]	Yes	Cotton	$HgCl_2$
Luckey	No	—	No	Yes	Glass wool and cotton	Steam
Gustafsson	Yes	200	No	Yes	Glass wool, asbestos, and Carborundum	Dry heat
Reyniers and Trexler	No	—	No	Yes	Glass wool	Steam

[a] See text for structure.

of the air compressor which was changed every 3 days. The air was passed through a fine mesh metal cage to catch oil droplets from the compressor. A cotton filter on the other side of the compressor was changed less frequently, and the final cotton filter attached to the germfree cage was never changed. Balzam (1938) also maintained a positive pressure of about 35 ml of water. His inlet filters were small boxes, 60 × 150 mm, filled with cotton and sterilized in an autoclave. The air flow in his system could be as high as 10 cubic meters per hour. The air system of Glimstedt (1932) was similar to that of Schottelius: two cotton filter bats, one 12 cm² and the other 9 cm² were separated by 5 cm of air between them. These were sterilized at 50°C with formaldehyde (diluted 1:3) sprayed into the apparatus. A special feature of the cotton filters was that they were dipped in either a 2% solution of quinosol ([$C_6H_3OH(CH_3)N$] $2H_2SO_4$) or a 1% solution of mercuric chloride, then dried; thus any moisture which was formed on the filters reactivated the germicide to kill microorganisms. The air treatment of Glimstedt included a series of calcium chloride drying tubes which were changed daily. In his later experiments (1936a) the air was pumped through a 13 cm long cotton filter attached directly to the apparatus. The air system used by Reyniers and Trexler (1943b) and by Reyniers et al. (1946b, 1949b) consisted of prefiltered air pumped through long glass wool filters. These filters were sterilized with steam and could be dried by steam introduced into special pipes running through the center of the filters. Usually small quantities of air were used, about 0.2–0.5 cfm. The prefilters of Luckey (1956a) were large tubes filled with cotton. The air was humidified as desired: high for chicks during hatch to prevent the sticking of the shell to the chick, and low immediately after hatch. As the early investigators observed, the more dry the apparatus, the less difficulty there is in maintaining sterility. The air was heated to 39°C during incubation and hatch (Fig. 3.28); following hatch, the temperature was reduced about 3°C each week. The air was next filtered through alternate layers of glass wool and cotton in a pipe. The air outlet was a ½ cm glass tube 40 cm long with a constricted end to allow the desired air pressure and air flow. A manometer placed over the end gave an index of both air flow and air pressure. Usually about ½ cfm at 3 psi.

Gustafsson (1948) used a prefilter with tightly packed glass wool and cotton wool to take out the small droplets from the air compressor. He (1959b) used a special air sterilizer which had asbestos

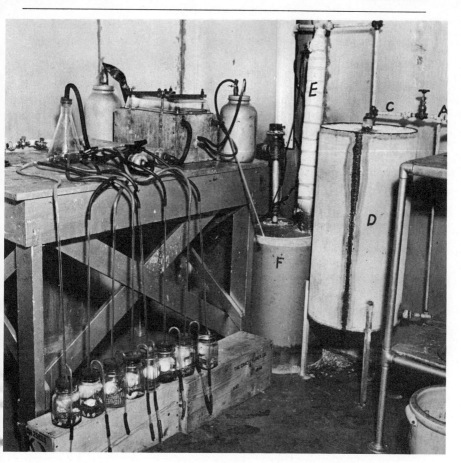

FIG. 3.28. Simplified system for rearing germfree chicks. Prefiltered air enters at (A) may go through the humidifier (D), or may by-pass this at (C) before it enters heater (E) and mixing chamber with sensing element (F). The air is sterilized in tubes which contain glass wool and cotton filters and goes into sterile chamber or into the testing jars via the manifold. Liquid media may also be sent through the manifold. Air exits through open tubes. Water and food in outside containers supply the chicks in the sterile chamber via rubber tubes. (Photo from T. D. Luckey, 1956, *Texas Repts. Biol. and Med.* **14,** 483.)

fiber, glass wool, and Carborundum embedded in it, with an electric heating element which was maintained at 300°C and heated the air to over 200°C. It is quite probable that most virus particles would become attached to the glass fibers by electrostatic attraction. However, thorough testing for virus holding ability has not been applied to any presently used filters. A. W. Phillips *et al.* (1960) used steam to sterilize the air filter on their plastic isolator. They used the low pressure Cambridge filter* for both inlet and exhaust. Trexler (1957) described the sterilizing systems for the plastic isolators. Dry heat was used to sterilize his air filter. The inlet filter (Fig. 3.29) had four layers of ½ inch glass wool filter (mst type PF-105)†. Reyniers and

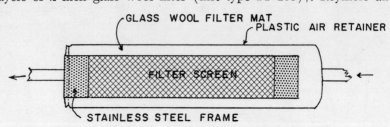

GLASS WOOL FILTER MAT

PLASTIC AIR RETAINER

FILTER SCREEN

STAINLESS STEEL FRAME

FIG. 3.29. Trexler simplified air filter. The prefiltered air which enters at the right must pass through two or more layers of glass wool filter mat, a large surface area of a porous filter bed designed to give efficient low pressure filtration.

Sacksteder (1960a) used only two layers of this filter down. Trexler preferred an outlet trap for the air rather than a filter since it reduced to a minimum the contamination due to wet, dirty, or plugged outlet filters, and it allowed a large air flow to be used. A floating cap may be calibrated to indicate the air flow. The trap contained triaryl phosphate ester solution as a sealing fluid; this had the advantage of having a high density and a low vapor pressure.

The air filtration system for the sterile room of Luckey (1960) (Fig. 3.23) has not been subjected to exhaustive breakdown tests of the individual components, but has functioned properly with no contamination detected from the air system for a period of several months. The outlet filter to the room was a Cambridge low pressure filter; the air also escaped from the door in large quantities when entrance or exit was made through the plastic flaps. No contamination could be detected which could be traced through this flap door system. As long as adequate quantities of sterile air were going through an opening without undue turbidity, the interior remained sterile.

Speculations on other systems for sterile air should include the chemical generation of oxygen at a controlled rate inside the chamber with the uptake of CO_2 by an alkaline bath in the bottom of the cage.

* Cambridge Corporation, Syracuse, New York.
    † The glass wool mat is obtained from the Owens-Corning Fiberglass Corporation, Toledo, Ohio.

Such a system would require no ventilation and no air filtration. Humidity could be controlled by a system such as that used by Cohendy: condensing water from the atmosphere. Water evaporated from excreta and metabolic water would comprise a major portion of the water required; therefore, if food with high moisture content were used, no connection with the outside environment would be needed for water, air inlet, or air outlet. Another system would be the symbiotic growth of *Chlorella* or other plant which would take up the carbon dioxide of the animal and produce adequate quantities of oxygen within a single enclosed system. It is suspected that the oxygen in a compressed tank of oxygen would be sterile. If aseptic connection could be made from this supply of oxygen to a germfree cage, this might be a good source of sterile oxygen for the cage. Another simple system would be one which would use large low-pressure filters on the sides of the isolators and would rely on diffusion for gaseous exchange: a modern version of the Schottelius system. The air centrifuge of Iinoya (1961) may be useful.

Food Sterilization

A wide variety of methods for diet sterilization have been used in the past (Table 3.4). Nuttall and Thierfelder (1897) boiled milk for 30 minutes on 3 consecutive days. Schottelius (1902) placed diet material into vessels and sterilized them in a Roerback steam sterilizer. Apparently the time required for sterilization was determined for each batch of diet. When sterility tests showed the diet to be sterile, the vessels was again placed in a sterilizer and resterilized before being taken into the cubicle. Cohendy (1912a) apparently sterilized diet in an autoclave for an adequate period of time. Küster (1914) boiled goat milk for 15 minutes on 5 consecutive days, Glimstedt (1936a) boiled milk in a steam bath at 100°C for 45 minutes in 3 days, and Reyniers and Trexler (1943b) sterilized their milk in an autoclave at 121°C for 20 minutes. The method which Gustafsson (1948) used for milk was similar. With milk or with diets to which water has been added to give a consistency of mush or gelatin, heat sterilization is most effective and the diets can be maintained in solid containers. Media is steam sterilized in culture tubes in routine manner with a minimum of problems with heat penetration or trapping of air.

Reyniers *et al.* (1946) established the methods which have been used for steam sterilization of solid diets in most subsequent work. A summary of this method is: The solid diet is wrapped in cloth bags in such a manner that the steam has no more than 1 cm to penetrate; i.e., 2 cm total thickness. This is placed in the sterile lock, vacuum is pulled for 5–10 minutes; then 5 minutes of free flowing steam is used to help "wash out" residual air before steam pressure is admitted. Thermocouples inserted in the food are used to register the fact that the diet is heated to 121°C for a period of 20 (17–25) minutes. As indicated in Fig. 3.26), the diet is hot for a longer period of time than

TABLE 3.4

DIET STERILIZATION PRIOR TO 1950

Investigator	Type	Agent	Time (min)	Temp. (°C)	Thickness (cm)
Nuttall and Thierfelder	Milk	Boiling	30[a]	100	—
Schottelius	Solid	Dry[b]	?	100	?
Cohendy	Solid	Steam	25	115	?
Küster	Milk	Boil	15[c]	100	—
Glimstedt	Milk	Steam	45[a]	110	—
Balzam	Solid	Steam	180	127	2.5
Reyniers and Trexler	Milk	Steam	20	121	—
Reyniers et al. (1949b)	Solid	Steam	20–25	123	2.5
Gustafsson	Solid	Steam	25	120	2.5
Luckey	Milk	Steam	20	120	2[d]
Luckey	Solid	Steam	20–25	123	2

[a] For 3 consecutive days.

[b] Diet material was sterilized in their own vessels, tested for sterility, and then resterilized.

[c] The milk was boiled for 5 consecutive days. Then only flasks which tested sterile were used.

[d] Solid diets were mixed with water to form a thick porridge and sterilized in the same manner.

is indicated by the sterilization maximum. It is emphasized that if the diet were packed too thickly or if the diet were too finely powdered, the steam could not penetrate properly and ineffective sterilization might result. To avoid this problem, thinner layers or a longer heating period would be necessary. Large quantities of pelleted diet may be sterilized since steam penetration problems are drastically reduced. It is not necessary to pull a vacuum following the diet sterilization since the saturated steam at the proper pressure does not leave more moisture present in the diet than was originally present.

The chemical changes induced in diets by steam sterilization are compared to those induced by radiation sterilization in Chapter 4.

New procedures using a high temperature for a short time are presently being evaluated for use in germfree routines.

Sterilization with agents other than steam was not used for diets until recently. One of the cleanest and least destructive methods for sterilization of solid diets is radiation, see Luckey *et al.* (1955c). γ-Radiation or electron beam bombardment with a potential greater than 2 million electron volts sterilized diets when over 2 million rads were used. Luckey (1960) and Miller (1962) used 2 million rads of γ-radiation. A. W. Phillips (1960) has used 3 million rads minimum and Horton and Hickey (1961) used 4 to 5 million rads. Since there was destruction of some nutrients with irradiation, higher levels are not to be recommended. Two million rads was adequate; therefore, a safety margin of 1 million rads is more than enough with the normal bacterial population found in most syntype diets. Satisfactory irradiation sterilization of fresh foods and of liquid diets is much more difficult owing to the excessive molecular ionization (see Hutchinson, 1961 for the effect of the medium upon the reactions obtained). Irradiation in the dry state was used routinely for heat labile materials as antibiotics and vitamin C.

Diets could be sterilized with chemicals but such procedures have not been used routinely for germfree animals. Colonies of mice and rats have been maintained on ethylene oxide (or carboxide) sterilized diets in a gnotobiotic condition for many months and through 2–5 generations. Ethylene oxide can be misused, as can steam sterilization or radiation. Ethylene oxide procedures have not been established for liquid diets because the compound is too reactive under these conditions and is very difficult to remove from liquid diets which contain fat. It is used to sterilize liquid media. Therefore, diets are usually steam or irradiation sterilized in packages before being taken into cages equipped for only germicidal trap or gaseous sterilization.

Filtration was used for heat labile materials in solution and was particularly useful for the sterilization of heat labile vitamins, such as thiamine and pantothenic acid. Filtration of cell-free tissue extracts has been used for sources of vitamins, antigens, and viruses. In each case bacteria-free material which could be used for the desired purpose was obtained. Material to be filtered into a germfree tank was usually prefiltered once and filtered twice again in two successive filters on the isolator. Many isolators have a plug in the sterile lock for filtration purposes. Since gravity flow is too slow and vacuum should not be used, pressure filtration is the method of choice.

One method for obtaining sterile food has not been exploited to date; namely, the presentation of sterile organisms to germfree animals. This method was used in a study in which sterile chicks were fed to germfree rats for the purpose of trying to find vitamins or nutritional factors which could increase lactation (presented in detail in the next chapter). Landy (1960) fed sterile bean sprouts to guinea pigs in an attempt to prevent an enlarged cecum, but this was not successful. The process of feeding extra males and old females from a sterile colony of animals to experimental animals would appear to be the simplest way to prepare antigen-free diets. Thus, excess animals from a breeding colony could be used to produce an "antigen-free colony." In order to minimize the number of foreign antigens the intestinal tract should not be used as food. Minerals, vitamins, fiber, and carbohydrates should be added to get the best utilization of the homologous protein. Springer (1959) suggests several possible sources of antigens in such a system (including possibilities from the animal itself). Although antigen-freeness approaches the infinite in cleanliness, an *antigenostic* (from *antigengnostic*) biological system with *only known antigens* may be possible.

Since soluble synthetic diets are available, it should be possible to filter a complete diet into the germfree cage. This process would be expensive in time and money but it might be worth the effort. Irradiation sterilization of the dry diet would be feasible. The steam sterilization of a synthetic diet in liquid form would be expected to lead to many reactions which have not been adequately studied. It should be noted that chickens do not feed easily from a liquid diet. They have some difficulty in getting enough food, and they have more difficulty in keeping themselves clean. In anticipation of the use of germfree chicks, the author (1943, unpublished) added water to a syntype diet and steam sterilized it in a thick soup consistency. When this mixture was fed to conventional chicks, it was found that diet dripped from the beaks of the chicks and got all over the feathers and the cage. First one wing would be glued to the body, next the second wing. Eventually both feet became glued to the bottom of the cage. In some cases even the beak was attached to the cage floor and the poor chicks were effectively immobilized. However, Reyniers *et al.* (1960a) found that such diets made into a Jello consistency could be used to feed germfree animals (mice and quails). The advantage of such a diet was that water did not need to be added separately.

Sterilization of Water and Other Liquids

Information has already been presented concerning the sterilization of water and other liquids. The use of biological water in a
recycling process is theoretically good: since no outside source is
involved, contamination is minimized. If the cage were kept relatively
dry and a cold finger or plate provided for condensation, approximately one-half of the water required could be caught. In Cohendy's
(1912a) experiments with moist air, more than enough water was
trapped by the cold finger and a place had to be provided for an
overflow after the water cup was filled. The amount of water con-
densed will depend to a large extent upon the humidity of the air
which enters. Dry air is preferred to moist because it is much easier
to sterilize. Wet filters invite fungal or bacterial growth to grow
through the filter. However, air below 10% relative humidity is too dry
for optimum biological conditions and leads to irritation of mucous
membranes, drying out of the skin, and dandruff. Therefore, a relative
humidity of 20–30% is preferable. Another way of introducing water
is to use a wet food: milk, a soup, Jello, or a mash the consistency of
agar will provide enough water for the animals so that little or no
other water must be provided. At the same time this is one of the
most efficient ways to sterilize the diet.

Water could be irradiated or sterilized with chemicals but these
methods have not been used on a practical basis. Since most compounds which are bactericidal are either harmful or distasteful to vertebrates, particularly mammals, the chemical would have to be neutralized or aerated to be removed. Filtration of water is feasible and has
been suggested for practical use, but none of the systems presently
operating use it routinely. The basic problem to be solved would be to
keep bacteria from growing through the wet filter over a period of
many months. Steam sterilization is routinely used for water. Water is
normally packaged in small containers up to 1 pint in size; sometimes
1 or 2 liters are used. For containers of 500 ml or less the usual steam
sterilization of 17 lb pressure for 20 minutes is adequate for liquids.
This can be done in a cotton-stoppered flask. Reyniers et al. (1946)
routinely used milk cans which were filled with water and soldered.
Trexler (1959a) recommended the use of presterilized water in containers which can be taken in with either gaseous sterilization or
through a germicidal trap.

Sterilization of Equipment and Utensils

Simple utensils, interior cages, balances, water, food, and small pieces of cloth can be steam sterilized during the initial sterilization of the cage. However, any complex apparatus which has porous surfaces or interlocking parts which would not allow steam to penetrate readily should be sterilized with dry heat. This is also true for large quantities of powder or grease or tightly wrapped cloth. These things should be wrapped in 2 layers of heavy paper and sterilized with dry heat. Routine use of dry heat sterilization indicates that material can be sterilized at a shorter time than is usually recommended in texts. However, a safety factor is needed since sometimes materials are encountered in which spores are difficult to kill. A graph taken from Reddish (1954) (Fig. 3.30) indicates the importance of size and shape in sterilization. Therefore, the use of thermocouples in any large package is recommended in order that the operator know that the temperature at the center of the large package of material was adequate for the prescribed time.

After being presterilized with dry heat the material is then taken to the sterile isolator and resterilized in a conventional manner. This may be done with chemical spray, liquid trap, or steam sterilization. In any case only the surface or wrapping needs to be sterilized; and even with a liquid trap, material can be taken into the germfree cage before moisture penetrates the two layers of paper.

When diets and other material are presterilized with radiation they are usually packed in three plastic bags. Immediately before being passed through a germicide lock or into a spray lock the outer plastic is taken off. The dirt on the outside bag never enters the germicide. The sterile second package can be readily passed through the trap into the germfree isolator. Inside the isolator the second package is discarded leaving the desired material in a single plastic bag with no germicide on the outside of the bag. This is particularly essential where the material is diet or is to be added to diet since no trace of germicide should be allowed in the diet.

Sterilization of Animal Surfaces

Nuttall and Thierfelder (1897) used 5% HCl dip followed by 1–1000 mercuric chloride solution in order to sterilize the eggs. Each day thereafter the eggs were sprayed with mercuric chloride solution. This was probably too great a dilution for adequate sterilization of eggs. They concluded that bacteria were already in the oviduct before and during the laying down of the shell and were established within the shell membrane: "We must stop using chickens in the study of the above problem. Unfortunately, it seems to us that the result also means relinquishing an experimental attack on the entire problem of

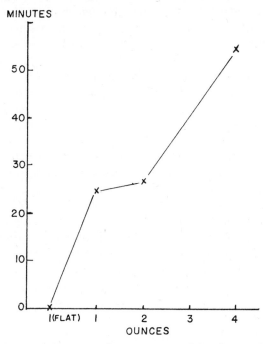

FIG. 3.30. Heat penetration. The time required for the powder to reach the sterilization temperature varies according to size and shape of the material. A 1-ounce petri dish reaches the sterilization temperature as soon as the autoclave is at required temperature. A 1-ounce bottle takes about 25 minutes, a 2-ounce bottle takes about 27 minutes, and a 4-ounce bottle takes approximaetly twice as long. From the data of Reddish (1954).

germfree life." This came after their unsuccessful attempt to rear guinea pigs in the germfree condition. They felt their conclusion substantiated the result of Zorkendorfer (1893) that indicated eggs were contaminated. Schottelius (1899) confirmed the work of earlier bacteriologists and showed that the egg interior was bacteria free although the shell was infected. He realized that if the membranes of the egg shell were kept intact and the egg were kept dry, the danger of infection would be at a minimum. The entry of bacteria and especially mold mycelium could be made through one of the fine openings of the wet or damaged egg shell. Schottelius knew the largest pores of the egg were found over the air pocket of the egg and the temperature of the sterilizing baths was most important; cooling of the egg would tend to draw air or moisture inside while a warm bath would cause little change in the temperature of the egg and therefore no major change in the gas pressure within the constant volume of the egg. He made a great number of pertinent investigations for a suitable method for disinfection of the eggs and developed a system which gave bacteriologically sterile eggs.

More recent studies on the bacterial infection of fresh eggs was reviewed by Haines (1939). The microbial population of inoculated eggs decreased with time during incubation. Studies indicated that sterilized or well cleansed egg surfaces contributed to the hatchability of the eggs. For this reason formaldehyde gas and detergent washes are sometimes used to increase hatchability in commercial hatcheries. Studies on the bacterial invasion of embryonated eggs after the death of embryos and the preparation of the egg shell for sterilization were presented by Reyniers et al. (1949b). The results confirmed work of Heneston and Hendrick (1947) which showed that a detergent wash of an egg gave a good percentage of sterilizable eggs. With no detergent wash 5–10% of the eggs were not sterilizable in 1% mercuric chloride. Forsyth et al. (1953) presented work on the factors affecting the microbial population of egg shells and showed that eggs properly washed soon after laying had 90% less microorganisms than those not treated. However, since improper washing "drives" the microorganisms inside the shell, it is much preferred that no treatment be given the eggs prior to their being received for germfree work. The experimenter then has at his command all of the procedures which are used to sterilize the egg surface.

Reyniers et al. (1949b) gave comparisons of different germicides, different concentrations, and different bath times on the sterilization of egg shells. Since mercuric chloride was as effective as any and better than most germicides, further detail was given concerning the effect of mercuric chloride dilution at different time intervals on the hatch and the sterilization of egg shells. Eggs were disinfected at 0, 18, 20, or at 0 and 20 days. In all cases germfree chicks could be obtained and in all cases the percentage of hatch was high.

Different procedures have been used in the procurement of sterile germfree chicks and other birds. Metaphen solution at 1–500 for 45 minutes gave sterile eggs. However, no hatch data was obtained. Since 2–20% of the eggs are contaminated even following sterilization it is obvious that setting too many eggs in a single isolator would result in a high number of contaminations. For this reason 4–10 eggs are a practical compromise for obtaining sterile germfree chicks. More than 20 eggs were never used at one time. Miller (1962) found that eggs washed with 5% solution of Dreft followed by treatment with Diaprene chloride gave sterile eggs when a 2.5% concentration was used for 5 minutes or when a 3 minute dip was used with a 10% concentration. The hatch was good in a large incubator.

Schottelius (1908a) used 0.5% HgCl₂ and brushed the eggs vigorously 1 day before hatch. After this washing he attempted to rinse the mercuric chloride completely from the eggs with strong saline and dried them with sterile cotton. The whole operation was maintained at a temperature of 40°C in order not to harm the embryo. The eggs were dried and the sterilization repeated. A high proportion of these eggs were sterile. Cohendy used 0.5% mercuric chloride solution and a saline rinse at 40°C before incubation. Cohendy (1912a) and Balzam (1937b) selected clean eggs as carefully as had Schottelius. Balzam (1937b) immersed the eggs on the 18th day of incubation in 1% mercuric chloride solution for 2 minutes at 40°C after which he brushed them vigorously. They were then wrapped in sterile cotton, placed in a germfree apparatus, and again dipped in 1% mercuric chloride. Lakey (1945) found a 1–1000 dilution of Roccal,* to be a satisfactory wash. Eggs were submerged in this solution at 40°C for 5 minutes. In his early work Reyniers followed the procedure of Balzam. In later work Reyniers et al. (1946) brushed 20 day embryonated eggs with a detergent in order to mechanically clean the surface and to permit the germicide to penetrate into the pores. The egg was placed not more than 1 inch below the surface of 1% mercuric chloride for 8 minutes and the germicide was allowed to dry on the shell. After further review of the bacterial content of eggs and the methods used to sterilize eggs, a standard method was adopted by Reyniers et al. (1949a). It is presented in detail in the section on obtaining germfree birds. Luckey et al. (1960) used essentially the same system for sterilizing turkey eggs except that the second dip was performed at 27 days, which was 1 day prior to hatch for the turkeys. Forbes et al. (1958c, 1959) immersed 18 day old embryonated eggs

* A 10% solution of alkyldimethylbenzylammonium chloride manufactured by Winthrop Chemical Corporation, New York.

for 2 minutes in a 0.15% detergent solution, PN-700 conditioner.* The
eggs were then dipped for 12 minutes in 2% mercuric chloride solution
at 37°C. These methods allow about 4 of every 5 experiments to
begin with germfree chicks.

Germfree mammals present more procurement problems than do
germfree chicks. One is the aseptic transfer of full term fetuses from
the sterile uterus of the conventional mother into the isolator. This
transfer requires the surface sterilization of the abdomen of the pregnant mother. Nuttall and Thierfelder (1896b) shaved the abdomen of
guinea pigs, washed them successively with soap and water, mercuric
chloride, and finally with alcohol and ether. The animal was then
wrapped in wet towels and introduced into a sterile tent, the rearing
cage and instruments were previously placed in the tent. Küster
(1914) washed the mother goat with warm 2% Lysol solution followed
by a warm water rinse. The operating room was thoroughly disinfected by the method of Liebermann: intensive rubbing with a clay
and soap (without water) followed by the laying down of a thick
layer of an aseptic paste using 95% alcohol. On the day of the operation
disinfection of the room was repeated and at this time the operator
disinfected himself with the Liebermann bolus method. The operation
was carried out under a spray of hydrogen peroxide. Glimstedt
(1936a) performed Cesarean operation on guinea pigs in a room
used only for this purpose under strictest asepsis. Reyniers and Trexler
(1943b) evolved the concept of a surgical unit attached to a germfree
cage. The abdomen was prepared by removal of the hair, detergent
wash, a bath in potassium mercuric iodide, and then treatment with
tincture of iodine solution. The abdominal surface was brought into
close contact with the cellophane membrane soaked with Merthiolate
1–1000† which divided the upper and lower chambers of the operating
cage. Details of the operation on the early work with guinea pigs and
on the first monkey experiment (Reyniers, 1932; Reyniers and Trexler,
1943b) have not been published. Their method used for guinea pigs
was similar to that used for rats by Reyniers *et al.* (1946) which is
described in the following section. Gustafsson (1948) also gave the
details of the Cesarean section on rats. The abdominal skin was cut
and pegged to a ring. This was sealed to the bottom of the operating
chamber and tincture of iodine (1:10) was used to bath the exposed
surface for 10 minutes. With this procedure no contact was made with
the outside of the skin and the operating area. The methods used for

* Service Industries, Philadelphia, Pennsylvania.
† Ely Lilly Co., Indianapolis, Indiana.

guinea pigs by Phillips *et al.* (1959) and for mice and rabbits by
Pleasants (1959), are very similar to the method of Reyniers *et al.*
(1946).

Obtaining Germfree Animals

Innately Germfree Animals

Although a good supply of some laboratory animals is now available from germfree colonies, this was not always the case. It is more
practical to obtain certain animals, such as birds, from the egg than to
maintain colonies of germfree chickens. Therefore, the first germfree
animals were procured from non-germfree, or conventional, animals.
However, even the first germfree animals which were obtained in
order to start colonies were innately germfree. The Cesarean operation includes transfer of the mature embryo from the bacteriologically
sterile uterus and placental membranes into a germfree isolator. In
the experiments of Nuttall and Thierfelder (1897), Küster (1914),
Cohendy and Wollman (1922), Glimstedt (1936a), and Luckey
(1960) the Cesarean operation was performed in a tent or room
which housed the germfree apparatus nearby. In each case an aseptic
transfer of the young was made to get the germfree embryo into the
germfree cage. No contamination is reported due to the aseptic transfer of the sterile embryo to the germfree environment. In the methods
of Reyniers *et al.* (1946a) and Gustafsson (1948) the aseptic transfer
was eliminated since the young were taken directly from the uterus
into the sterile cage and the sterilized surface of the dam made a
direct connection with the germfree operating cage. Contamination
from the embryos, the operation, and the transfer occurs in less than
1% of all experiments.

Theoretically, it should be possible to cleanse a mother prior to
parturition and place her in a sterile nest. As the young are born,
they can be transferred from the reach of the mother into a germicidal
trap and then into a sterile cage while still in the amniotic sac. The sac
and placenta can then be discarded and the young should be sterile
because each has been in a complete envelope until this was ruptured
in the sterile environment. This procedure should not be technically
difficult because the mother would be in somewhat of a trance, apparently a natural narcosis, during the birth of multiple young.

The whole operation is somewhat simpler when egg-laying species
are involved since the embryo within the egg is normally sterile. It is
a simple problem to collect clean eggs and sterilize the outer surfaces

before passing each egg into a germfree tank which can be used as an incubator. However, this procedure is less reliable than the direct procurement of germfree animals from the mother, as shown by the contamination rate which varies between 2 and 20% at the time of hatch.

Since it is known that some diseases are transferred *in utero* or in the oviduct, sources of animal stock must be obtained which are free from such diseases. The status of virus diseases is still not clear, but in virus diseases as in bacterial diseases, it must be recognized that the introduction of young is the biggest break in the germfree system. All parts of the germfree apparatus should be physically tested for the passage of particles which would exclude bacteria, fungi, rickettsia, or viruses. But assurance of germfreeness must also come from biological barriers when the first germfree animals are taken into an isolator.

Acquired Germfree Status

It appears to be at least theoretically possible that the chick embryo, at least the inside of the egg, could become contaminated and the natural defense mechanisms of the egg could render the embryo and the egg sterile. Since the egg shell with all its membranes and different layers represents a good bacterial barrier, destruction of microbes within the egg would be a real step toward effective preparation of the egg interior for the development of a sterile embryo. The shell of an egg is usually sterile before the egg is laid (Stuart and McNally, 1943) and it is rarely contaminated when it passes through the cloaca (Haines, 1939) unless the hen has diarrhea.

Although very little work has been done on the decontamination of laboratory animals this must be considered as an important procedure since it would give animals which have a full complement of well developed microbial defense systems without the presence of living microorganisms. Such an animal should be important in theoretical biology, particularly in the study of defense mechanisms, and could be a source of germfree colonies. The work which has been done on this problem is reviewed in Chapter 6.

Techniques for Rearing Germfree Animals

Fish

Although germfree fish have never been raised, they have been obtained by several workers; the only problem which remains is to work out proper nutrition. (Published details were presented in Chapter 2.)

Amphibia

O. Metchnikoff (1901) reared germfree tadpoles by gathering freshly laid eggs and placing them in sterile water. The outer surface of the eggs were thoroughly cleaned with sterile water to remove the slimy soft layer which was permeated with bacteria and algae. The inner layer was difficult for microorganisms to penetrate partly because of mechanical impermeability and probably because of bactericidal activity. The inner layer was normally found to be germfree. After thoroughly cleaning the eggs until the outer surface was gone and the inner surface was clean, Metchnikoff kept the eggs in flowing water, which had been sterilized through a Chamberlain candle, until embryo movement could be seen. These mature eggs were then thoroughly cleaned again in sterile water and the jelly layers teased apart with sterile needles. The individual embryos were placed in sterile wash water and then transferred to individual glass vessels which contained diet sterilized at 120°C. Moro (1905) repeated the experiment of Madame Metchnikoff using essentially the same procedures but with greater amount of aeration for the hatch and rearing. Material and all eggs were gathered in 1% boric acid solution and cleaned, then the outer jelly solution was mechanically removed and the eggs were vigorously washed in flowing water. A second transparent jelly coating was removed and the eggs, which were now surrounded by only a thin transparent membrane, were disinfected in a 0.3% boric acid solution. Eggs treated in this manner were found to be germfree from both aerobic and anaerobic bacteria and the frog larvae hatched 46 days after this treatment.

Birds

Reyniers *et al.* (1949b) described the following standard for the sterilization of eggs for germfree research. Fresh clean eggs are allowed to assume room temperature, then brushed vigorously in a 1% Dreft solution in distilled water at 38°C. This solution should be flowing in order that one egg does not contaminate another. The eggs are then submerged 1 cm under the surface of 2% mercuric chloride solution for 5 minutes at 38°C. The germicide is allowed to dry on the shell and the eggs placed in an incubator at 38°C. The eggs are turned automatically several times a day for 18 days. At 20 days the eggs are candled and an appropriate number with active embryos are placed in a narrow nylon coarse mesh sack and submerged for 5 minutes at 38°C in the 2% mercuric chloride germicidal trap of the germfree tank. They are maintained 1 cm under the surface to keep hydrostatic pressure low until they are taken into the cage. They are then taken into the germfree tank which is maintained at 38°C until the chicks hatch within a few hours: infrared lamps, a heating blanket, or a 38°C room may be used. If the germfree cage has a steam jacketed sterile lock, steam may be introduced with a steam proportioning control* to maintain 38°C in the sterile lock through the hatch. The egg shells are removed from the space available to the chicks and the germfree chicks are tested for sterility.

Horowitz et al. (1960) used peracetic acid to sterilize egg surfaces at 19 days incubation. They simply placed the nonsterile eggs in a nonsterile plastic tank and sterilized the tank in the usual manner with the chemical. The eggs were placed on a sterile mesh so that peracetic acid could completely envelop them, individually sprayed at the beginning of the process, and turned at least twice during the sterilization period.

Mammals

Time of Parturition. The weight and maturity of the young at birth is an important variable in the success of hand-rearing of germfree mammals. It is essential to obtain the young at full term. The fast rate of development of rats *in utero* is illustrated in Fig. 3.31. These mammals doubled their weight every 2 days during the last week *in utero*. During the last day they gained 68 mg per hour: a 1% increase in total weight every 5 hours! Therefore, many methods have been used to predict the exact time of parturition prior to the Cesarean operation. The simplest method of determining the time of parturition is to count the days from a known breeding date. This was done in rodents simply by separating the sexes until the breeding day desired. The method of vaginal smears has been used, but it was laborious and the examination upset many of the females. A more efficient method was to examine the female rats on the night 21 days before the operation. Those in heat (showing lordosis when the back was stroked) were placed in the cage with two males. Immediate submission of the female confirmed the heat; the females were left with the males for 1–6 hours. Observation of a vaginal plug the next

* Minneapolis Mail Order Co., Philadelphia, Pennsylvania.

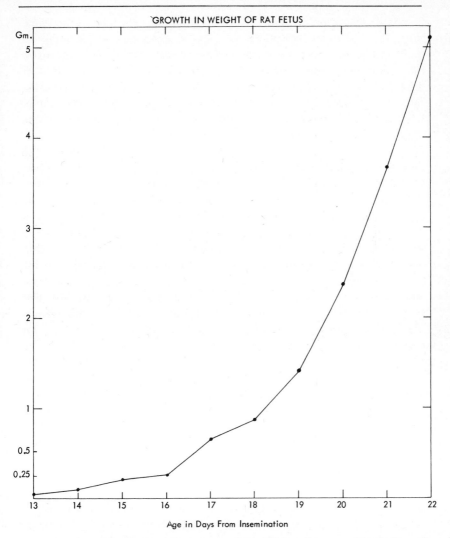

GROWTH IN WEIGHT OF RAT FETUS

Age in Days From Insemination

FIG. 3.31. Weight increment in rat fetus. Curve from combined data of Stratsenburg (1915), Angula and Gonzales (1932), and Hamilton and Bewar (1938).

morning confirmed insemination. About 80% of these cast litters on the predicted day. The gestation period for many species is given in standard references such as Spector (1956) and may be determined more definitely by astute observation of an inbred colony maintained under constant environment. Glimstedt (1936a,b) set the time of

Cesarean operation in guinea pigs by breeding several at the same time, the Cesarean operation was begun when one of the mothers delivered young by natural birth. Since guinea pigs and large mammals may have more than 1 day variation in the gestation period of different individuals, neither of the above methods is entirely satisfactory. Methods for estimating the time of parturition based upon individual characteristics are preferable. The development of the mammary gland or the time of expression of milk have been used, but are not reliable enough indices. Much better is the eye of the master to evaluate things as size or weight increase, general mobility, the change in muscle tonus and stretching of the abdominal muscles, the placement of the uterus, size (determined by palpation) of the embryos, movement of the embryos, the bursting of the placenta, and most particularly the nesting activity of the dam. The action of the undisturbed rat immediately preceding parturition is significant; labor movements with lordosis may be seen for a variable length of time (up to 1 day); there is usually an increased nesting activity with considerable nervousness exhibited. A few minutes before the first birth the mother-to-be calms and often appears to sleep; this trance-like quiescence develops into a natural narcosis. A useful method for the determination of parturition date has been developed by Bruce Phillips and Patricia Wolfe (1959). They followed the spread of the symphysis pubis; when it reached 1 cm, parturition time was near. When the rate of diastasis increased rapidly to 2–2.2 cm, the Cesarean operation was performed. After much time and effort in measurements of this change and many X-ray analyses, they learned that Glimstedt (1936a) had used this method to advantage two decades previously.

The ultimate method for mammals which have large litters was worked out by Bud Teah and J. A. Reyniers and was used for years in our work at the University of Notre Dame. The repeated report of "germfree" from M. Wagner in the bacteriology laboratory showed the method to be practical. Four or five rats were bred 21 days before the operation day; on the due date, the rats were watched constantly until one gave birth to the first of her litter. She was quickly stunned or anesthetized and the remainder of the litter were delivered by Cesarean birth into the germfree cage within 5–7 minutes. This method regularly gave germfree young which were vigorous and mature at birth.

A combination of these methods was used to determine the proper time to operate on sheeps and pigs. Ewes have added characteristics which are helpful: the abdomen drops perceptively between the thighs 1 or 2 days prior to parturition and the perivulvular area protrudes prominently. Since most lambs are born in the early morning hours, preparations for the Cesarean operation can be performed without undue hurry during the day.

Operation. The germfree Cesarean section formerly began with the presentation of anesthesia. If it is given, it should be used much as Gustafsson (1948) used it: the mother was given a light ether narcosis, after which the spinal cord was cut at the 6th cervical segment. This allowed the ether to be dispersed before the young were delivered, and provided complete surgical anesthesia in the area of the operation. The fast Teah-Reyniers operation was used in most experiments by the author for rearing germfree rats. When the first embryo was delivered by natural birth, the mother was sacrificed by a blow on the head, quickly tied to an operating board, the abdomen shaved with electric clippers and scrubbed with 1–1000 Zepherine chloride. The prepared animal was then inserted into the operating trap of the germfree operating tank (Fig. 3.12) and raised until the abdomen made tight contact with the plastic membrane which separated the operating trap from the operating space above. The plastic was wet with Zepherine chloride (1–1000) and the operating area draped with sterile towels. The epidermis and the plastic was picked up at the center line with small forceps and a 3 inch incision was made through both the skin and the wet plastic using a cautery brought to red heat. The edges of the skin, the sterile towel, and the plastic were secured with hemostats and layed back to give an operating area. The muscle and fascia were moistened with germicide; the operating area at this point looked very similar to that of Gustafsson (1948). Incision was next made through the dermal layers using a cautery protected by a mosquito hemostat by sliding it underneath the cautery. The edges of the abdominal wall were separated with retractors. The exposed uterus was clamped off with hemostats at each ovary and at the cervix, and extirpated. Several germicide-treated towels were quickly placed over the exposed interior of the dam and the young were delivered from the excised uterus. The amnion was removed from each of the young and the umbilical cord was cut after being clamped with a hemostat. The nose and the mouth of the young were wiped clean from all mucus and the young were encouraged to breathe as needed by a gentle massage; then the hemostats were removed. Approximately 6 minutes following the normal birth of the first young, the rest of the litter had been delivered by Cesarean birth into a germfree cage. The young were placed in a cloth-lined container and passed from the operating cage through the sterile lock into the rearing isolator. The inner door of the rearing cage was then closed and the feeding and care of the young germfree rats became the important issue.

Larger animals with few young present more difficulties (Luckey, 1960). Pregnant ewes judged to be carrying twins were sheared closely, the abdomen was shaved and washed with tincture of iodine, and the mother was tied on an operating cart and draped with plastic. The uterus was extirpated, rinsed in 2% Diaprene chloride, and passed into the sterile room through the "air trap" (the blast of sterile air leaving the sterile room through the tent flap door). The operator inside took the young from the uterus and thoroughly wiped the mouth and nose before taking the young from the placental membrane. The umbilical cord was tied and cut. The young were dried and placed in a pen in the sterile room. This operation was also very fast: 30 seconds from the time the uterus was extirpated, the young were freed in the sterile room, breathing sterile air. The operator in the sterile room must use a heavy gown or apron and gloves while handling the lambs, since any germicide from the suit burned the mouth and made the lambs refuse food.

Levenson et al. (1960b) and Landy (1961) pioneered the sterile operative technique with large animal and human patients. The order of procedure for Cesarean section on pregnant gilts was quite similar to that used for human appendectomy and other abdominal surgery. The work of Landy (personal communication) will be described for the Cesarean operation of pigs; it is illustrative of the method used for sterile surgery on patients. The germfree delivery unit is a previously sterilized 1/1000th of an inch thick vinyl tent, equipped with sterile cautery knife, large knife, clamps, and a sterile source of air. The skin is carefully shaved and scrubbed for 10 to 15 minutes with Hexachlorophene soap. Then three coats of 7% iodine solution are administered. The plastic hood is raised from the table and the bottom surface is sterilized with 2% peracetic acid. A sterile plastic adhesive is applied to the bottom of the plastic unit and to the skin. This is allowed to dry briefly and the operating unit is lowered into the abdomen with even pressure, sticking the two together. Sodium thiamylal, 10 milligrams per kilo, is injected through a long needle into the vena cava for anesthesia. Incision is made with a cautery knife through the floor of the isolator and through the epidermis of the abdomen. Then a large sterile knife is used to complete the incision into the perineal cavity. The embryos are taken from the uterus and fetal membranes. Then the newborn pigs inside the surgical unit have the umbilical cord clamped and cut. They are then passed from the operating unit into the rearing unit. Mucus is aspirated and artificial respiration given as needed and the young pigs are thoroughly dried. This operation is successful and most pigs begin to walk and eat shortly after the operation.

Microbial Testing

Theory

Large beds of quicksand exist along the path of each new scientific development. If one does not cross these areas quickly, one may bog down indefinitely. In the development of germfree techniques as a major tool for biology, the beds of quicksands can be identified as: (1) instrumentation; (2) nomenclature; (3) technical details—testing any one experiment for absolute sterility could be a major research undertaking; and (4) theory—the theory of testing for microbial sterility must rest soundly upon the concepts of life and the characteristics of living organisms.

A chamber may be sterilized by heat, gas, chemicals, ultraviolet light, or other irradiation and still have certain characteristics of living organisms. The contents may still contain many molecules of cellular origin and usually a number of whole cells which may impart immunologic and other response to living organisms placed in the sterile chamber. M. Wagner could not understand what had happened in one "germfree experiment." His cultures were negative, while repeated examination of feces revealed a quantity of bacteria equivalent to that of conventional chicks. The phenomenon was easily explained when he learned that the diet contained about 10% of a commercial residue from a bacterial fermentation. The experiment was germfree, but the animals and microscopic tests showed bacteria. The dead bacteria were abundant in the feces and had given the chicks a good oral vaccination of antigen. This illustrates one example of the need for different categories of "germfreeness."

Virus present another problem, as discussed in the introductory chapter. Most workers agree that viruses should not be the cause of diseases in germfree animals. In this sense *germfree* would mean free from symptomatic viruses. Virologists suspect that the germfree animal of this decade may harbor nonsymptomatic viruses. As our understanding of the basic characteristics and limitations of life is increased we may devise improved detection of such unwanted material in gnotobiotic research. Our present state of ignorance is such that we think of living organisms as being a bundle of self-duplicating DNA (deoxyribonucleic acid) molecules with accessories which play the tune of life with variation in a genetic fugue. All of this is wrapped at least part of the time in a cellular package. The wrapping may vary considerably; the accessories, those dynamic enzymes and metabolites, are usually strikingly similar in all cells (cellular variation is mostly "cell wall" deep) with minor variation in the energy theme; and the basic rhythm of life is continuously beat by the nitrogen bases sitting in the DNA row. Until we can understand the complexities of variation in which DNA and accessories can survive, differentiate, and duplicate, we cannot define life. Until we can define life we cannot hope to devise tests to detect all variations of life nor to clearly distinguish one from another. This is exemplified by the viruses, which defy the cellular morphology of classic biology.

Intracellular parasites and viruses sometimes require special techniques for detection. The organisms may be present in the sperm or eggs before fertilization. Other endogenous contaminants must penetrate the uterine barriers. Such organisms are more difficult to separate from the host than exogenous contaminants which may enter through a break in the microbial barrier.

From a practical viewpoint we may simplify and almost ignore the theoretical concepts with their inherent problems. The experimental procedure defines the limits of our ability to detect living forms be they microbes, viruses or worms. Thus, the concept of germfree research changes with time as tests are improved. As Wagner (1959a) pointed out, commercial culture media are good and can be made suitable for many fastidious microorganisms. The best detector for microorganisms which cannot be cultivated is the germfree animal itself, a good culture medium. If the organism were active in the animal, it would give evidence of its presence by the numbers of foreign cells present, immunologic response, cytopathology, or overt symptoms of disease in the host. Motile forms are easily detected by microscopic observation of wet mounts. Most routine testing includes:

(a) a search for cellular organisms by microscopic examination of fecal material and sputum; (b) an attempt to culture a wide variety of microorganisms using a variety of media and environmental conditions, (c) spot checks for fastidious microorganisms, (d) observation for symptomatic virus, (e) sporadic checking for occult viruses, (f) visual observation for leaks and mold, and (g) olfactory examination of the exhaust air. The sampling procedure is a most important part of the cultural examination (Fig. 3.32). Multiple swabs or samples are routinely taken from: (a) saliva, (b) rectal feces, (c) excreta from the floor, (d) skin, (e) food, (f) water, (g) air, (h) walls, and (i) glove surfaces. Experience has shown that at least one animal in each cage should be thoroughly examined by autopsy and samples obtained for the microbial test from the cecum, lungs, ileum, liver, and other tissues.

Basic assumptions are made in the testing procedures which are disturbing to all who contemplate germfree work. First is the assumption that no microbes are present if they cannot be detected by the prescribed procedures. The microbe is absent until proven present. It is difficult to evaluate the error involved in this assumption. In the ceca of rats slow growing organisms have been found (Wagner, 1959a) which were probably present in other rats thought to be germfree. These were pleomorphic organisms which never accumulated in large number and were therefore not easily detected by direct examination. Second is the concept that contamination in one animal in a cage implies that all were contaminated. In a closed environment, it is difficult to imagine that part of an isolator is germfree and part contaminated. Yet it is not infrequent that viable organisms are present in some part of the cage which houses germfree animals. In such situations it is best to *let sleeping bugs lie*. For example, it is known that most germicides are not 100% effective. If the mercuric chloride, used to sterilize eggs, is neutralized, viable spores can sometimes be recovered. Mercuric chloride is effective for two reasons. It is not washed off the egg shell; therefore, any time that enough moisture to activate spores is present, that same moisture reactivates the germicide. Second, when bits of egg shell are fed to germfree chicks, they do not become contaminated. This is true even when the egg shell has been inoculated before germicide treatment. A startling example can be reported from rat work with the big tank at the University of Notre Dame. Microbial sterility of the rats in their small cages was established and was maintained during the time one rat got loose, was

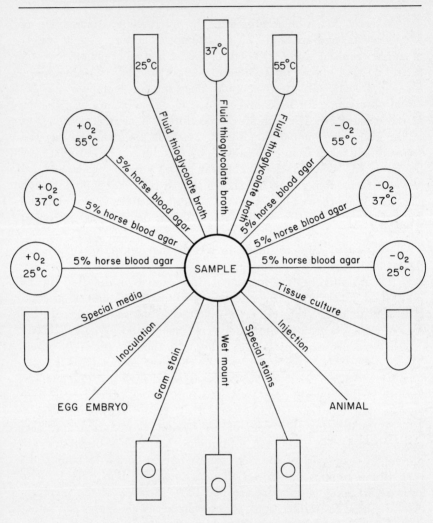

Fig. 3.32. Summary of bacteriological testing procedures. General scheme provided by M. Wagner (1959, *Ann. N. Y. Acad. Sci.* **78**, 90.)

recaptured from the floor of the big tank, and was found to be contaminated. The caged rats and the sides of the tank continued to test germfree. (Jokingly, it was suggested that a loose rat be considered standard procedure for sterility tests.) Another difficult situation was that of Waterhouse (1959) who wished to determine whether or not the intestinal flora of the wax moth contributed to its digestion of wax. The medium was particulate so it was impossible to detect any but massive infections.

Wagner (1959a) suggested two phases in the determination of germfree status: (1) Organisms held under maximum security should be searched exhaustively for contaminants of all kinds. Microorganisms which were endogenous, introduced from prenatal contamination, may be very difficult to grow for a variety of reasons. Virus and rickettsia must be shown to be absent or not active. (2) A simplified search for contaminants in animals or plants which have been removed from the area of maximum security into isolators in the ordinary laboratory. Exogenous contamination from accidental breaks in an isolator should rarely involve fastidious organisms without also involving the readily cultivated types which are ubiquitous. In many circumstances the animal is its own best criterion of sterility in germfree experiments. It is continually sampling food, water, and air and it is a good medium in which many fastidious microorganisms can develop. The state of the lymphatic system and antibody development in young animals may be used as evidence with most diets. A third consideration becomes apparent in gnotobiotic research which involves a germfree host which has been inoculated with 1, 2, 3, or more known microorganisms. Details are presented in Chapter 6. Microscopic observation and special media become particularly important. In dibiotic experiments the presence of microorganisms may mean nothing, and development of the lymphatic system is expected. Specific antibody titration should still be useful in gnotobiotic monitoring.

The term, *germfree*, indicates a negative quality or state. Negative results in the test for contaminants are the only proof of the state of germfreeness. Philosophically, any test which indicates the absence of contaminants may be open to suspicion, while any test which shows the presence of microorganisms (or other contaminants) is adequate. In this paradox, the more ways in which one looked for contamination, the more likely he was to find his was not a gnotobiotic experiment. This view is useful in the evaluation of the adequacy of the criterion of germfreeness used by workers throughout history.

Limits of Knowledge and Interpretation

The term *gnotobiotic* can be criticized in its literal meaning because one can never *know life completely*. The term gains stature from this criticism because until life is known completely one cannot be sure that he has defined life adequately to exclude strangers from the forms he wishes to study. Gnotobiosis thus becomes a philosophic goal in itself and the actual meaning of the word denotes the high improbability of reaching that goal. We use the term to the extent that we define our measure. This problem acquires importance in the detection of living forms. Until we agree on what is life, it will not be simple to detect all second living forms in gnotobiotic experimentation. Viruses are the obvious *pièce de résistance* of today; tomorrow the viruses may be as simple to detect and count as are most cellular forms today, but there will be then more subtle forms to be evaluated and more difficult decisions to be made. Should infective DNA be considered? Once again laboratory procedures can lead us until we know more definite answers. This is reason enough for the adoption of a nomenclature with absolute standards; otherwise, the term *germfree* will mean something different after each major advance in our understanding of bacteria, virus, protoplasts, transduction, and mutation.

Historical Review of Sterility Tests

Man's first concepts of the presence of microorganisms came from two separate actions: infection and fermentation. These concepts received a common and factual basis in 1675–1680 when van Leeuwenhoek described various microorganisms and Robert Boyle stated that disease could be best understood by one who understood fermentation. This prediction was fulfilled two centuries later when Pasteur showed that certain diseases were the manifestation of specific microorganisms. Armed with this philosophy and the new isolation techniques of Koch and others, microbiologists learned to detect the presence of a stranger microbe in a "pure culture" of bacteria, plants, or animals.

One method for the detection of microbial contamination is visual inspection of the sterile area. This method works nicely in research with tissue or virus culture where the nutrient media used would allow vigorous growth of many microorganisms. This method was used with germfree animals as the simplest and least effective part of a proper examination for contaminants. On rare occasions an organism (usually a mold) has been seen growing in a remote part of the germfree cage before it has been picked up with cultural tests. Historically the method was important. Visual inspection was the only test mentioned by Nuttall and Thierfelder (1897) in their chick experiments which were found contaminated by organisms growing on the egg white used for food. In their experiments with germfree guinea

pigs they used both microscopic and cultural methods in which samples of the alimentary canal, excrements, and food picked up from
the bottom of the cage were inoculated onto agar, gelatin, and sugar
agar, and incubated aerobically and anaerobically.

Schottelius (1899) gave clear descriptions of his methods for
testing the sterility of egg surfaces, chicks, and cage. One-third of the
eggs used for each experiment were washed free of germicide and
placed in nutrient gelatin to test the disinfectant. The sterile room
and chick cage were tested for sterility with each entry. The test was
conducted by placing gravel, egg shells, sand, food, water, excreta,
feathers, etc., in tubes filled with liquid gelatin. The chicks were
treated much as the other material in the cage. Some of the chicks
were chopped up and tested for anaerobic bacteria (apparently the
organs were placed in deep tubes with gelatin over them). Schottelius never found any contamination in experiments in which feces
had already been examined with no bacteria being found. The main
criticism of Schottelius' testing was that no special media were used
for yeasts or fastidious microorganisms, and he used only 37°C incubation. Examination for viruses was not carried out although this was
several decades after the etiology of some of the virus diseases had
been elucidated.

While Cohendy (1912a) was at Freiburg, his methods for testing
for contaminants were very similar to those of Schottelius. When he
returned to the Pasteur Institute, Cohendy used gelatin plates and
bouillon tubes placed under the condensing coils. In each experiment
he made inoculation of feces, food, water, and bits of many organs
into anaerobic and aerobic gelatin tubes. These were incubated 5 days,
examined grossly and microscopically. Then the vessels were inoculated to demonstrate the ability of the media to support growth.
Cohendy noted that feces of germfree animals contain dead microbial
cells. He also used the odor of the exhaust air as an indication of
sterility. This worked well for some organisms and was worthless for
others. Although the methods of Cohendy were as good as those of
Schottelius, his lack of specialized media, the limited incubation temperatures used, and the short incubation period could be criticized.

Küster (1914) ensured sterility of the milk by aseptic collection
followed by heating on five successive occasions and direct observation for 6 months before use. He examined the rearing chamber and
his germfree goats thoroughly. Samples were taken of the skin, hair,
umbilical cord, and various body tissues. These were maintained aero-

bically and anaerobically in bacteriological media. Jars with agar and bouillon were left open in the chamber at the end of the experiment. Feces and urine were collected daily and bacteriologically examined with agar and bouillon in aerobic and anaerobic conditions. Every 10 days blood samples were examined microscopically and serologically. The serological examination was made to test for antibodies against goat coliforms and hay bacilli. The dead goats were left in the chamber 10 days and re-examined by cultural and histological examination.

Balzam (1937b) checked for sterility by placing feces on a mixture of 0.6% peptone, 1% glucose, and 1.5% agar in meat broth. He also noted that feces from germfree chicks had a honey scent while that of infected birds smelled sour. He immersed one chick in an open beaker of peptone water placed in the cage throughout the experiment. The clarity of the peptone broth indicated the absence of most microbes. The lack of variety of samples and media (particularly blood agar and thioglycollate), the use of limited range in incubation temperature and the disregard of internal organs for sampling left much to be desired in the bacteriological studies of Balzam. He apparently learned little from the more astute bacteriological examinations of Cohendy and Küster.

The samples examined for bacteria by Gustafsson (1948) included: (1) cloth and cotton used in the Cesarean operation, (2) placenta, (3) milk, (4) feces each week, (5) bedding, (6) urine, (7) other refuse, and (8) dead animals. At the end of the experiment samples included: (9) washings from the whole animal, (10) colon contents, (11) cecum contents, and (12) ileum contents. Some dead animals were left in the apparatus for a period as long as 2 weeks to serve as substrate for bacteria. These samples were placed in the following media: (a) placental broth with 0.1% glucose, (b) placental broth with 0.1% glucose and 0.2% agar, (c) malt extract agar (for the detection of fungi), (d) Tarozzi liver broth to give anaerobic conditions, (e) 4% horse blood with 2% agar, and in later work (1959), (f) thioglycollate broth, and (g) Sabouraud's agar. These samples were incubated at room temperature and at 37°C. Natural specimens and stained specimens (Gram and May, Grunwald, and Giemsa) were examined using both the phase and regular microscopes after 1, 2, and 14 days, and in later work, 21 days. Fecal smears were examined microscopically. This careful work might have been made more reliable by the use of a high temperature (51 or 55°C.) for incubation and possibly the use of more glucose in one of the media. Gustafsson (1959b,c) has recently begun testing for viruses using tissue culture of HeLa, amnion, and kidney cells.

The early methods of Reyniers (1932) were adequate for many bacteria but they did not include special tests for a variety of other microorganisms. Later Reyniers, with several students, studied the problem of the sterility of the germfree animal in a thorough and systematic way. His rigidly built apparatus received exhaustive tests before and during use. Contaminations during transfer of cultures were found to be greatly reduced when performed in a sterile enclosure rather than an open laboratory or even a transfer room (Ervin, 1938). Various parts of the testing procedures were evaluated bacteriologically by Cordaro (1937). The efficiency and effectiveness of glass wool air filters was determined by A. W. Phillips (1941b) using both spores and droplet nuclei. Reyniers and Trexler (1943b) reported they studied "breakdown" tests for the air filters, gaskets, and gloves, and repeated testing of diet sterilization procedures. Sterility of the cage sterilization was tested by seeding with heat resistant spores.

Further details of the method used at Lobund were given by Reyniers, Trexler, and Ervin (1946). The samples included food, water, and swabs from the following sources: cage and gloves surfaces, nasal, oral, anal, aural, and genital cavities, feces, urine, hair, skin, blood, and isolated organs as available. Tissues were examined either *in toto* or after grinding. The whole animal was sometimes placed in Tyrode's or a peptone solution for incubation. Samples were incubated in Tryptone or Neopeptone* media both aerobically and anaerobically. Reyniers, Trexler, and Ervin later used thioglycollate media and 5% horse blood in brain-heart infusion agar. At 1, 2, 3, 7, 21, and 28 days the cultures from 25°C, 37.5°C, and 50°C were examined in wet mounts and stained material. If contamination was suspected, solid, semisolid, and liquid media were used in subculture. The system was checked by deliberate inoculation of the animal in order to be sure it could be detected. Some inoculations were made in eggs and live animals in a search for virus in germfree animals. The methods reported by Reyniers *et al.* (1949b) differed from those reported in 1946 mainly by the increased refinement for virus cultivation. This was not a routine examination. Attempts were made to propagate virus by passage of minced germfree feces, brain, spinal cord, and

* Baltimore Biological Laboratory Products.

other organs via cerebral and other routes into other germfree animals, conventional animals, and the chorioallantoic membrane and the yolk sac of embryonated eggs. No viruses were found nor were symptomatic viruses suspected.

The bacteriological examination conducted by Miyakawa *et al.* (1958a) involved microscopic examination, virus examination, routine cultivation, and special cultivation procedures. Tanami (1959) used thioglycollate medium to incubate samples taken from amnion, gauzes from the swabbing of the animal and the tank, feces, and diet. The tests by Reyniers *et al.* (1960a) were expanded by incubation of cultures at 55°C as well as 25, 37, and 50°C. The methods proposed below were based upon the work of Wagner (1959a), B. P. Phillips (1960), and Reyniers *et al.* (1960a).

Summary of Methods

In practice the important control being exercised in gnotobiotic research is that over the physical contact of living microorganisms. As long as *intimate physical contact* is prevented between the species under consideration and all other species, the condition is gnotobiotic. Macroscopic, microscopic, symptomatic, and cultural evidence must be accumulated in order to establish the gnotobiotic state of the species being studied.

Sampling

Microbiological theory and experience suggest that all individuals in a small confined area, such as a germfree cage, would have similar exposure and contamination by any microorganisms within the area. The microorganisms may survive or establish colonies in the individuals at different rates depending on many biological and physical factors. A simple example would be the oral inoculation of *Escherichia coli* into a single rat in a germfree cage. There would be a measurable time lapse before that organism could be detected in the feces of the other rats in that cage. However, unless the distance or microbial barriers which separate individuals within a single enclosed unit is great, the time factor is negligible in practical considerations and a single individual may be considered to be microbiologically equivalent to any other individual of the same species in the same cage receiving similar diet and treatment.

Samples taken for direct microscopic examination and bacteriological culture are usually collected on swabs moistened with saline prior to use. While expressed feces are useful for routine parasitological examination, a thorough examination demands the sacrifice of one animal in each cage. Many parasites and some bacteria maintain active colonies in the cecum, ileum, or tissues of the body without abundant evidence showing either externally or in the blood, saliva, urine, or feces. Virological examination requires samples of fresh tissues from a variety of sources. The death of an animal offers a golden opportunity for tissue samples because most contaminants will flourish in a weakened animal. However, both Cordaro (1937) and Ervin (1938) concluded that simple tests to determine bacteriological sterility were as effective as whole animal tests. Autopsy and collection and manipulation of multiple samples is best done within the germfree cage to minimize possibilities of outside contamination. If this is not possible, a hood and transfer room should be used.

Sources of samples are:

a. Tank surfaces should be routinely wiped with moistened swabs. This should include separate swabs for rubber, plastic, or glass and metal surfaces in order to avoid the oligodynamic effect of heavy metals. Large tanks need to have media sprayed on representative surfaces for adequate coverage. This could be incubated in the cage before sampling.

b. Food and water should be sampled each time a fresh supply is taken in. Samples of food should be procured from the center of the new supply and from any moistened part of the food which has been in the cage for some time. Fluid food is itself an excellent bacterial culture medium. The most conservative investigators routinely tested their food for contamination before admitting it to the cage where animals were kept. Since the water is continually catching dust particles from air movements and spilled material (such as food and excreta), and washes part of the animals as they drink, the water gives a good reflection of the presence of most microorganisms in the cage. Since the water container is not cleaned thoroughly each day, low osmotic pressure is not a problem: this is the theoretical foundation for the semi-automatic "bactytester" used in recent models of germfree chick cages (H. T. Miller and Luckey, 1962).

c. Feces and urine samples are important because they give a regular index of the internal status of the animal without need for sacrifice. Fresh feces may be expressed in mammals to give adequate samples for parasitology. Swabs are used to obtain rectal or cloacal samples. Urine samples are readily available if mammals are placed in metabolism cages. Otherwise, a cloth or sponge may be placed under the animals for collection purposes.

d. Body surfaces. Moist swabs are rubbed over the skin and feathers or hairs of the animals. The swab should be manipulated under the fur or feathers to obtain direct contact with skin. A few hairs or a small feather should be included in the sample in order to obtain sampling from both dermis and epidermis.

e. Secretions. Samples of saliva, nasal fluid, tears, genital fluids, and mucus from the rectum are readily obtained by appropriate manipulation of the swab. Sweat is not usually a serious consideration in bacteriological sampling and is adequately covered by the samples obtained from the skin.

f. Blood and biopsy tissue from living animals is sometimes taken for experimental work. A part of this is available for microbiological examination.

g. Whole animal culture was used by several investigators because it was the simplest and best sampling device of all. The animal is continually collecting material from the air, water, cage surfaces, and other animals. The animal is the *raison d'étre* of all germfree life. Viable spores found in the cage on the germicide-treated egg shell are of little importance when they do not contaminate the animal. Dead animals are sometimes left in the cage for several days, or weeks, in order to give opportunity for microorganisms to grow. Whole animals have frequently been placed in nutrient broth or gelatin for bacteriological evidence of the germfree status of the experiment. While this is good evidence, it may tell little about the conditions in the tissues or body cavities. Therefore, body cavities should be opened to expose different organs and tissues (lungs, brain, heart, lymph nodes, liver, stomach, intestines, kidney, and muscle) before the animal is placed in nutrient media. A better practice is to place small cubes of a variety of tissues into nutrient media: these would include the above tissues, blood, and intestinal contents.

h. Other samples may be useful depending upon the operation being performed. Material gathered from the floor represents a mixture of food, feces, urine, water, skin sloughings, and air. This is used when open flasks are exposed in an isolator. Placental tissue is used to test sterility of Cesarean operations. Special instruments, bedding, and parts of the cage, such as air filters, should be checked routinely by samples from wet swabs. The author routinely includes packaged bacterial spores* inside the diets for bacteriological control.

Media

Fluid thioglycollate media is the most accepted single medium for sterility testing. The swab containing the sample or the samples is introduced into a deep tube. The top few millimeters will allow the growth of aerobic organisms while the bottom will allow anaerobic organisms to grow. This medium is enriched and made more anaerobic when small samples of tissue are introduced. The placental broth media are especially good for fastidious microorganisms.

Brain–heart infusions agar with 5% sterile defibrinated horse blood is most useful as a solid medium. The swabs are streaked across this surface while tissues and other samples are aseptically placed on the surface. These should be maintained in aerobic and anaerobic condition. Bray dishes are used to obtain the desired CO_2 tension.

Other media include dead animals which are allowed to stay at room temperature in the cage, liquid diet, a mixture of water, food, and excreta which sometimes accumulates in the cage. Embryonated eggs, cells in tissue culture, chicks, and mice are used for inoculation in attempts to grow virus from germfree tissue homogenates. Living germfree animals should be most useful as media in the virus search. Special media for specific organisms may be used as deemed necessary.

Incubation

The earliest workers used ambient temperatures of the germfree cages as the main temperature to incubate cultures. Later this was used with other samples being cultured at 37°C. Since thermophilic organisms grow best at higher temperatures, the Lobund group used 50°C incubation with those at 25°C and 37°C. Even this was not considered high enough for some thermophilic organisms. Therefore, the three temperatures presently recommended are 25°C, 37°C, and 55°C. Sometimes 40°C is preferred to 37°C when testing for microorganisms in birds since most avian species have a higher body temperature than large mammals.

The incubation period may last 2–4 weeks. The cultures should be observed at 1, 2, 3, 7, 14, 21, and 28 days.

* Spordex: 100,000 spores of *Clostridium sporogenes* in small plastic bags from American Sterilizer, Erie, Pennsylvania.

Macroscopic Observations

Direct observation of germfree animals is informative for gross invasion by debilitating organisms. As long as the animals look healthy, no virulent infectious agent has established itself. Clinical symptoms are the main evidence used routinely for assuming that symptomatic viruses are absent. Since germfree rats and mice may die in 5–7 days when placed directly in a conventional stock colony, direct observation is good evidence for massive inoculation with a wide variety of ordinary, potentially virulent organisms. The operator should make careful observations to make certain that no break in the physical system has occurred. Wagner (1959a) emphasized that the value of continuity of cumulative negative findings in the biological testing for contamination rests upon the continued integrity of the isolation barriers under positive air pressure. Breaks in the physical barrier may occur without a contamination of the germfree animals (surprisingly large breaks in gloves have occurred without contamination of germfree rats), but the continuity of the system for those animals, the *gnotobiotic* pedigree, is broken and evidence for germfreeness must be judged by subsequent testing.

Direct observation of the cage contents may, on rare occasions, reveal a mold growth which has not yet been indicated in the bacteriological routine. More often, close observation of the cage leads to improved practices which will avoid impending breaks in the system. Olfactory examination of the outlet air of the cage will sometimes detect microbial contamination of a germfree experiment.

The culture plates and tubes are observed by direct vision at 1, 2, 3, 7, 14, and 21 and 28 days. Growth in an occasional tube or plate may be expected from transfer or incubation in nonsterile rooms. A pattern of growth in several of the cultures is good evidence for a contaminant. Absence of observable growth leads only to closer examination. Cultures which are negative should be inoculated to show that the medium will support growth and that no antibacterial material has been added with the sample. As C. R. Phillips and Hoffman (1960) pointed out, this step was most important in testing a wide variety of inanimate objects.

Microscopic Observation

If gross examination shows no growth in the cultures, the plates are carefully scrutinized with 50× magnification before they are considered negative and the liquid media are used to make smears for examination with a high resolution microscope.

Direct microscopic examination of the samples is a part of the bacteriological routine. Gustafsson (1948) used phase microscopy on wet mounts. Fecal smears are checked for motile bacteria and protozoa since the mere presence of microbial cells has a much different meaning than the presence of *living* microbial forms. The photomicrographs (Fig. 3.33) illustrate the appearance of typical fields at high magnification. Dead microbial cells are routinely seen in germfree animals. Organisms in the diet are killed during the sterilization procedure, but the cells are concentrated during the passage of food through the gastrointestinal tract by the action of digestion and absorption of the major foods to a much greater extent than any destruction of the cells. This phenomenon of concentration by taking other material away, via absorption, has been called *bioincrassation* (Luckey, 1958). If the diet has bacterial products added, the amount of cells found in fecal smears approximates the quantity found in feces from contaminated animals. For this comparison, photomicrographs of smears from feces of mono-inoculated animals and conventional animals are presented.

Other preparations of the samples fixed on slides are stained by the Gram, Wright, acid-fast, or Machiavella stains, depending upon the need. Wright-stained tissue sections and blood smears are also used to supplement the bacteriological routines. The absence of microbial forms in teeth plaques, tonsils, or blood is useful evidence for the bacteriologist. Since germfree animals usually have a lowered white cell count and their phagocytes respond poorly to the usual stimuli, the number and state of white blood cells is pertinent. Further morphological evidence might accrue from examination of the intestinal lymph nodes. In germfree animals these are only about one-third the size of those in conventional animals.

Other tests which may be performed are specific antigen-antibody reactions for one or more suspected microorganisms.

Protozoa Detection

While wet mounts are being examined for bacteria, they are routinely scrutinized for protozoa, yeasts, molds, worm eggs, and larvae. Preparations made from fresh intestinal contents, particularly the cecum, are the most useful for this purpose. The smears are fixed and one of several suitable stains is applied. Schaudinns fixative fol-

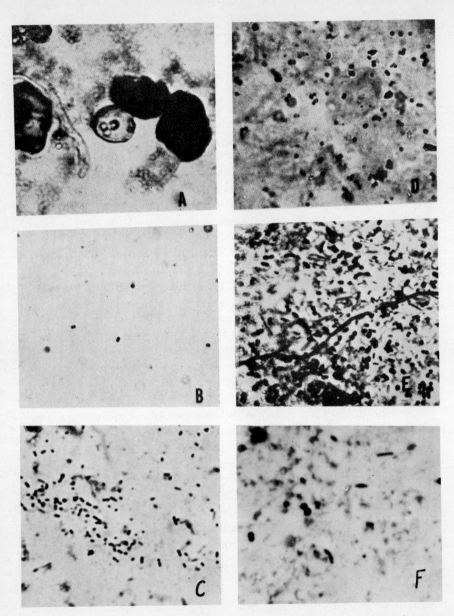

FIG. 3.33. Photomicrograph of fecal smears with gram stain. A. Fecal smear from germfree chick fed autoclaved syntype diet. Remains of dead microorganisms are frequently seen. B. Low incidence of *Diplococcus* in fecal smears of a germ-free chick. (No culture could be grown.) C. Fecal smear from chick inoculated with a nonadapted strain of S. *faecalis*. Food and water culture were positive and fecal culture was negative. D. Abundant micrococci in fecal smears of mono-

194

lowed by Heidenhain's iron-alum hematoxylin was reported to be useful by Wagner (1959a). Centrifugation in zinc sulfate is used to concentrate possible protozoan material. Wright's stain of the blood elements is also useful in the search for parasites in germfree animals. Protozoa, plants, and insects are the three major divisions of living forms which are not expected as contaminants in germfree animals. Wagner (1959a) reported seeing no protozoan contaminants in thousands of fecal smears from rats, mice, rabbits, guinea pigs, or chickens. The inoculation of germfree guinea pigs (Phillips *et al.*, 1958) with *Amoeba histolytica* resulted in no permanent establishment of colonies in the absence of other microorganisms. They could be established by traumatizing the inoculation area. Other protozoa are easily established, as reported in Chapter 6.

Parasite Detection

The parasitological survey of germfree animals of B. P. Phillips (1960) agreed with data obtained by other workers. His data from multiple tests showed that no parasites were found in germfree birds or mammals excepting dogs. The majority of dogs delivered by Cesarean birth into sterile environment have carried larval nematodes. Glimstedt found worms in germfree dogs, and in the author's experience at the University of Notre Dame only 1 out of 6 germfree pups were wormfree. All others carried *Toxocara canis* and one had *Ancylostoma caninum* larvae. Although adult *Toxocara canis* were found, no signs of nematode reproduction were seen in "germfree" dogs. Excluding the dog work and experiences wherein parasites were inoculated into animals (see particularly the work of Newton and co-workers), no other reports are known in which parasites were found in germfree animals.

Examination of material for parasites (see B. P. Phillips, 1960, and a standard text for details) entails dissection with macroscopic observation for the presence of large parasites and for pathology or other abnormality which may suggest parasitic activity. Fresh samples from different levels of the gastrointestinal tract are diluted with Locke's solution and scrutinized microscopically for the presence of

contaminated chicks. E. Fecal smear from conventional animal fed autoclaved syntype diet. Note the variety and frequency of microorganisms. F. Low incidence of a nonadapted strain of *Escherichia coli* in chicken fecal smear. Culture of food and water was positive; culture of feces was negative. (Photomicrographs courtesy of M. Wagner and H. Miller.)

ova or parasites. Zinc sulfate flotation methods are used to concentrate not only protozoan cysts but also ova and small larvae. Microscopic examination is made from thin and thick smears of peritoneal fluid and blood and impression smears of liver, brain, and spleen stained with Giemsa. Samples of all tissues are minced and digested in artificial gastric juice for 24 hours at 37°C. The sediment from this material is examined microscopically for ova and parasites. Samples of lung, spleen, liver, brain, kidney, lymph nodes, muscles, and intestine are fixed in 10% formalin (buffered), embedded in paraffin, sectioned, and examined microscopically after staining with hematoxylin and eosin. B. P. Phillips (1960) also recommended pressing diaphragm samples between pressure plates for examination for encysted larvae.

Arthropods

A germfree tank is one place one would not expect to find the ubiquitous insect. Gnotobiotic animals are routinely examined macroscopically for evidence of infestation of lice, fleas, and mites. Observations reported to date give no arthropod contaminants in germfree isolators. However, this problem is both practical and serious in disease-free animal colonies. In one gnotobiotic colony, where a colony had been started from germfree rats, only eleven species of microorganisms were present until a wild mouse gnawed his way inside bringing anthropod and other contaminants.

Rickettsiae

Routine search for rickettsiae *per se* has not been conducted by any group working with germfree animals. The microscopic, bacteriological, and histological examinations have revealed no evidence of the presence of these forms either directly (through observation of the cells) or indirectly (diseased animals). Wagner (1959a) reported finding no rickettsiae in spot checks on intestinal contents or impression smears from the spleen and other organs. He used the differential stain of Macchiavella according to standard procedures.* Methods used in the search for viruses in germfree animals constitute useful evidence for the rickettsiae-freeness of germfree animals.

* Manual of Methods for the Pure Culture Study of Bacteria (Biotechnical Publication, Geneva, New York, 1951).

Virus

The detection of viruses, which can neither be seen by microscopic examination of tissues nor be grown on simple culture media, presents special problems in gnotobiotic research. The classic method of detection for viruses, the observation of pathology caused by a filterable virus, is valid for germfree animals. As will be seen in this section, germfree animals are probably more susceptible to virus infection than are conventional animals. Therefore, the classic system for virus detection is more sensitive in germfree animals than in polycontaminated animals.

Gustafsson (1959a,b,c) reported that no viruses were present in his germfree rats according to examination of feces for agents which were cytopathic for human amnion, HeLa, and monkey kidney cells. A. R. Taylor (1959) found no evidence of any cytopathogenic agents when germfree Bantam chick tissue was observed through four passages of monkey kidney, amnion F180, human heart, and Detroit-6 tissue culture cell lines. Wagner (1960) and Reyniers (1959b) found no virus in spot tests of several germfree animals. T. G. Ward (1959) reported that about 25% of the cecum samples from germfree animals exhibited filterable agents which were tentatively classified in the ECHO group. Wagner (1959a) pointed to the possibility that these viruses may have resided equally well in the donor and the recipient. Until tests are confined to germfree or virus-free animals, inoculation data are not convincing. Further evidence on the question of the presence of virus in germfree animals was presented at the VIIth International Congress for Microbiology. Fitzgerald and Habel (1959) commented that after extensive search of germfree animal tissue, one agent which would grow in rabbit kidney was found in the salivary glands of rats. The Japanese groups, employing the usual techniques, have found no virus (Miyakawa, 1959c) and the group at Lund, Sweden, had found no viruses to that date (Gustafsson, 1959a). Preliminary studies by Dr. Thomas G. Ward (1961, personal communication) with 8 mouse virus antigens indicated that the sera of approximately 250 germfree mice did not show the presence of demonstrable antibodies to the antigens. Very few possible examples of symptomatic virus have been found throughout the history of germfree research; none were proven to be a viral agent. In one, Gordon *et al.* (1959) reported a *jitters* in chicks which had some symptoms of a virus infection. Attempts to transfer a filterable agent were not successful. Another possibility of a spontaneous symptomatic virus seen in germfree animals was a lung consolidation in newborn rats, but no good evidence was reported to indicate it was transmissible agent. Wagner (1959a) commented: "Other unpublished evidence indicates that respiratory disease of presumably viral nature may at times have been carried in rats and guinea pigs that were taken by Cesarean section and that tested free of bacteria and fungi." Miyakawa (1955a) and Iijima (1950) also expressed this belief. Reyniers and Sacksteder (1959b) and A. R. Taylor *et al.* (1959) reported a filterable, transmissible agent was found in germfree chicks following carcinogen induced tumor formation. The particles obtained were stated by Taylor (1959) to be what "We have been accustomed to call virus or viruslike." It seems probable that such experiments showed the way to look for viruses in germfree animals: stress the germfree animal using chemical, physical or psychological means to develop conditions under which inapparent viruses may assert themselves in overt action or provirus may be transformed into virus. Phillips (1961) has suggested a virus etiology for respiratory disease in germfree animals.

Needed Methods

Standardization of the microbial detection system is needed for the increasing number of laboratories entering germfree research. Historically and presently (when compared in different laboratories) the term *germfree* has many meanings. Macroscopic and microscopic examination for invertebrate parasites is simple and effective. The search for eggs and larvae of nematodes, cestodes, and other metazoan parasites should be carried out with fresh fecal material and from cecal contents of recently sacrificed animals. No serious need is known for a means of detection of protozoa, excepting for the suspected intracellular parasites found in insects. The fastidious nature of these and many other microbial forms presents a challenge to search out new ways to grow and identify the forms which presently defy our cultural methods. If these forms reproduce within the germfree animal, the number of individuals seen upon microscopic examination is evidence that viable fastidious forms are present. The extent to which disease is not seen is evidence that certain virulent forms are absent. The absence of respiration disease in old rats and mice is presumptive evidence for the absence of those pleuropneumonia-like organisms which can cause such symptoms. Germfree animals should be used in a thorough study of the detection of fastidious micro-organisms following their inoculation into a germfree animal. If a specific microorganism were suspected, it might be detected by the antibody titer of the "germfree" animal.

A systematic survey of the serum of germfree animals for antibody specific to a wide variety of known viruses should be inaugurated. T. G. Ward (1959) suggested that inoculation of blood, tissues, urine, or feces should be made into chick embryos of different ages by various routes of inoculation. One-day old mice and tissue cultures would also be useful. One of the most useful hosts is the germfree animal itself. T. G. Ward suggested four methods by which latent viruses might be unmasked in germfree animals: (1) study older germfree animals which have allowed more time for any symptoms to develop, (2) search for spontaneous tumors—when found they may be induced to release a latent virus, (3) have strict accounting for all individuals in a colony in order to note those dying of unde-termined cause, and (4) examine tissue cultures, preferably with germfree tissues within the system.

For standard routines, examination should be made for one virus or several viruses which are most likely to inhabit the species being reared gnotobiotically. A more complete survey of the colony or system can be made as special virological problem from time to time. Serological reactions to one or several viruses common to the species being used should be inaugurated as a routine test. A certifica-tion of the viral status could be added that of the bacterial status for a *pedigree* of a given line of animals from the laboratory.

Contamination

Accidental contamination of a germfree experiment is usually sufficient cause to stop that experiment and start a new one. This is the prime factor which makes germfree research time and patience consuming. If the break in the gnotobiotic system is obvious and if the experiment has matured enough to provide usable data, immediate use of the animals might salvage part of the time and effort put into the work. Delay of more than a few minutes would allow too much time for infection to start and myriad uncontrolled reactions to begin to change the germfree or gnotobiotic animals into useless material.

Positive pressure inside the germfree cage, cleanliness, and liberal use of germicidal solutions and powder in routine operation combine to allow minor breaks without contamination. Such accidents include

TABLE 3.5
EGG STERILIZATION

Investigator	Temp. (°C)	Brushing	Detergent	Germistat	Concentration	Time
Nuttall and Thierfelder	—	No	No?	HgCl	1:1000	Every other day
Schottelius	40°	Yes	No?	$HgCl_2$	1:200	20 days
Cohendy	40°	Yes	No?	$HgCl_2$	1:200	0 days
Balzam	40°	Yes	No?	$HgCl_2$	1:100	20 days
Luckey et al.	39°	Yes	Yes	$HgCl_2$	1:100	20 days
Reyniers et al.	38°	Yes–no	Dreft	$HgCl_2$	1:100	20 days

TABLE 3.6
CLASSIFICATION OF CONTAMINANTS 1939–1947[a]

Source	Organism
Egg	*Streptococcus faecalis*
	Paracolobactrum sp.
	Escherichia coli
Gloves	*Staphylococcus aureus*
	Staphylococcus epidermidis
	Micrococcus epidermidis
	Lactobacillus sp.
	Micrococcus sp.
	Penicillium sp.
Filter	Mold
Sterilization	*Bacillus subtilis*
Unknown	*Sarcina* sp.
	Alcaligenes sp.
	Micrococcus sp.
	Gram-negative rod

[a] Reyniers *et al.* (1949b).

small leaks in a gasket, pin pricks, or small tears in rubber gloves which can usually be patched without contamination.

The contamination data from several years' work with germfree chicks illustrates the main sources of contamination and the species of microorganisms usually associated with each type of breakdown (Table 3.6). Most breaks are small and often a single species is found. Fecal organisms are often found whenever the eggs are not completely sterilized. *Bacillus subtilus,* or other spore-forming organisms, may be found following incomplete sterilization of the apparatus. Molds may grow through the filters (particularly the outlet filter) if they become wet and/or dirty. Glove breaks usually allow species of *Staphylococcus* or *Micrococcus* to enter. Some idea of the amount of contamination for chicks, turkeys, guinea pigs, mice, and rats is given in Table 3.7.

Production, Maintenance, and Repair Problems

Most of the technical aspects of rearing germfree animals have been presented in this chapter as individual entities. There remain

TABLE 3.7

CONTAMINATION IN GERMFREE RESEARCH

	Chicks[a] (1939–1948)[d]	Turkeys[b] (1950–1954)[d]	Guinea pigs[a] Aug. 1952– Nov. 1957)[d]	Mice and rats[a] (Mar. 1955– Oct. 1957)[d]	Rats[c] (1956–1958)[d]
No. Isolators	—	4	—	6	—
No. Cesarotomies	—	—	298	—	—
Total animals	128	—	963	767	—
Total experiments	11	8	114	—	41
Average length of experiments (days)	117	35			56
Experiments, germfree	10	4	98	—	
Experiments, contaminated	1	5	16	1	5
% Contaminated	9	56	86		12
% Germfree	91	44	14		88

[a] Reyniers (1959a).
[b] Luckey et al. (1960).
[c] Gustafsson (1959b).
[d] The first date indicates the start of the experiment, the second indicates the end.

problems of production of germfree animal colonies, maintenance of the germfree units, and repair problems. The material to follow presents an accumulation of experience and helpful suggestions in the practical aspects of raising germfree animals. The historical view will not be presented; rather we will assume an exemplar cage which has both a sterile lock and a germicidal trap. Definitive methods for the operation and maintenance of germfree equipment have not been published for a variety of reasons. References which are helpful in discussing some of the problems are papers by Horowitz *et al.* (1960), Snow and Hickey (1960), Reyniers (1959a, 1960a), and Gustafsson (1959b).

Whether a tank is new or has been used, the same procedures are involved in preparing it for sterilization and use. The first step is the disassembly of the apparatus and thorough cleansing of all parts. A detergent should be used because any dust or dirt which remains gives an increased load of bacteria which must be killed during sterilization. Also adhering particles might be impervious to steam, and therefore, would not be adequately sterilized. Second, it is necessary to inspect all gaskets, joints, and rubber gloves, and replace or repair any defective parts. Third, is the reassembly and loading of the rearing cage or sterile lock. During assembly it is important that all sides of a gasket be equally tight; therefore, all nuts must be brought to the same tension with an indicator wrench. The loading should be done according to the principles of loading as autoclave, namely, no dead air spot should be blocked off, no closed containers should be used which have not been presterilized, and contact between two surfaces should never be over a broad area which might prohibit steam from penetrating. For repairs and replacement it is worthwhile to have a full time mechanic available for 10 or more cages. When more than this number of steel cages are used, a machine shop is needed.

The search for leaks in the unit is done with vacuum, pressure, or special gas. Gustafsson (1948) filled the chamber with ammonia and used moist indicator paper to detect leaks in his system. Another method is simply to close the isolator with adequate pressure to make the gloves extend horizontally. As long as the ambient temperature remains constant the gloves should stay at the same level. If there were a leak it would quickly be detected as the gloves slowly descend. A useful method is to exert pressure in the tank and cover the tank with a layer of liquid soap or detergent. If leaks were present, bubbles would be made at the site of the leak. This method is not satisfactory for the low pressure (about 1 cm water pressure) plastic isolators. When using the heavy steel cages a vacuum may be exerted and maintained for an indefinite period during which the pressure changes could be noted on a pressure indicator. Leak detectors, such as the Freon leak detector* are most sensitive. Freon is added to about 10% of the volume of the isolator and all orifices closed. This concentration is not harmful to animals. If any Freon escapes, the electronic detector indicates and locates the leak. The major sources of leaks are newly soldered connections, gaskets which are old, worn, or improperly seated, and rubber gloves. After the cage is thoroughly tested and in operation, the rubber gloves become the weakest part of the system. They are particularly susceptible to oxidation. Most contaminations result either from the rubber gloves or from outlet filters during operation. Experiments are too valuable to be ruined by cigarette ashes, rings, brooch pins, or cuff links tearing, destroying, or making a pin-point hole in the gloves; therefore, personnel must obey strict rules to protect these weak links in the system.

Details of different methods of sterilization were given previously.

Space

In order to maintain germfree animals in a germfree cage, it is necessary to provide service functions, utility, and a variety of needed accessories. Standard isolators have approximately 1 cubic meter of space which must be efficiently arranged with adequate room for arm movement with a minimum possibility for glove tears. No equipment or storage can be close to the gloves. The isolator which sits on benches of the normal laboratory is less costly in space than one which has its own stand, for the simple reason that the bench may be used for storage while the cage is sitting on it, and used for other things while the cage is being serviced. On the other hand, the cage having its own rack has the advantage of mobility. Of particular interest in this regard is the Fisher-Horton Isolator which is a self-sufficient unit. The isolator may be used in any room having an electric outlet. Everything on the cage is automatic, including the switch to battery operation in case of electric failure. Obviously nothing would be saved by putting this cage on a bench because all the space underneath the cage is efficiently used.

A good incubator and hatching unit must be available for birds. Having germfree mammals in a cage implies that space for a stock

* General Electric Co., Schenectady, New York.

colony of animals must be available, since there is no commercial source for germfree animals at the present time. Normally at least two cages would be required for a colony and a third cage needed for use as a spare to be cleaned and made ready for transfer of animals from one cage to another. Since a variety of different types of isolators may be used in one laboratory, it is highly desirable that cages be standardized as far as the sterile lock appointments are concerned. Adapters, called "dutchmen" in laboratory parlance, can be made; but it is preferable that any isolator may be connected directly to another.

Space is also required for the sterilization equipment. Cages are normally moved to a sterilizing area where steam, vacuum, and air pressure are available in one place. In order to be most efficient in taking in food, water, and utensils, a sterile lock system was devised which would service three cages at one time; the space required for this setup is approximately 10 square feet. Space is also required for cleaning isolators; one end must be taken off for cleaning. Everything must be taken out and cleaned thoroughly and an area must be available where parts can be stored. A store of food and water and small replacement parts, such as light bulbs, nuts, bolts, gaskets, spare cages, metabolism cages, breeding cages, bedding, parts for the air filter, and gloves must be available. Many items such as the bedding must be presterilized and a store of presterilized material should normally be available. Since items such as gloves are not readily available, a large supply should be maintained.

The space requirements of supporting services must be considered: diet preparation, microbiological testing, autopsy, and development. Although diets may be available commercially, most of them are not adequate following steam sterilization. If radiation were used for diet sterilization a means of transporting the diet to and from the radiation facility without undue heating of the diet would be required. Since rancidity is a big problem, diets require refrigeration and protection from air. Usually a room is needed for a mechanical mixer and storage of pots, pans, and large quantities of protein, carbohydrate, fat, salt, and fiber. Microbiological testing requires a minimum of 3 incubators, a transfer hood, storage for tubes and plates, and areas for staining and microscopic observation and for preparation of media, and washing and sterilization of glassware. The autopsy requirements may be minimal, but they should include a deep freeze for dead animals, an instrument cabinet, a small table, and sectioning and staining equipment. The space requirement for development is most variable, but it may be anticipated that in any long term experimentation certain modifications will be desirable. If soft plastics are used extensively, an electronic sealer should be provided.

Decontamination

The decontamination process is the reverse of inoculation, conventionalization, or contamination. The essence of the process of interest here is to make a gnotobiotic system. This might involve the identification of one or more species present which were previously unknown to the investigator, or it might involve reduction in the number of microorganisms species in the system. Gnotobiotization may be accomplished in several ways. One is to determine that a system is indeed germfree. This process occurs at the beginning of germfree experiments, when laboratory procedures and observation of the material show the experiment to be free from all demonstrable living contaminants. This process is decontamination from the viewpoint that germfree young were obtained from a non-germfree mother. The second process is similar to the first. If a gnotobiotic experiment or colony becomes contaminated, identification of all species of contaminants will readmit the system to the world of gnotobiosis with a greater number of gnotobiotes than were present before the contamination. Inoculation of gnotobiotes with a pure culture would give a different gnotobiotic system. The fourth method is of interest here.

Decontamination, the method of gnotobiotization pertinent to this discussion, is the active process of elimination of microbial species from intimate contact with the host. Preliminary work has given promising results. Kijanizin (1894a,b, 1900a,b) fed sterile food to animals and noted that the intestinal flora was usually simplified. Absolute sterility of the environment was not observed. Nelson (1941) placed a young guinea pig in a sterile cage and gave it sterile food, water, and air for 1 year. It was regularly transferred to a fresh sterile cage. The animal exhibited autodisinfection to the extent that only three species of microorganisms could be found in the cage. One, a mold, could not be found inside of the animal. All except two species, one streptococcus and one diplococcus, were eliminated from the animal. Reback (1942) confirmed and extended this work. Weaned rats fed autoclaved diets in a nonsterile environment were found to have a simplified intestinal flora. When the animal was fed sterile diet and transferred biweekly into a sterile cage, most enterococci were lost within 1 month. After 3 months no fission yeasts, no cocci except lanceolate cocci, and almost no gram-negative rods were present in the feces. Some true yeasts and a mold were present and gram-positive rods were most abundant. When the experiment was repeated with sulfadiazine in the water, no yeasts and no spore-bearing rods were found, cocci and mold were rare, while numerous fission yeasts, coliform rods, and aciduric rods were seen. The rod forms were both anaerobic and aerobic. Reyniers (1946a) summarized this work by suggesting that animals in a closed environment fed sterile material have a fixed flora which become stabilized with only one or two kinds of microorganisms. The intestinal flora of the white rat also became simplified with the exclusion of lactobacilli and yeasts when a complete anal block was affected (Wagner, 1946). Before such rats died at 10 days, the total microbial population was greatly diminished. The hypothesis that the death of rats was caused by intestinal infection or toxins produced by the microorganisms was effectively denied by unpublished experiments of Wagner and Reyniers (1946) in which germfree rats with a complete anal block were found to die with similar clinical symptoms, and at about the same time as did conventional rats.

The above results and the possibilities of using new germicides and antibiotics suggested the feasibility of obtaining germfree animals by this approach. If the autodisinfecting ability of the animal could be confirmed, decontamination would have real potential for future use. The following studies by J. Pleasants and the author were conducted on decontamination over a period of 3 years (1949–1952) at the University of Notre Dame. A three-hole hood was built to accommodate the mouth parts of three jars as shown in Fig. 3.34. The churn jars were adapted for maintaining germfree rats for a short period of time. The cap had a sterile air filter on it, and sterile food and water were introduced with each transfer. Weekly transfers were made after sterilizing the hood and jar surfaces with a germicide spray. The center jar contained a germicide for bathing the animal during the transfer and the right-hand jar was the new sterile cage for the newly washed animal. Thus, aseptic transfers could be accomplished simply, without access to airborne contaminants from the outside. Experiments were made with contaminated rats fed a marginal diet (L-222) for 4 weeks. The fecal cultures indicated the flora to be 95% yeast, 2% lactic acid organisms, 1% coliform organisms,

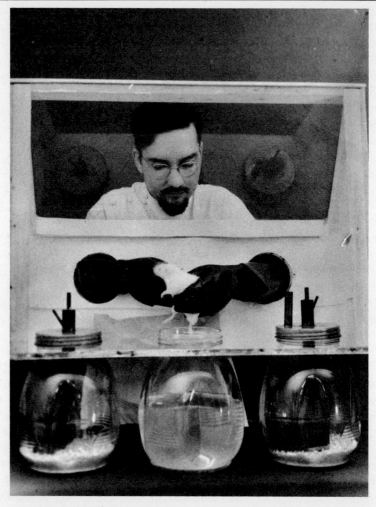

Fig. 3.34. Decontamination hood for gnotobiotic rats. The rat is taken from the used jar to the left of the operator (J. Pleasants), bathed in germicidal solution in the center, and passed into a sterile jar on the right.

and about 2% unknown microorganisms. In the second experiment 10% Thalamyd was included in the diet. The rat on this diet lost weight, 90 grams in 25 days, had severe diarrhea and died. Bacteria were still present in the feces.

In an attempt to obtain germfree rats by decontamination, a

pregnant rat which had been maintained with a lactobacillus mono-flora was placed into the jar system and treated with streptomycin. The cage became contaminated during the 5th week. A gram-positive spore forming rod and two gram-negative bacilli were found in the cage. The diet (L-109) was supplemented with 0.5% chloromycetin and the rat bath was 1–500 Roccal and 1–10,000 mercuric iodide. After two transfers no microorganisms were found in the rat. Three weeks later only the gram-positive rod was found; therefore, the contaminants had been eliminated and the experiment ended as it had begun, with one gram-positive rod. In the 2nd, 3rd, and 4th experiments with the jar system no progress was made. In the 5th experiment a pregnant rat was obtained from a contaminated germfree experiment which had only one contaminant, *Bacillus megatherium*. Diet L-109 with 0.5% chloromycetin was fed. When the young were born 5 days later, the chloromycetin was eliminated from the diet. A gram-positive rod was found at 16 days and both a large bacillus and a diplococcus were seen. At 1 month 0.3% chloromycetin was added and 3 days later the fecal smear showed very few rods. After 1 week with chloromycetin the fecal smear tested negative and no growth could be obtained from any cultures, with or without neutralization of the drug. Chloromycetin was taken from the diet and 2 days later the fecal smear was still negative. Decontamination was complete. The animals were bacteriologically sterile for a short time. Nine days later, with no drug in the diet, a large gram-positive spore-forming anaerobe was found which was definitely not *Bacillus megatherium*. It was obvious that the jar system was not bacteriologically safe; therefore the work needs to be repeated with standard isolators. Since the experiments with the jar system gave every promise of success, it should be combined with the preliminary work of Nelson and Reback to decontaminate a conventional animal by feeding effective germicides in the diet in a sterile environment.

The success of H. Sauberlich (1961, personal communication from Fitzsimmons General Hospital, Denver) in maintaining a sterile intestinal tract in men fed antibiotics, combined with current experiments in aseptic surgery and patient care by Levenson (1961, personal communication from Walter Reed Army Research Center, Washington) and Landy (1961, personal communication from Arkansas University Medical Center, Little Rock) indicate good possibilities that gnotobiotic techniques are applicable to man and hospital practice.

Summary

The methods used in germfree research have been presented with a theoretical viewpoint and examined from an historical approach. The usefulness of each work resided in the methods promulgated and in the results of testing. If germfree animals were obtained, the methods were good; if contamination occurred, the method left something to be desired. In theory, each germfree cage was simply a complete mechanical barrier separating the contaminated environment from one that is controlled with respect to the species present. Inside the barrier a sterilization procedure cleared the interior environment of all living microorganisms; as long as the barrier remained intact, the interior was sterile. The biological barrier must also be considered because living organisms must be introduced into the sterilized isolator. A mechanical barrier cannot keep out indigenous organisms introduced with the proposed germfree animal; therefore, the background of the animal colony and the cleanliness of the individuals introduced was of importance. The biological barrier can not be ignored.

The practice of germfree research today shows the variety, size, and shape of the germfree cage could be varied in infinite pattern (Table 3.1). The main barrier may be steel, brass, hard plastic, soft plastic, rubber, or wood. The isolator may be small, as in the transfer jars which have air enough for only a few minutes life of the animal; or it can be as large as a sterile room or sterile building. The attachments on the cage may be equally varied; therefore, adequate instrumentation of germfree research is a major factor in gnotobiotics. The main isolators used today are those of Reyniers, which can stand steam sterilization, and the plastic isolators of Trexler, which are inexpensive and easy to operate. The thin metal wall cage of Gustafsson, the rigid plastic tank of Phillips, and the small isolator of Luckey and Miller are used less extensively.

Irrespective of size, shape, and complexity, everything in the cage must be microbiologically sterile. Everything taken into the cage must be sterilized by one means or another. The most effective method and the most used method is steam under pressure for food, water, and equipment and filtration with incineration for air. Steam pressure is an efficient killing agent and has good penetration, although it mixes less well with air than some of the chemical gases such as ethylene oxide. One of the most desirable methods for sterilization of dry diets is radiation. γ-Rays or high energy electron beams are very efficient in killing bacteria and could be used effectively for solid diets and other material. Radiation is less useful for liquid diets, milks, or fresh foods. Dry heat is useful for inanimate material, instruments, cloth, and powder, and is most useful for presterilizing material. The intermittent sterilization of foodstuffs is not practiced extensively although it is a reliable method. Its drawback is the time involved and the reactions which occur at room temperature during the long sterilization time. Filtration is an effective method for sterilization, but it is not useful for large quantities or for viscous fluids. With few exceptions the great arsenal of chemical germicides have not been used extensively. Ethylene oxide is useful in gnotobiotic research despite its toxicity to biological material and its reactivity in producing derivatives from vitamins in the food. Each method of sterilization has characteristics which are desirable and others which are less desirable. The undesirable characteristics are more obvious with ethylene oxide, but they are also present in all other methods of sterilization. Peracetic acid is the most widely used chemical sterilizing agent for cages and other inanimate objects. Mercuric chloride has been used extensively to sterilize egg surfaces. Surfactants are most useful in preliminary washes to reduce the microbial density on material to be sterilized. Other germicides, exemplified by a few quaternary nitrogen compounds, have proven to be satisfactory in practice despite theoretical and laboratory testing handicaps.

Germicides used by early investigators for sterilization of cages, diets, eggs, abdominal surfaces, and for the air were reviewed. The general impression gained was that sterilization of material was solved during the controversy on spontaneous generation in the 19th century. Therefore, in the early germfree experiments, sterility was not a serious problem when compared to adequacy of diets. For this reason, the sterilization of food was considered in more detail.

Methods used to obtain germfree animals by past investigators and recommended procedures practiced today were presented. Since the maturity of the young at birth is of great importance in raising animals by hand, the various methods of determining parturition time within a very few hours for large animals and within minutes for rats and mice were reviewed.

Methods of testing for contamination comprise one of the most important activities in gnotobiotic research. The limits of the operator's ability, the limits of practicality, and the limits of knowledge and interpretation are considered. An historical review of the methods used by early workers with some evaluation of the adequacy of their methods gives insight into the character and need of germfree research and suggests recommended methods for the detection of bacteria, fungi, worms, protozoa, and viruses. Needed methods are suggested and a consideration is given to contamination rate, sources, and identification. When all is said and done, the animal itself provides one of the best tests for sterility. The gnotobiotic animal provides constant sampling of the food, water, air, and cage surfaces, and gives a concentration of any microbes picked up. It provides incubation at body temperatures with food and moisture always present in the intestinal tract. The germfree animal is an ideal place to grow contaminants since there are no microbial antagonists present and body defense mechanisms are undeveloped. Clinical, morphologic, and chemical reactions of the germfree animal provide excellent criteria to supplement bacteriological routines for the detection of contamination. Practical problems of production, maintenance, space requirements, special attachments to the door, operation of the sterile lock, and the need for accessories such as gloves, cages, and gaskets were briefly presented.

Finally decontamination has been appraised as one of the important areas to be developed in the future.

CHAPTER 4

Nutrition of Germfree Animals

General Considerations

Nutrition was the focus of the theoretical *raison d'être* in early considerations of germfree life, and nutrition has played the leading role in the development of germfree research. Many investigators entered the field to solve nutritional problems. For example, Bogdanow began in 1898 to raise germfree fly larva because he suspected that the fat formation reported by Hoffmann (see Bogdanow, 1906) resulted from bacterial decomposition of the food rather than from metabolic action of the larva. The serious failures in the attempts to rear germfree animals can be attributed more to poor nutrition than to unresolved problems of contamination. The pioneer guinea pig experiments of Nuttall and Thierfelder (1896a) indicated apparent nutritional deficiency. Schottelius' (1908a) decade of failures with germfree chicks probably was a result of nutritional inadequacies. The varied diets used by Cohendy (1912a) were apparently more nearly adequate than those used by his predecessors. Küster (1913b) maintained germfree goats satisfactorily for a short period of time. In his limited experiments he obtained some data regarding the nitrogen and cellulose utilization by goats in the germfree state. Whereas Metchnikoff (1901) and Moro (1905) had failed, Wollman (1913) found germfree tadpoles could be reared if they were fed properly. Guyenot (1913d) indicated that sterile meat fly larvae grew satisfactorily only when yeast extract also could be substituted for whole yeast.

The nutritional requirements of animals are inversely proportional to their biosynthetic capacity. In ruminants this biosynthetic potential includes the synthetic abilities of the microorganisms within the rumen. The extent to which microorganisms of monogastric animals contribute their biosynthetic potential to that of the host is one of the major questions in nutrition to which research with germfree animals can contribute. Pasteur (1885) considered the question from the viewpoint of the aid to digestion and the breakdown of natural materials given the host by the intestinal microflora. His consideration of this potential symbiotic activity of the microorganisms was the main reason he stated that life should not be possible without bacteria. Almost three decades elapsed before a young man in the Pasteur Institute, Cohendy, was able to show that life was possible without bacteria. Since subsequent investigators have amply substantiated this finding as far as artificial foods are concerned, the question of survival has been answered. Regarding the question of digestibility, it will be seen that germfree animals do have most of the normal digestive enzymes attributed to mammals. The role of microorganisms in the breakdown of cellulose will need to be investigated carefully since it has been shown by Conrad et al. (1958) and Johnson et al. (1960) that radioactive C^{14} cellulose is partially digested by the conventional rat. They did not present radioactive cellulose to rats which were restrained from coprophagy; therefore, this experiment should be repeated without coprophagy, and in germfree animals. This would help interpret data which indicate that beavers (Currier et al., 1960), rabbits (Cools and Jeuniaux, 1961), and a marsupial (Moir et al., 1956; Calaby, 1958) utilize cellulose.

Another major question was raised by Nencki (1886): namely, the ability of intestinal bacteria to produce toxic compounds. Depending upon the extent to which this occurred, the host was subjected to toxins from the microflora; therefore, the growth of conventional animals should be retarded. Comparison of the growth rate of germfree and conventional animals shows there was probably very little retardation either directly or indirectly by microorganisms in the tract: the exception in chickens has been elucidated by Coates et al. (1952).

Intestinal Synthesis Theory

Is the synthesis of nutrients by the intestinal microorganisms an important contribution to the dietary requirement of the monogastric host? Germfree animals and monoinoculated animals are most useful in obtaining direct evidence on the intestinal synthesis theory. The intestinal synthesis theory may be presented in the following component parts: (1) A wide variety of species of microorganisms exist in large quantities within the intestinal lumen; they grow, metabolize, and reproduce therein. There are ample bacteriological data to support this part of the thesis. (2) The microorganisms of the intestinal tract can produce nutrients required by the host. There is sound evidence that many microorganisms can synthesize certain B vitamins; other microorganisms require B vitamins. This was reviewed by Peterson and Peterson (1945). There is little doubt that the production of B vitamins does occur by microorganisms while living in the gastrointestinal tract. However, some intestinal microorganisms require B vitamins. The balance between microbial synthesis and utilization is not known. Part of the evidence was the high concentration of B vitamins found in the feces. Data to be presented in this chapter will indicate that the same phenomenon occurs in germfree animals. The better evidence regarding this point is the animal balance studies which have been made. Unfortunately, most do not indicate whether the vitamin was produced by the microflora or released from the tissues of the host. The site of production is still open to direct evidence. (3) The nutrients produced by the microorganisms are either excreted by the cell, extracted from the cell, or the cell bursts to release nutrients into the intestinal lumen before the host can utilize them. Some vitamins are known to be released from cells, although other studies indicate that vitamins may be taken up in greater quantities than they are released, depending upon the conditions of the intestinal tract and the microflora present. (4) The last part of the intestinal synthesis theory is the assumption that B vitamins or other nutrients produced in the intestines of monogastric animals are absorbed and utilized by the host *before* they are excreted in the feces. While there is much indirect evidence, there is no direct evidence that such does occur.

Most of the indirect evidence ignores any action of drugs on the host tissues. Even the evidence from germfree animals to be reported herein is indirect. There is evidence that some of the material produced by the intestinal microorganisms normally reached the host by way of coprophagy. This is outside the intent of the intestinal synthesis thesis. A further point to be considered would be that if nutrients produced by the intestinal microflora were utilized, the question remains of *how much* are utilized and what proportion of the nutritive requirements can be met by this system. The evidence on this topic is either lacking or indirect.

A germfree ruminant would be of tremendous interest in nutrition. Such a study was approached with the idea that if all the nutrients provided by the microflora were put into the diet, the germfree ruminants should survive and grow as well as conventional ruminants.

This becomes, in essence, both a test of the present state of knowledge of nutrition and a search for unknown factors.

Diet and Microorganisms

It may be noted that most of the diets used in germfree research have been purified diets. A few practical diets have been used, but thus far no synthetic diets have been fed to germfree animals. The use of synthetic, chemically defined, diets in germfree animals would advance the standardization of germfree animals as a biological tool. Satisfactory diets have not been worked out and the expense of such diets would prohibit their extensive use.

Since bacteria and other microorganisms are part of the nonsoluble portion of the intestinal contents, they might act as the equivalent of fiber in the diet. Since they are of colloidal dimensions they probably play an important physical role in digestion and absorption phenomena in the intestine. The quantity of (dead) microorganisms present in purified diets is usually very low but not low enough to provide an antigen-free diet. Micrococcal forms are found in the diet; some come from the hands of the operators and some are indigenous in the materials used. Much needed antigen-free diets are being developed at the present time; their use would give a better base line for immunological studies and would be another contribution toward standardization of this biological tool.

It is probable that microorganisms of the intestinal tract help the host in ways not considered a part of classical nutrition; i.e., contributing to muscle tonus or peristalsis of the cecum and stimulating the development of defense mechanisms. One role of microorganisms might be a secondary factor in nutrition, i.e., they challenge the body's defenses continually; energy of the body is used in fighting myriad micro-infections which can cause serious damage to the lumen of the intestinal wall or the metabolism of the host. Another action, which has been shown by Wagner (1959b), is that of oral vaccination. In time, most germfree animals did show immunological responses to the very low level of dead microorganisms in the food. Likewise, larger quantities of dead microorganisms or their products could be added to the food and elicit good immunological responses. Specific actions found include the stimulation of globulin formation, increased lymphatic development, and bactericidal power of serum. Finally, it is proposed that microorganisms can produce toxins in the food. According to the history of food poisoning, most of the action of the microorganism occurs before the food is swallowed. This differs from the growth depressing compound(s) produced by *Clostridium perfringens* (*welchii*), where direct inoculation of the animal resulted in growth depression (assuming no coprophagy). The postulation has been made by Coates *et al.* (1952) that bacteria can cause a depressing action in the well-being of the host; this has been proposed in one explanation of the action of antibiotics in stimulating growth. These effects can be disregarded once germfree animals are used.

The presence or absence of living microorganisms has little to do with the function of diet in the animal *per se*. The energy and essential nutrients of the diet are used to make the same armament of essential metabolites in germfree and polycontaminated animals. Only the germfree animal can give reliable data on the quantitative nutritive requirement of the animal with no microbial contribution. Germfree animals inoculated with known microorganisms will give a clear picture of the importance of microorganisms in nutrition. All nutrients which are required by the host must be available in adequate quantities, and in available form. Each nutrient must be present in quantities such that it is not harmful and it should be present in proper balance with other nutrients for the species involved. The thesis of nutrition as a common denominator in biology, proposed by Luckey (1957), indicated that a single diet could be used for a wide variety of organisms. The same thinking should apply to germfree animals. A diet which is adequate for germfree chicks can be expected to be adequate for germfree mice, rats, or dogs (see Luckey, 1960), although consideration must be given to the special requirement of some species; for example, the guinea pig must have in its diet a supply of vitamin C which most other mammals can synthesize. Diet L-356 illustrates this concept; it has been fed to germfree rats, mice, rabbits, and chicks.

The diets used in germfree research might thus be expected to vary more according to its purpose than for the species involved. Diets with high sugar content and hard particles, to help abrade teeth, are useful in dental caries. Antigen-free diets will be required for definitive studies on innate immunity. Liquid diets are used for hand-feeding newborn mammals before a colony is started. Simple, inexpensive diets are needed to maintain breeding colonies. Synthetic diets are needed to help define all the parameters of nutrition and to eliminate diet as a variable in research.

Innately Sterile Foods

Germfree animals of one species have been fed to germfree animals of another species and sometimes cannibalism has occurred in germfree cages. Innately sterile foods have not been exploited because a variety of good, simple methods is available for sterilizing diets. The use of innately sterile food would significantly reduce the amount of microbial contamination present in the original ingredients. Although this would not be an antigen-free diet, it would provide monobiotic animals in the strict definition of the term (which implies the absence of microorganisms or their biologically distinct products). Antigens from known species only would be present. If the protein and other macromolecules came from the species being fed, antigen formation should be at a minimum. Thus, the excess from stock germfree mice could be used as protein for antigen-free mice.

Few specific examples of the use of innately sterile foods can be cited: Landy (1960) fed sterile grass to germfree guinea pigs and Luckey (unpublished) fed germfree chicks to germfree rats. Once a colony of mammals is started, the germfree mothers provide sterile milk to the young. The quality and quantity of proteins in colostrum of sterile mammals should be compared with that of colostrum from contaminated mammals.

Diet Changes during Sterilization

Last, but not least in the nutrition of germfree animals, is consideration of the changes in diets during sterilization. The effects of the sterilization procedure upon the diet are not too well known. In many cases it was obvious by visual observation that changes had occurred in the diet. Tremendous numbers of reactions are accelerated which would not normally have occurred to an appreciable extent: destruction of vitamins and amino acids (Table 4.1), denaturation of proteins, caramelization of carbohydrates, and penetration of the fat into the container. Steam is one of the most destructive of the agents used to sterilize diet, although it is not as drastic as dry heat or nascent oxygen, iodine, or chlorine which are used for utensils and other material. Material is elevated above room temperature for more than 1 hour during the "17 minutes" steam sterilization. In solid diets, the main reaction seen was the browning reaction between carbohydrate and protein. As will be seen, this gave a lowered biological value for the protein; the reduced carbohydrate utilization was less well studied.

TABLE 4.1
DESTRUCTION OF NUTRIENTS (μg/gm) DURING STERILIZATION

Nutrients	Diet L-109[b]						Diet L-245				Diet PD 56227[d]				
	Theory	Found	Ray sterile	Steam sterile	Steam and store	% Loss[a]	Theory	Found	Steam sterile	% Loss	Theory	Found	Steam sterile	Steam and store	% Loss[a]
Thiamine	60[b]	64	—	14	14	88	50	27.6	3.9	86	16.0	14.3	1.5	2.1	90
Riboflavin	30	27	32	28	—	0	20	13.2	9.4	29	16.0	8.1	6.4	4.8	21
Niacin	100	101	118	106	—	0	100	98	83	15	50	66	47	47	29
Pantothenic acid	300	298	298	211	—	29	100	40	30	25	44	20	11	15	45
Choline[d]	2.0	—	—	—	—	—	2.0	—	1.94	(3)[e]	2.0	1.45	1.28	—	12
Pyridoxine	—	—	—	—	—	—	20	—	16	(25)	12.0	10.9	7.0	4.8	36
Biotin	1.0	5.8	—	6.1	5.1	0	0.50	0.48	0.38	21	0.40	1.6	1.5	1.4	6
Folic acid	10.0	6.2	5.9	4.1	5.8	34	20	3.8	2.5	34	5.0	3.3	1.2	1.1	64
Vitamin B12[c]	—	20.2	—	5.8	—	71	20	12.3	9.9	20	—	—	—	—	—
Vitamin A	—	—	—	—	—	—	—	200	133	34	17	6.5	4.6	4.0	29
Vitamin C[d]	2.0	1.6	—	0.8	—	60	1.0	—	0.8	30	—	—	—	—	—
Vitamin E[d]	—	—	—	—	—	—	—	—	—	—	0.7	1.08	0.58	—	46
Protein (%)	—	—	—	—	—	—	26.2	23.6	23.2	2	35.3	—	—	—	—
Tryptophan[d]	—	—	—	—	—	—	—	—	—	—	4.5	4.0	3.7	—	7
Lysine[d]	—	—	—	—	—	20	—	—	—	—	21.6	25.0	29.5	—	0
Fat (%)	8.0	7.8	—	6.2	—	0	—	—	—	—	—	—	—	—	—
Dry wt (%)	(95)[e]	93.4	—	93.6	—	—	—	—	—	—	—	—	—	—	—

^{a} % loss $= 100 - \left(\dfrac{\text{steam sterile}}{\text{found}} \times 100 \right)$

[b] Diet L-120 data for thiamine and fat.

[c] mμg.

[d] mg/gm.

[e] Values in parentheses are estimates with little data (usually one determination).

If the carbohydrate were starch, the heat might improve the carbohydrate utilization. One property of starch was definitely improved
by steam sterilization; it was less pasty after heating than before.
Some diets which before sterilization caked in the mouths of chickens
were quite satisfactory after sterilization.

Caramelization was one of the undesirable changes in heat-treated
diets. The group at the National Institutes of Health, under Dr. Floyd
Daft, learned to sterilize sucrose by heating a supersaturated solution.
When cool, the crystallized sucrose could be mixed into the rest of the
diet which had been sterilized separately. Sterilization by γ-rays is

TABLE 4.2
MINERAL REQUIREMENTS OF RATS

Element	HMW Salts (mg/5 gm)	Salts IV (mg/6 gm)	Required (mg%)	Recommended (mg%)	Luckey Salts I (mg/6 gm)
Ca	1100	910	600	900	821
P	250[a]	650	550	800	590 (200 in casein)
K	600	730	150–500[b]	500	607
Na	140[a]	340	70–500[b]	500	509
Cl	500	510	50	200	180
I	0.3	3	0.01	0.2	3.4
Mg	50	50	6	25	45[c]
Mn	0.8[a]	10	8	10	18.5
Fe	30	16	2.5–50[b]	50	59
Cu	2	1	0.5	5	5.8
Co	—[d]	—	0.004?	1	0.7
Zn	—[d]	7	0.6	2	1.4
F	3	—[d]	—[d]	0.5	0.7
B	—[d]	—[d]	?	0.1	0.1
Al	0.05	—[d]	?	0.1	0.3

[a] These are below the required amount.

[b] The high value was used in reproduction or lactation experiments when the low
value was found to be too low.

[c] This was placed high so that the mixture may be used for chicks and guinea pigs
as well as rats.

[d] None was added.

excellent for diets containing large quantities of glucose and/or
sucrose. The salts used in different diets are compared to the requirement of the rat for each element (Table 4.2). No thorough study
has been made of the changes in mineral composition of diets during
sterilization.

In the author's experience, the major problems with sterilizing liquid diets include coagulation, broken emulsions, and precipitates of inorganic and organic material. The reactions obtained depended primarily upon the ingredients and the pH of the final mixture. The pH must be adjusted carefully for optimum results with liquid diets (see Fig. 4.1). The optimum pH for most diets was 6.2. When natural milks were sterilized, similar problems were seen. The addition of acid phosphates to adjust the pH and dilution of milk diets decreased coagulation and other undesirable reactions. Preparation of the liquid diets required homogenization to obtain smaller fat particles than in natural milk because the heat treatment increased the particle size.

The use of both liquid and solid steam sterilized diets presented the common problem of vitamin and amino acid destruction. A good idea of the loss of specific nutrients can be obtained from the data in Table 4.1. The destruction of vitamins in the three syntype diets during steam sterilization was usually similar. However it was surprising that no riboflavin, niacin, or biotin was found to be destroyed in diet L-109. About 25% of the riboflavin and niacin were lost in the other diets. Most of the thiamine (up to 90%) and 25–45% of the pantothenic acid were not recovered following steam sterilization. Very little biotin and choline were destroyed. A reliable estimate of vitamin B_{12} destruction was not obtained. About one-half of the pyridoxine, folic acid, vitamin A, vitamin C, and vitamin E was lost during steam sterilization. Very little change was seen in the protein or lysine or tryptophan during steam sterilization. The dry weight of these diets was not changed appreciably. The loss of fat in diet L-109 was expected because lipid often impregnated the wrapping.

Many of these changes were measured by chemical or microbiological tests (Luckey *et al.*, 1955a), but it is suspected that more changes are not known than are known. Therefore, it has been the practice to feed conventional animals sterilized diet for several generations *before* that diet was used for germfree animals.

With all the nutrients studied in dry diets, radiation sterilization was considerably less destructive than was steam sterilization. The appearance of the diet following electron beam sterilization or γ-radiation sterilization (from spent fuel sources) was very similar to that before sterilization. The 2 million rads used with dry diets were less destructive of nutrients than were lower levels used for fresh foodstuffs. No destruction of vitamin C was found when crystalline ascorbic acid was sterilized with cathode rays. Where sufficient flux

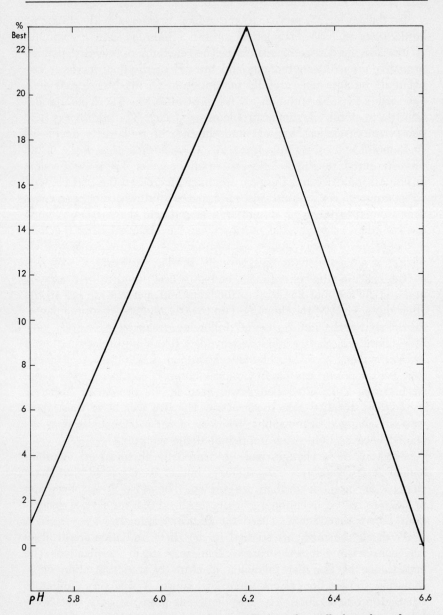

Fɪɢ. 4.1. Optimum pH for sterilizing milk formula. Milk formula and synthetic milks cannot be sterilized satisfactorily at any pH. The most usable product is obtained at about pH 6.2 more often than at any other pH.

of γ-radiation is available, it is the agent of choice for dry diet sterilization.

The loss in potency of antibiotics sterilized by different methods is given in Table 4.3. The losses were estimated by analysis of the preparation following sterilization and assay after the sterile antibiotic was mixed into the diet inside the germfree cage. Based upon these data, the method adopted (Luckey et al., 1956) was that of electron beam sterilization of the antibiotic diluted in 1 gm lactose.

Colonies of conventional mice and rats have been maintained on ethylene oxide sterilized dry syntype diets (L-109 and L-128) and practical animal feeds. However, attempts to maintain rats fed ethylene oxide sterilized milk have not been successful. The rats apparently found something distasteful and starved to death. It was possible that not all of the ethylene oxide was removed following the sterilization or that harmful compounds were formed.

It is emphasized that each method of diet sterilization is useful and adequate for its purpose. Each method could be misused, a point which is not well appreciated in the developmental stages of a sterilizing procedure. While Hawk and Mickelson (1955) and others indicated that ethylene oxide could be toxic and suggest that ethylene oxide sterilized diets would be inadequate, it is emphasized that ethylene oxide *can* be used to sterilize diets in a *proper* manner and such diets will support colonies of animals. The author, in collaboration with J. A. Reyniers and M. Wagner at the University of Notre Dame, maintained a gnotobiotic colony for over 8 months with ethylene oxide (carboxide) sterilized diets. Viable *Bacillus stearothermophilus* was not recovered from diets that had been inoculated with spores of this organism and then sterilized with ethylene oxide. Several generations of rats and mice were maintained on this diet with no evidence of harm. A similar example may be seen in the radiation sterilization of diets; improper radiation sterilization could produce harmful compounds in diets as can ethylene oxide. However Luckey et al. (1955c) showed that radiation sterilized diets were adequate for a mouse colony reared through several generations.

In order that the diets be complete following sterilization an excess of heat labile nutrients was added. Since it was expected that approximately 50% of the pyridoxine, folic acid, pantothenic acid, and riboflavin might be destroyed, the quantity of these vitamins added was doubled. Variations in constituents, moisture, and temperature during the sterilization cycle gave different rates of vitamin destruction. In

4. Nutrition of Germfree Animals

TABLE 4.3

PERCENTAGE LOSS OF ANTIBIOTICS DURING STERILIZATION

Antibiotic	Loss by electron radiation sterilization in starch	Loss by steam sterilization in diet	Loss by other methods of sterilization	Loss by mixing with diet	Total loss	Assay method
Aureomycin	—	100	2[a]	—	—	Microb.
Bacitracin	30	—	—	83[d]	88[d]	Microb.
Chloromycetin	—	58–66	—	40–45	58–66	Microb.
	—	42, 48	—	—	42, 48	Color
	—	—	0[e]	—	82, 83	Alcohol extraction
Procaine penicillin	42	—	—	—	—	Microb.
	0	—	—	0	0	Microb.
	0	—	—	—	—	Microb.
	0	—	—	—	—	Chemical
Penicillin G (K salt)	37–48	—	16[b]	—	36	Microb.
	—	—	99+[b,c]	—	—	Microb.
	—	—	—	—	—	Microb.
Terramycin	0	—	—	—	—	Microb.
	—	95.5+	—	—	—	Microb.
	—	—	98[f]	—	—	Microb.
	—	—	40[g]	—	—	Microb.

[a] Dry heat at 110°C for 10 to 30 hours.
[b] Dry heat at 170°C for 1 hour
[c] Autoclaved 25 minutes at 15 psi in acetic acid, heated in oven 3 hours at 140°C.
[d] Adsorption to diet may be counted as lost.
[e] Autoclaved in solution.
[f] Autoclaved dry in plugged tube.
[g] Seitz filtered.

some diets 90% of the thiamine was destroyed; in others, 95% was lost. Therefore 20 times the required amount of thiamine was used. These quantities give no evidence of toxicity from either the vitamin or its products.

The First Colony of Germfree Mammals

Several mammals have been reared by hand-feeding techniques with little or no colostrum or natural milk. Reyniers (1946a) experienced no difficulty in rearing Cesarean-born germfree monkeys. Albanese et al. (1948) have reared human babies on a variety of syntype diets with apparent success. Guineas pigs were reared through more than one generation by Luckey (1954a) and Read (1958) with syntype diets. Germfree rabbits have been reared from birth on syntype diets by Luckey and Teah (unpublished) and Pleasants (1959). A lion (Luckey and Hittson, 1952), pigs (Luckey, 1954a and Landy, 1961), kittens (Luckey, 1961a), sheep (Luckey, 1960), and germfree goats (Küster, 1913b) have been reared with little or no colostrum. The ease with which larger mammals could be reared contrasts with the difficulties encountered in rearing rodents with no colostrum. The failures and sporadic success in attempts to rear mice, guinea pigs, hamsters, and rats uncovered many nutritional problems which needed to be solved before consistent success was to be attained in rearing germfree mice (Pleasants, 1959) and rats (Pleasants, 1959; Gustafsson, 1959a) by hand. These successes were based upon knowledge summarized herein. Two factors of vital importance to the rearing of germfree rats (and mice) were: (1) the finding of Reyniers and associates (1946) that Cesarean born must have their genitalia stimulated for proper elimination to prevent uremic poisoning; the frequent baths given the rats of Gustafsson (1948) also accomplished this; and (2) the methods developed by Glimstedt (1936a,b) and Teah and Reyniers (1948, personal communication) for obtaining mature young by Cesarean section.

The weight and maturity of the young at birth was an important variable in the success of hand rearing of rats: those with a birth weight below 4.0 gm were rarely weaned, while those at 5 gm or more had the best possibility of survival. No real advantage was found in starting with rats having a birth weight over 6 gm. However, it was essential to obtain the young fully developed. The fast rate of body development near the time of birth was illustrated by the increase in body weight noted by Stratsenburg (1915), Angula and Gonzalos (1932), and Hamilton and Bewar (1938) in Fig. 3.31.

The effect of anesthesia of the dam upon the health and survival of the young was an unknown variable. Deep ether anesthesia of the dam made the young difficult to revive. Barbiturates were much better; the young from barbiturate-anesthetized dams were often quite lively a few minutes after birth. The young seemed to be the most healthy when the dam was sacrificed following a blow to the skull prior to the Cesarean operation.

Another problem studied was the optimum temperature for rearing newborn rats. The body temperature of the newborn rats was 33° ± 1°C (oral) and 35°C (rectal) and gradually rose to 37°C (rectal) during the next 10 days. The nest under the young was 28–32°C while the temperature of the young under the dam was 36 ± 2°C (skin temperature). The growth of normal born rats taken from their mother at 1 day and hand-fed diet L-185 in nests at different temperatures is given in Fig. 4.2. Growth and survival were better at 35°C than at either 30° or 38°C. Thereafter, newborn hand-fed germfree rats were maintained at 35–36°C by directing infrared lights on the cage. The skin of the young rats usually appeared dry at this temperature, so the humidity was increased with the "wick in a bottle" system.

The main problem was defined in terms of the growth and survival of the hand-fed rats as compared with that of the normal born, dam-suckled rats. Unlike the growth curve of most newborn mammals, the growth curve of dam-suckled rats (Fig. 4.3) showed no decrease in body weight the first day. The mother rat was found on the nest 90% of the time during the first 2 days. Most of this time the young were found to be connected to the teat tightly enough that they were sometimes lifted bodily when the dam was picked up. The lower curve represents a successful experiment with germfree rats (Reyniers et al., 1946). The hand-fed rats ate for only 2 minutes in each 60, usually lost weight during the first few hours, and thereafter gained slowly.

A syntype diet (L-135) was formulated to contain all the nutrients known to be required by rats and other vertebrates. The ingredients were such that they could be mixed with water and fed as a "synthetic" milk (see Appendix III for the components). In order to verify that the diet was adequate it was fed to weanling rats; one group was fed the diet as a liquid and another group received the diet after it had been lyophilized. Both groups of rats ate the diets

readily and grew well (Fig. 4.4). When newborn germfree rats were
hand-fed diet L-135 they grew at a very slow rate and survival was
not good. The diet appeared to be adequate for weaned rats but
hand-fed suckling rats did not consistently survive on it.

Another possibility for the many early failures in hand rearing of
rats was the special nutritive value of colostrum which was denied

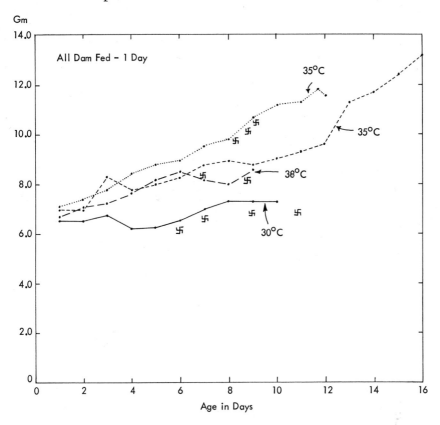

Fig. 4.2. Growth of hand-fed rats at different temperatures.

these hand-fed young. Except for the globulin fraction which provided
the newborn with a supply of antibodies before its own tissues were
able to make them, the exact compounds which were needed were not
well defined. Reyniers (1946a) reported that newborn rats could not
be foster suckled to mother rats which had lactated 7 to 21 days. This
posed the question: how much colostrum did the young rat require?

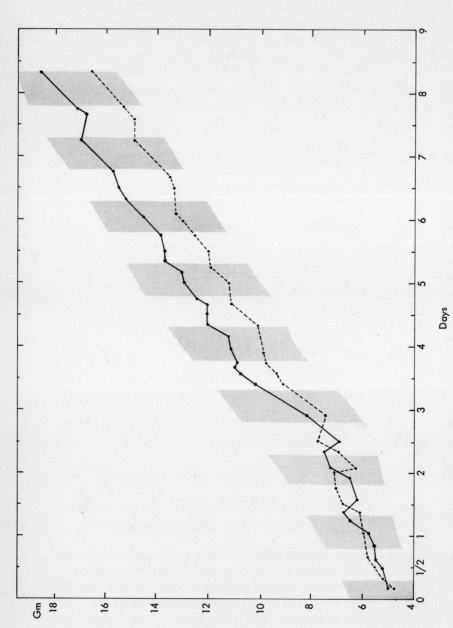

FIG. 4.3. Growth of suckling rats weighed every 2 hours. Obtained with the collaboration of A. Loranc at the University of Notre Dame. The stippled area represents gains during the night. Each line represents the average weight of one litter of 8–10 young rats.

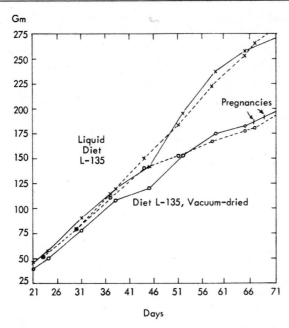

FIG. 4.4. Growth of rats fed synthetic-type milk diets through reproduction. The open circles represents females, the x's represent males. The solid line represents the liquid diet being used while the dashed line represents vacuum dried, L-135.

Newborn rats were allowed to feed from their own mother for 48 hours and then switched to a foster mother of 10 days lactation. They survived when the foster dam would accept them. The colostrum feeding period was shortened until, as shown in Table 4.4, the rats were taken with no colostrum, the last group also survived. The results

TABLE 4.4
COLOSTRUM REQUIREMENT OF YOUNG RATS

Date and expt. no.	Day lactation: foster dam	No. start	Age start (in hr.)	No. survive
7.16.48 I	10	10	48	10
7.16.48 II	10	10	24	10
7.16.48 III	10	10	8	10
7.16.48 IV	12	6	2	6
11.28.52 V	9	10	0[a]	9

[a] Cesarean birth, weight at 21 days is 30.1 gm.

were verified by successfully foster suckling Cesarean-born rats to mother rats of 9 days lactation. The difference between success and failure was the manner in which the foster dam was induced to care for the newborn rather than in any specific compound in colostrum. Subsequently rats and other mammals were routinely raised by hand-feeding in the germfree cage following Cesarean operation.

Since Reyniers (1946a) had suggested that the germfree rat required vitamin C, it was normally included in the diet (5 mg/100 ml) and special study was made of the vitamin C metabolism in rats (Meeks, 1950). Brain tissue contained a high concentration of vitamin C which decreased markedly (on a per gram of rat basis; Fig. 4.5) at

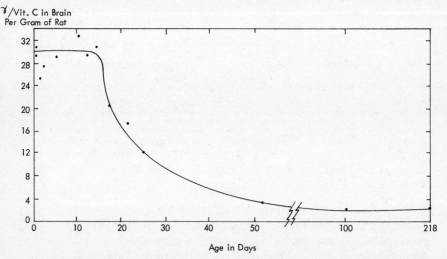

FIG. 4.5. Vitamin C concentration in rat brain using normal suckled rats. Data of Meeks (1950).

about 15 days of age, when the rat began to eat solid food. The vitamin C in the liver of newborn rats (Fig. 4.6) indicated that the ratio of reduced to oxidized vitamin C changed dramatically from birth to 10 days. Germfree rats fed no vitamin C were much lower in both reduced and oxidized liver ascorbic acid than were dam-fed rats. When ascorbic acid was added to the diets of germfree rats, the liver content of total ascorbic acid was much higher than that of dam-fed rats. Analysis of rat milk for vitamin C and estimation of the amount of milk consumed per day allowed an evaluation of the amount of this vitamin received by the suckling rat from his mother. When this

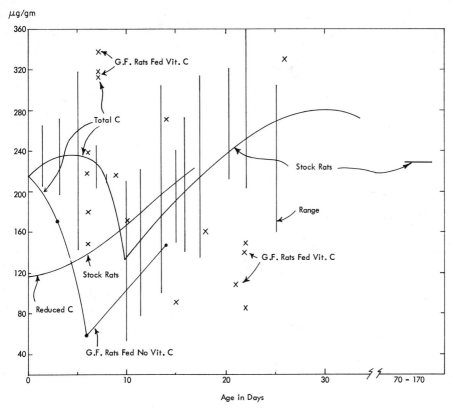

FIG. 4.6. Vitamin C content of rat liver. The germfree rats are noted by x. The total vitamin C is high at 0 days, although reduced vitamin C is low. The difference between the total and reduced indicates the oxidized vitamin C. The x marks the vitamin C content of the liver of Gf rats fed vitamin C. The vertical lines represent the range of values from which the curve for the stock rats was derived.

was added to the total amount present in the carcass at birth, vitamin C was found in greater quantities in the total carcass than the rats had received (Fig. 4.7) showing that dam-suckled rats could synthesize vitamin C. This agreed with evidence from mature rat liver tissue slice experiments by Smythe and King (1942).

Analysis of newborn and 4 day old rats (Table 4.5) showed the hand-fed rats had gained little weight and little nitrogen while the dam-fed rats had doubled their body weight and tripled their nitrogen content. Crude fat determinations indicated that the hand-fed rats lost

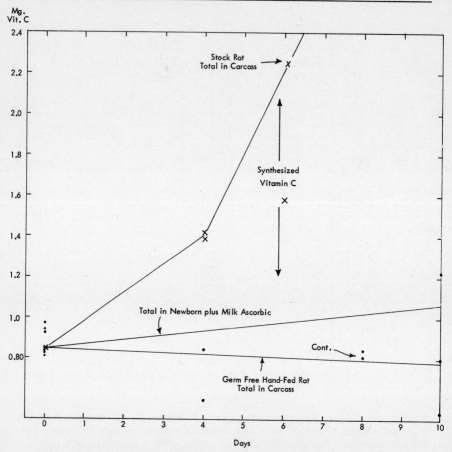

Fig. 4.7. Evidence for vitamin C synthesis in suckling rats. The lower curve indicates that the hand-fed rats did not show a total increase in ascorbic acid in the carcass. The middle curve is obtained by adding to the initial body store an estimate of the quantity of vitamin C obtained from rat milk. The difference between the top curves indicates the quantity of vitamin C presumed to be synthesized.

85% of the fat they had at birth while dam-fed rats increased their total fat content by 3½ times. At the same time the germfree rats had fatty livers; the fat content of the liver of germfree rats was 2–3 times greater than that of dam-fed rats.

The quantity of milk to be fed was difficult to estimate. The different methods used gave very different results as shown in Fig. 4.8. Brody (1945) obtained much greater values than any given here.

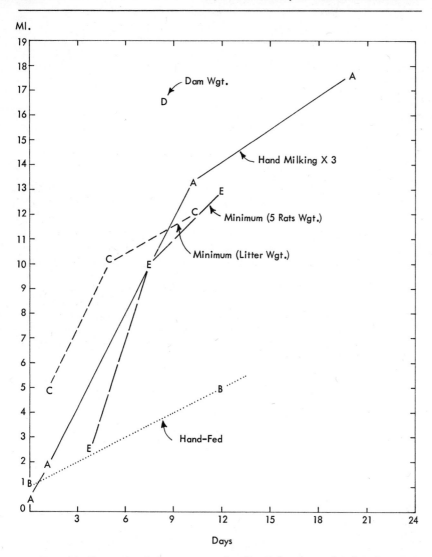

FIG. 4.8. Estimates of the amount of milk produced per day by the rat. A represents three times the amount obtained during the best hand milking of rats. C represents a minimum obtained by weighing the litter every day. E is obtained the same way with a different litter. Both of these represent minima and one might expect to multiply this by a factor of at least two for the food efficiency factor. Point D was obtained by weighing a mother before and after lactation during the day. This method was used by Brody (1945) to obtain much higher values.

TABLE 4.5

GROSS ABSORPTION IN SUCKLING RATS

	Age (days)	Weight (gm)	Total N₂ (mg)	Total fat (mg)
Newborn	0	5.2	5.93	68.3
Germfree[a]	4	5.3	6.42	9.1
Stock	4	10.0	16.7	252

[a] Hand-fed.

Finally, an analysis of rat's milk was undertaken by Luckey *et al.*
(1954b). Quantities of 0.1–0.5 ml of milk were obtained by pooling
the yield from 12 teats of a single dam during the colostrum period
while 4–8 ml could be obtained later. Both rat milk and colostrum are
opaque, white, watery fluids. There was no sour (butyric acid) odor
of the curdled rat milk in the stomach of suckling rats, while stomach
contents of rats fed cow's milk or formula had a strong odor. This

TABLE 4.6

COMPOSITION OF RAT MILK AND EARLY COLOSTRUM

Component	Colostrum	Milk
Dry weight (%)	32	22
CHO (%)	2.9	3.7
Fat (%)	22	9.3
Protein (%)	9.0	8.7
Casein (%)	7.3	7.2
Globulin (%)	1.6	0.9
Albumin (%)	0.48	0.05
NPN (%)	0.092	0.08
Ash (%)	0.45	1.4
Calcium (%)	0.10	0.27
Phosphorus(%)	0.14	0.25
Potassium (%)	0.093	0.11
Sodium(%)	—	0.14
Iron (%)	—	0.0007
Magnesium (%)	—	0.030
Copper (%)	—	0.0007
Chlorine (%)	—	0.12
Zinc (%)	—	0.006
Vitamin E (mg%)	—	0.27
Vitamin A (μg/gm)	—	9.2
Vitamin C (mg%)	—	1.0
Thiamine (μg/gm)	—	1.4
Riboflavin (μg/gm)	2.21	2.6

TABLE 4.6 (*Continued*)

Component	Colostrum	Milk
Niacin (μg/gm)	20	18
Pantothenate (μg/gm)	2.9	5.5
Pyridoxine (μg/gm)	—	0.76
Biotin (μg/gm)	0.09	0.08
Folic acid (μg/gm)	0.30	0.33
Vitamin B_{12} (mμg/gm)	—	170
pH	6.3	6.7
Specific gravity	0.997	1.04
Osmotic pressure ($\cong$ molar NaCl)	0.10	0.16
Viscosity (centipoises)	—	6.4
Surface tension (dynes/cm)	—	50
Butyric acid (% of fat)	—	0.0
Caproic acid (% of fat)	—	0.0
Caprylic acid (% of fat)	—	3.8
Capric acid (% of fat)	—	6.3
Lauric acid (% of fat)	—	4.0
Iodine no. of fat	—	48.5
Saponification no. of fat	—	220
Glycine (% of protein)	—	1.7
Valine (% of protein)	—	5.0
Leucine (% of protein)	—	5.5
Isoleucine (% of protein)	—	4.7
Proline (% of protein)	—	7.8
Tyrosine (% of protein)	—	3.9
Phenylalanine (% of protein)	—	3.8
Tryptophan (% of protein)	—	4.6
Aspartic acid (% of protein)	—	5.8
Glutamic acid (% of protein)	—	20.2
Arginine (% of protein)	—	3.4
Histidine (% of protein)	—	2.5
Lysine (% of protein)	—	5.3
Threonine (% of protein)	—	4.5
Cystine (% of protein)	—	4.0
Methionine (% of protein)	—	1.9

was explained by the absence of butyric acid in rat's milk (Table 4.6). During lactation the pH, osmotic pressure, specific gravity, and viscosity of rat milk increased. These changes were partially explained by the chemical changes which occurred during this period. The gross constituents of rat milk underwent dramatic change during one lactation cycle (Fig. 4.9). Colostrum is two thirds fat on a dry weight basis. The fat content dropped rapidly from 22%, wet basis, during

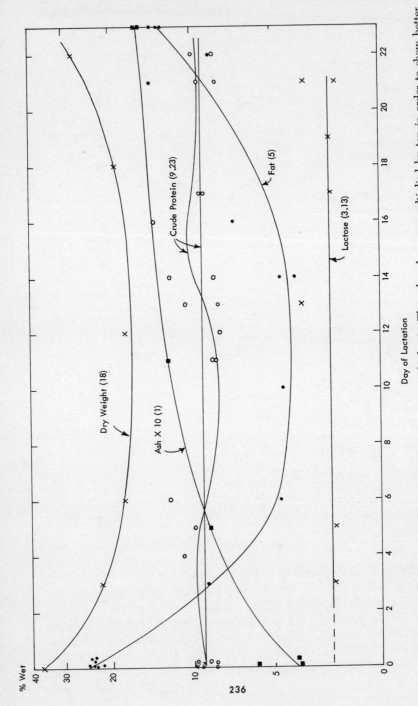

Day of Lactation

FIG. 4.9. Gross composition of rat's milk on a wet weight basis. The ash values are multiplied by ten in order to show better the differences obtained. Two curves might be drawn for the protein content depending upon the use of the scattered data. The dry weight was obtained experimentally and agreed well with the sum of the other major ingredients. Data from Luckey *et al.* (1954b).

the first week to about 9%; then it rose during the last week of lactation.

Armed with this data, investigators formulated many new diets: high fat diets for the complete suckling period, high fat diets for the early period, followed by lower fat, etc. Egg yolk diets were compared to cream base diets. Water was fed before the diets or alternated with diets. One fact was outstanding—the survival rate of the hand-fed rats increased remarkably when high fat diets were used. Skin color and texture were improved markedly and more rats were weaned. Obviously the young rats fed the low rat diets had not received enough energy. However, success in rearing these Cesarean-born babies to weaning remained erratic. The dip in the growth curve was eliminated, but the growth rate remained slow (Fig. 4.10). Nothing could be cor-

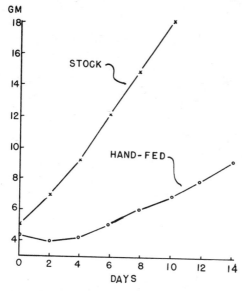

Fig. 4.10. Growth of suckling rats.

related to either the success or the failure. One year (progress was measured in years) the summer months would be good and seasonal factors would be suspected. Most disturbing were the results from feeding hand-expressed rat's milk to newborn rats: they grew no better than when fed the man-made diets (Fig. 4.11). It appeared to be obvious that the young rats were getting enough to eat because one could see the curd of milk through the abdominal wall. A great variety of different methods of feeding were tried. The crescendo of exotic experiments stopped abruptly when, in 1954, Dr. Tom Mende inaugurated a simple change: feed more food. The baby rats were fed

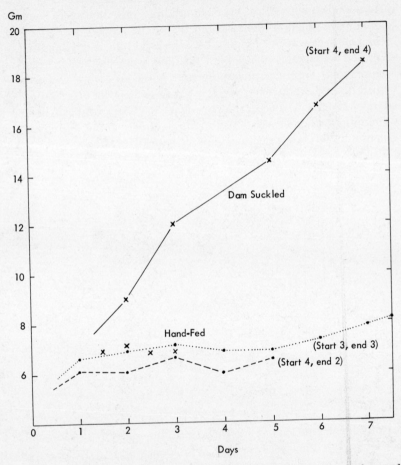

FIG. 4.11. Nutritive properties of rat's milk directly from the mother and expressed rat's milk fed by hand.

a prescribed amount through a nipple attached to a syringe. Immediately, the weaning of hand-fed rats became a routine, stable procedure. Many of the diets tried previously were then found to be quite adequate when fed in proper amounts. Apparently, the rats had been starving although milk was constantly in their stomach. The effect of the application of this new knowledge on the half-life of newborn, hand-fed rats is shown in Fig. 4.12. Making the diet simulate the high fat food of the mother rat increased the half-life to about 10 days. The Mende "overfeeding" technique increased the half-life well passed weaning. Gustafsson (see Wostmann, 1959a, p. 182) found he could increase the weaning weight of hand-fed rats to 20 gm by using high

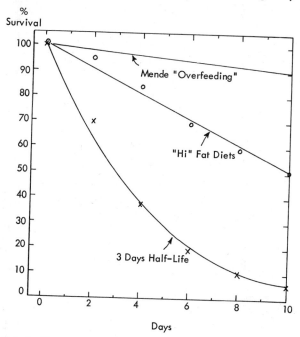

Fig. 4.12. Suckling rat survival. Survival of rats fed a low energy diet, high energy diet, and greater quantities of diet.

fat diets. The fruition of germfree research owed much to this successful venture in the hand-feeding of newborn rats. As soon as Julian Pleasants (then in charge of rearing rats) had weaned a substantial number of rats, he successfully turned his efforts to rearing mice—one-fifth the size of rats.

When hand-fed rats first learned to eat solid food, at about 12 days, they gorged themselves. At 12–14 days some rats developed cataract and alopecia, and some exhibited a spontaneous fracture, as illustrated by the extra leg "joint" in Fig. 4.13. Consequently, analyses of the bone ash, bone calcium, and bone phosphorus were run on rats of this age

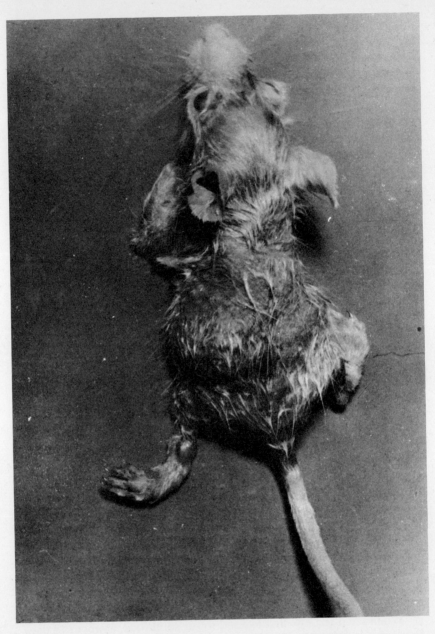

FIG. 4.13. Spontaneous fracture in hand-fed rats. Hand-fed gremfree rats ate voraciously when they learned to eat solid food. The abdomen would distend and the hind legs of rats of 13–15 days old would bend or break. The rats could not walk; they pushed themselves along the floor. The enlarged abdomen, enlarged cecum, and the protruding eyeballs indicate malnutrition.

under germfree and dam-fed conditions. The data (given later under mineral requirement) indicated that the bone calcium was apparently normal and the bone phosphorus of the germfree hand-fed rats was much below that of normal rats. Rather than change the 1.5:1 calcium-phosphorus ratio in these diets, the problem was approached by restricting the food available to the young rats when they first learned to eat. This prevented the development of the rotund figure and eliminated the spontaneous fracture.

Each success introduced a new problem! Almost all rats which were weaned developed an enlarged cecum. The cecum mass would become 25–35% of the body weight and rotate in a counterclockwise direction. This rotation twisted the attached intestine at the junction of the ileocecal valve until the passage of almost all material stopped. The animals became sluggish and showed lordosis with increasing frequency. This syndrome prevented the animals from breeding, although they were fed sterile diets (l-103 and L-128) which had been shown to be adequate for conventional animals. Most germfree rats died prematurely from the intestinal block. Therefore, the assumption was made that living microorganisms stimulated the intestinal mucosa for proper elimination, and it was surmised that fiber might fulfill this function in germfree conditions. Fiber (3% alpha cell) was added (diet L-109) and fed to young germfree rats. The cecum was reduced to acceptable size and breeding activities began. Food restriction was helpful in rats and was used effectively in guinea pigs. Neither fiber nor food restriction was adequate to allow germfree rabbits to survive. J. Pleasants at the University of Notre Dame obtained rabbits of good appearance and breeding activity by ligation of part of the cecum. It should be noted that this problem was not seen in germfree chickens or turkeys.

Although many gestations were completed through parturition, the germfree rats failed to lactate properly. While conventional rats fed the same sterilized diets would rear their young quite properly through several generations, pregnant germfree rats would make good nests, cast their young, and care for them for only 1 or 2 days; milk could be expressed from the mothers, but the young were not fed. Liver powder and yeast powder were added to the diet of the mother rats; next fresh liver and fresh meat were given once a week (by sacrificing germfree chicks in the cage and feeding first the fresh liver and then the carcass); and finally, a killed *Lactobacillus* culture was added to the diet (milk, after heavy fermentation with lactic acid organisms, was dried to a powder) and no young survived 3 days. Just a few days before casting the fourth litters in this experiment, the rats became contaminated. All 3 mothers raised litters in the new animal house. This evidence suggested that bacteria were indeed needed for lactation! Then came a most pleasant surprise. Rats left in the quiet of unmolested germfree cages reproduced, March 31, 1951, mothered their young, lactated properly, and reared the second generation rats to begin the first colony of germfree vertebrates. Apparently, *too much "help" had upset the motherly instincts.* Thus, was it dramatically shown that peace and quiet were more important than bacteria for successful motherhood.

Diets and Feeding

Since reference is made throughout the monograph to a wide variety of diets used to raise germfree animals, the compositions are given in Appendix III. The following summary indicates which diets have been used for different species of germfree animals.

Fish

Diet has apparently been the main deterrent in rearing germ-free fish. Baker and Fergusson (1942) attempted to rear platyfish free from bacteria in the germfree state but were thoroughly unsuccessful. Reyniers and Trexler (1943b) and Reyniers (1946a) also attempted to rear germfree fish with limited success. Shaw (1957) approached the problem with the idea that omnivorous fish should be used, and he obtained germfree guppies quite simply. However, he did not attempt to feed them.

Chickens

Almost all the published work with chickens has been concerned with steam-sterilized diets. A composition of diets used by early investigators is indicated in Table 2.6. The first diets prepared for germfree chicks were chopped eggs, but were not fed since the chicks of Nuttall and Thierfelder (1897) were not obtained in the germfree state. The mixtures used by Schottelius (1908a) and Cohendy (1912a) were given in Chapter 2, but are not to be recommended. Balzam (1937b) and Reyniers et al. (1949b,d) used practical diets which were adequate at those times.

When the author fed germfree chickens or conventional chickens

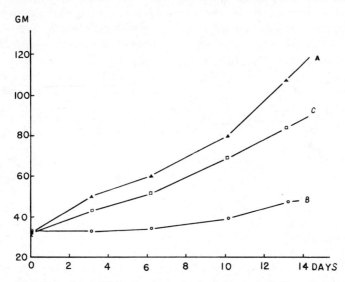

FIG. 4.14. Growth of White Leghorn chicks fed practical diets. A. Nonsterile diet. B. Sterile diet with added vitamins fed to germfree chicks. C. Steam sterilized diet with added vitamin and protein fed to germfree chicks.

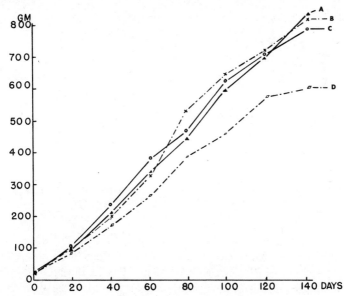

FIG. 4.15. Growth of Bantam chicks fed steam sterilized diets. A. Conventional bantams (average of 43). B. Germfree chicks (average of 33). C. Nonsterile diet. D. Broiler ration.

243

a steam-sterilized practical diet, the chickens failed to grow (Fig. 4.14). Since vitamin destruction was suspected, vitamins were added. The chickens grew no better. Protein was added to the vitamin supplemented diet and the chickens grew at an acceptable rate. Therefore the destruction of both protein and vitamins must be considered with practical diets. Practical diets which have been used successfully with germfree chickens are numbers L-124 and L-389.

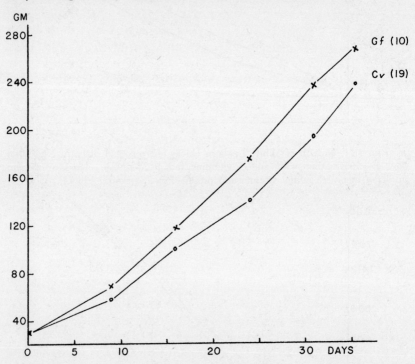

Fig. 4.16. Growth of Leghorn chicks fed a complete syntype diet, L-245. Gf = Germfree chicks (average of 10). Cv = Conventional chicks (average of 19).

Growth rates were similar for conventional and germfree Bantam chicks fed diet L-137 (Fig. 4.15) and for conventional and germfree White Leghorn chicks with diet L-245 (Fig. 4.16). These syntype diets were composed of crystalline vitamins and salts, purified corn oil, extracted casein as a protein, and starch for the carbohydrate source. Obviously there was a potential for small quantities of known and unknown vitamins in the casein starch and corn oil. These diets were very similar to those used during the past two decades of nutritional work and were comparable to those used for determinations of quantitative and qualitative vitamin requirements of conventional animals. Springer (1959) found antigens in such diets and suggested that even synthetic diets could not be antigen free. Chemically defined diets have not been used extensively in germfree research with vertebrates. This is a goal in nutritional research which has been attained with a limited number of protozoa and invertebrates. Greenstein et al. (1957) used a synthetic diet in solution which should be tried for germfree mammals. However, as the author learned in experiments with sterile diets in 1944, chicks have difficulty eating liquid foods: they literally got stuck in their cage by the glue-like material.

Other Birds

The main use of turkeys in germfree research has been the work with antibiotic stimulation. Diet number L-318 and syntype diet L-420 have been satisfactory. The growth of germfree turkeys fed L-318 was somewhat greater than that of conventional poults (Fig. 4.17; see Luckey et al., 1960 and Forbers et al., 1958c). The basic diet used for rearing germfree quails was diet T-105F, a fortified practical diet (Reyniers et al., 1960b). It is anticipated that any of the above diets would be satisfactory for other birds.

Guinea Pigs

The fact that guinea pigs can eat independently after birth was a deciding factor by Nuttall and Thierfelder (1895–1896) in their choice as the first animal to be used in germfree research. These workers fed sterile cow's milk, obtained by a combination of collecting it aseptically from teats that had been washed with $HgCl_2$ and rinsed with sterile, distilled water, and expressing it through a wet towel by a "sterilized hand." Sterilization was completed by heating of the milk on 3 consecutive days. In subsequent experiments Nuttall and Thierfelder (1896b) fed biscuits containing 7% N_2, 9% fat, 17% sugar, 0.2% cellulose, and 58% NFE (nitrogen-free extract). The guinea pigs showed no consistent growth in their experiments.

More recently, germfree guinea pigs have been reared and maintained on both syntype diets and practical diets developed primarily by Phillips et al. (1959). Phillips diets No. L-412 and L-445 gave the best results. Landy et al. (1961) used a mixture of aseptically grown Mong bean sprouts with Phillips diet L-445. The sprouts were not

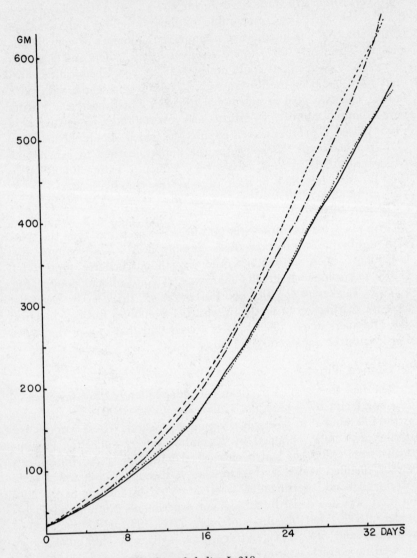

FIG. 4.17. Growth of turkeys fed diet L-318.
KEY: Germfree, - - - - - - 10 males; . . . . . . 11 females.
     Conventional, —•—•—• 31 males; ————37 females.

thought to be essential. Wostmann (1959a) simply added vitamin C to the rat diet L-465 to obtain a diet adequate for germfree guinea pigs.

Reproduction has recently been obtained in germfree guinea pigs by Teah in 1959 and Newton in 1960 but dietary problems such as the enlarged ceca, remain to be solved.

Rats

The later diets used for suckling rats were based upon analysis of rat milk (Luckey *et al.*, 1954b). Gustafsson (1948) used diet A-105, Reyniers *et al.* (1946) used diet 24N, Pleasants (1959) used diet L-420, and diet L-285 was found to be most successful in the author's experience. Of the many diets for weaning rats, the following are

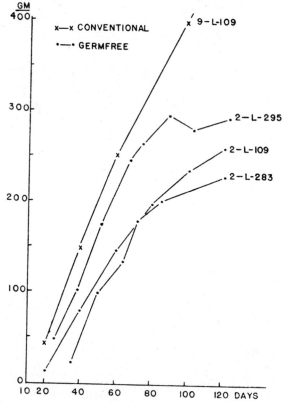

Fig. 4.18. Growth rates of germfree and conventional male rats fed steam sterilized syntype diets. The number of rats and the diets used are indicated following each curve.

useful: diet L-356, a practical diet fortified with vitamins and protein used to rear colonies of germfree rats; diet L-109 was the syntype diet employed as a standard to study growth requirements and other characteristics of germfree rats (Fig. 4.18). Gordon (1960b) suggested that improved caging and decreased crowding would obliterate the difference in growth rate between germfree and conventional male rats.

Mice

Very little has been published on the rearing of germfree mice. The diets used for mice were very similar to those used for rats both before and after weaning. Once germfree mice were reared, new strains were introduced by foster suckling. It was not found feasible to foster suckle mice onto rats, although Mrs. E. Holzman (personal communication) of Madison, Wisconsin, has accomplished this after a very few days of hand-feeding. The feeding methods of Pleasants (1959) are summarized. Two feedings of sugar-free Tyrode's solution preceded the feeding of 0.04 ml of diet L-420 plus quercetin every 2 hours. The quantity fed, given by syringe, was increased by 0.01 ml each day. At 2 weeks the mice were fed milk in an open container and they were weaned to solid food at 25 days. Although the milk formula was deficient in minerals, a few mice were weaned successfully.

Solid diet L-256 has been used for stock colonies of both germfree rats and mice by Wostmann (1959a) for 10 generations with no accumulative deficiencies being observed. About 80% of the normal born, dam-suckled young were weaned at 21 days. The general appearance of these animals was that of good health. The practical diet L-462 has been used successfully for Swiss albino mice and for mice of the C3H strain.

Rabbit Diets

Syntype diets for rabbits have been developed by Woolley (1957), Luckey (1954a, 1961a), and Wostmann and Pleasants (1959). The liquid diets fed to germfree rabbits were similar in composition to those used in the rat work. A comparison of the growth of conventional rabbits fed diets before steam sterilization and after steam sterilization with the growth of germfree animals fed the steam sterilized diets is given in Fig. 2.14. These diets have been used to rear rabbits through reproduction under conventional conditions. Unfortunately, rabbits in germfree conditions appear to have an unsolved dietary problem related to an enlarged cecum. Pleasants (1962, personal communication) has obtained good general appearance, good growth, and limited success with reproduction in germfree rabbits. He used diet L-449 G-El and must ligate part of the cecum before rabbits would reproduce.

Monkeys

The diet fed germfree monkeys by the group at Lobund (Reyniers, 1942a; Reyniers and Trexler, 1943b) was modified milk formula which simulated monkey milk supplemented with vitamins. Later the survivor was given oatmeal puree, vegetable puree, sliced apples, turnips, and carrots, with other vegetables and fruit. These authors state that the monkey was the most easily reared germfree animal they had tried.

Ruminants

During the work with germfree goats, Küster (1913b) appeared to have less trouble with diet than he had with contamination. He fed colostrum from the recovered mother goat for the first feedings 12 hours after the operation. He used both goat's milk and cow's milk, supplemented with rice water, oatmeal, and sometimes sugar water or clay. The latter materials were used to try to control the consistency of excreta. The sugar water was soon discarded and even feeding clay did not stop the diarrhea. The animals reared to 1 and 2 months of age appeared to be healthy.

In a study of comparative nutrition, Luckey (1961a) found that lambs were difficult mammals to rear on syntype diets. The diet finally developed for rearing conventional lambs was diet U-3. Success in rearing conventional lambs suggested that germfree lambs should be attempted. Germfree lambs were reared for a short time using diet U-3 (Luckey, 1960) sterilized by γ-radiation and fed as a mixture to young obtained by Cesarean operation. Smith and Trexler (1960) also attempted to raise lambs and kids in the germfree state. The diet used was cow's milk adapted for the purpose. At 60 days the germfree and conventional lambs both weighed about 9 kg while at 120 days the conventional lambs weighed 16 kg and the germfree lambs weighed 14 kg.

Pigs

Landy and Sandberg (1961) have obtained germfree pigs and fed them supplemented homogenized milk (Landy Diet No. 1) and report (personal communication) that growth is satisfactory for a short period of time. Dr. D. N. Walcher (unpublished) at Indiana University has obtained excess shoats from Cesarean operations (performed in order to obtain disease-free stock) and reared them for germfree experiments.

Other Mammals

Although other mammals such as dogs, hamsters, and cats have been obtained in the germfree state, no sustained work has been done with them and no success in rearing has been reported to date.

Nutritional Requirements

Feed and Water

Sterilized diet found to be adequate for conventional animals was usually found to be adequate for germfree animals. When the diet was presented *ad libitum* the germfree animals ate with habits characteristic of their species. The chickens were found to be pecking their diet most of the day. The rats ate two or three times a day, as do conventional rats maintained under experimental conditions. If they were fed in the morning, they ate a light breakfast. They usually ate again toward the end of the day when the lights were turned off. Their large meal was eaten shortly after midnight when they were the most active. Since the amount of food and water varied so much with the condition of the species, the amount wasted, and the composition of the diet, the values below are general estimates. White Leghorn chicks ate about 12 gm of a syntype diet per day and drank (plus waste) about 20 ml of water during the first week. At 1 month they ate about 30 gm and drank about 40 ml each day. As they matured the chickens needed over 100 gm of food and 200 ml of water per day. These feed values should be doubled for most practical or commercial diets which have more fiber and less calories. The quantities given might be reduced by 50% for Bantam chicks or quail, doubled for heavy breeds of chickens and trebled for turkeys. Guinea pigs eat about the same amount of dry food as did White Leghorn chicks during the first 2 months of life; the quantity needed by nonbreeding adults was about 40 gm per day. If the food included fresh greens and vegetables, guinea pigs ate 100–200 gm per day. Albino rats each ate about 8 gm of a syntype diet per day at weaning, and about 15 gm when mature. A newborn ate about 2 ml of milk per day. Germfree rats have a water intake somewhat greater than that of conventional animals, about 20 ml per day. They drank less distilled water than tap water, and they drank very large quantities (100–150 ml/day) of 5% sugar water when it was presented to them. Mice eat about one-third as much as rats, and rabbits eat about 10 times more than rats. Newborn germfree lambs were fed 500 ml of a synthetic milk per day and this was increased to about 800 ml by the end of the first week. Küster (1913b) fed about 1 liter of milk per day to goats at 1 month of age.

Starvation

Germfree animals appeared to withstand the ravages of starvation as well as did conventional animals, according to Schottelius (1908a), Shaw (1957), and Levenson (personal communication). Detailed studies on starvation have not been reported.

Digestion, Absorption, and Excretion

Using the concept of the grams gain per gram food, Forbes *et al.* (1959, Forbes and Park, 1959) found the food efficiency in germfree chicks was 0.37 when fed a syntype diet and 0.23–0.24 when fed a practical diet. These values agreed with the data of Balzam (1938) given in Table 4.7. A balance study with rats was made on several

TABLE 4.7
GERMFREE CHICKS BALANCE STUDY[a]

	Germfree	Conventional diet and cage control
Age at start (days)	13	13
Sex	3♂, 2♀	1♂, 4♀
Initial weight (gm)	680	800
Weight increase (gm)	1050	840
Food given (gm)	3500	3500
Feces (dry wt gm)	1120	1170
Gm gain/gm food	0.30	0.24

[a] Balzam (1937b).

occasions. It will be noted (Table 4.8) that the germfree rat ate a quantity of food equivalent to that of conventional rats when compared on a body weight basis.

One of the most interesting aspects of germfree animals has already been considered without really presenting the major point. What happens to the intestinal contents in the absence of microorganisms? First might be considered the total volume of the material. Assuming that more than 50% of the intestinal contents of conventional animals consists of bacteria or microbial products, it is reasonable to suspect that the total volume of the feces would be reduced by 50%. This suggestion is without basis in fact. Germfree rats and chicks ate about

TABLE 4.8

METABOLISM OF GERMFREE AND CONVENTIONAL RATS

	Germfree	Conventional	Germfree	Conventional
Diet	L-120	L-120	L-283	L-283
Age (days)	179	130	165	146
Days studied	22	10	21	21
No. and sex	1 ♀	2 ♀	2 ♂	2 ♂
Weight (gm)	223	273	221	324
Wt-change (gm)	+4.2	−3.3	−0.53	0.6
Food intake (gm/day/rat)	10.0	12.5	16.5	15.4
Food (gm/day/100 gm rat)	4.50	4.57	—	—
H_2O intake (ml/day)	21.9	21.3	33.9	18.7
Urine (ml/day)	13.8	22.9	9.8	9.6
Feces (gm/day)	—	—	1.98	1.21
Feces, dry (gm/day)	0.703	0.609		
Feces (% dry wt)	64.9	85.3		
Feces (% N_2)	4.22	3.05		
Feces (mg N/day)	41	32		
Urine (mg N/day)	186	295		
Excreta (mg N/day)	227	327		
Food (mg N/day)	352	440		
N balance	+	+		
Feces (% fat)	4.58	5.58		
Feces (mg fat/day)	19.1	37.2		
Food (mg fat/day)	580	700		
Fat retained (%)	96.8	94.6		
Urine (% fat)	0.205	—		

the same quantities (Table 4.8) as did conventional animals harboring myriad microorganisms; germfree mammals generally have more ingesta in the intestines, but the quantity excreted was approximately the same per unit body weight. Therefore, it appeared that the presence or absence of living microorganisms in the intestinal tract does not greatly modify the quantity of material ingested, present, or excreted. The enlarged cecum present in germfree mammals is not pertinent in this consideration because the size of the ceca of germfree birds is quite within the range found for conventional birds. If the quantity of ingesta is the same, there certainly must be a difference in composition. By bacteriological methods, there is the tremendous difference that no living microorganisms are found in the germfree animals, while up to one billion microorganisms per gram of contents are found in conventional animals. Microscopic examination shows that conventional animals have tremendous numbers of bacterial and microbial cells in the intestinal contents and feces, while the germfree animals generally have very few intact cells; these few are microorganisms which were killed during the sterilization of the diet. Comparison of the chemical composition of the intestinal contents, presented later, indicates that there are no differences in major constituents despite the tremendous biological differences between animals in the two categories.

Except for the B vitamin studies reviewed herein, little has been published on the absorption of material in the germfree animals. Küster (1913b) found that the gross utilization of sugar and fat was 98% in the germfree goat (Table 4.9) while no fiber was utilized.

TABLE 4.9
FOOD UTILIZATION IN GERMFREE GOATS[a]

Study		Milk	Feces
Sugar	Total milk (gm/day)	1350	27.5
	Dry wt (gm)	—	5.42
	Sugar (gm/day)	60.75	1.397
Fat	Total milk (gm/day)	1000	25.3
	Dry wt (gm)	—	6.7
	Fat (%)	—	16.4
	Fat (gm/day)	40	1.0
Cellulose	Total bran (2 days)	20	—
	Crude fiber of feces 3 days following	—	2.77% (2.60–3.01)
	Crude fiber (%)	4.34% of bran	—
	Crude fiber (total gm)	1.736	1.716

[a] Küster (1913b).

Wagner (1959b) showed that oral vaccination was quite effective in producing antibody response in germfree chicks and rats. Presumably protein antigens from the dead microorganisms were absorbed intact in order to produce antibody response. His data showing bioincrassa-

tion of *Mycobacterium smegmatis* in germfree animals are given in
Table 4.10. Since dead microorganisms in the diets were not digested,

TABLE 4.10

BIOINCRASSATION: THE CONCENTRATION OF DEAD *M. smegmatis*
IN GERMFREE ANIMALS[a]

Material	Average no. *M. smegmatis* per 100 microscopic fields
1. Basal ration	0
2. Feces from 1	0
3. Basal ration plus *M. smegmatis*	131
4. Feces from 3 after 7 days	870
5. Feces 3 days after *M. smegmatis* feed was discontinued	3
6. Feces 4 days after *M. smegmatis* feed was discontinued	0

[a] Data of Wagner *in* Reyniers *et al.* (1949b).

the intact cells were concentrated via the absorption of other diet
ingredients. This is the classic example of bioincrassation.

Requirements for Protein, Energy, Roughage, and Minerals

Very little is known about the actual requirements for protein or
energy in germfree animals. Protein destruction occurred during
ethylene oxide sterilization and steam sterilization of diets; therefore
extra protein is usually needed in diets fed to gnotobiotic animals.
Evidence of destruction of protein in practical diets is presented in
Fig. 4.14.

The roughage requirement of germfree animals deserves special
consideration. Although exact and controlled experiments have not
been performed, the clinical evidence suggested a requirement for
roughage in germfree rats. Most germfree rats could not be brought
to maturity nor could mature rats be maintained until roughage was
added to the diet. When 3% roughage was added, a fourfold reduction
in the cecum size occurred, and adulthood, maturation, and reproduction were attained. Detailed studies have not been reported to determine whether or not higher quantities of roughage would further
decrease the cecum's distension. Fiber in the diet has not eliminated
cecal distension as a major problem in germfree quinea pigs and
rabbits.

The mineral requirement of no germfree animal has been studied

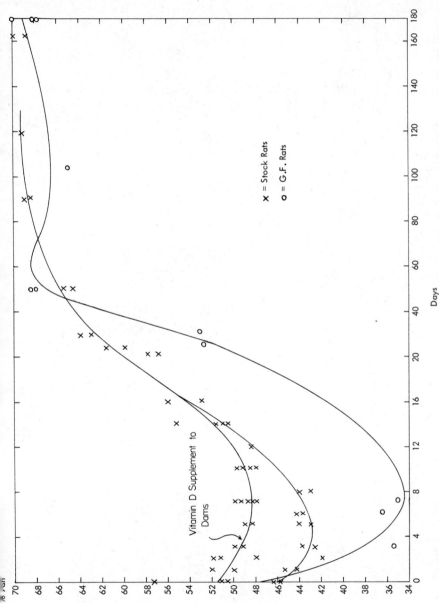

FIG. 4.19. Bone ash in rats (dry basis). The middle curve is obtained when the conventional colony was maintained on a stock diet. The upper curve was obtained when the stock diet was supplemented with fat soluble vitamins. The lower curve was obtained with hand-fed rats: a mineral deficiency was indicated.

in detail. Mineral deficiencies have been of particular interest since apparent phosphorus deficiency was seen in hand-fed germfree rats. The poor growth and spontaneous fracture illustrated in Fig. 4.14 in hand-fed rats were studied. It was necessary to determine the cause of this syndrome and to attempt to alleviate it in order that the hand-fed germfree rats could be properly weaned. The bone ash of dam-fed newborn rats decreased about 5% after birth (Fig. 4.19). The data for the upper curve were obtained by feeding the breeding stock a supplement of fat-soluble vitamins. Although the dip in the bone ash of germfree hand-fed rats amounted to about 25% of the mean value obtained at zero days, no difference between the two groups was noted for the muscle ash values (Fig. 4.20). Muscle phosphorus values

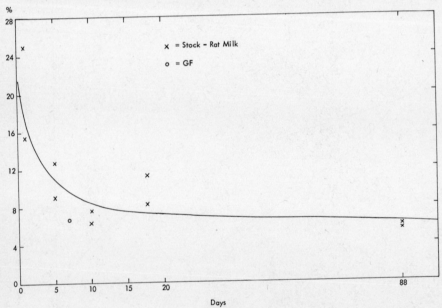

FIG. 4.20. Muscle ash in albino rats (dry basis).

in germfree hand-fed rats were about the same as those found in conventional dam-fed rats of the same age (Fig. 4.21). The dip suggested by the limited data for bone phosphorous (Fig. 4.22) was accentuated in the hand-fed rats at 7 days while no such effect was seen in the data on calcium. Although some of the milk diets may be low in minerals, solid diets are not. Thus plenty of phosphorus and calcium were available as soon as the rats began to eat solid food at 12–13 days. Most of the syntype diets used to date in feeding germfree animals have been so high in minerals, usually 8%, that they have invited diarrhea.

Vitamin Requirements

Although little attention has been paid to other nutrients, the vitamin requirement of germfree animals has been of special interest.

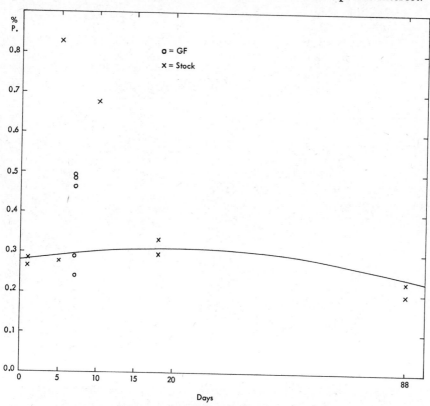

FIG. 4.21. Muscle phosphorus in albino rats (wet basis).

The vitamin requirements of germfree chicks have been studied systematically. What data are known for other species will also be summarized.

Vitamin A

The growth rate of germfree White Leghorn chicks fed diet L-245 with the vitamin A omitted was distinctly greater than that found in the conventional chicks (see Fig. 4.23). Some of the germfree birds

weakened and died while 5 of the 8 birds in one experiment continued
to grow and had a satisfactory appearance. Many exhibited leg weakness and ataxia. Conventional chicks appeared to be weaker than
germfree birds, gained no weight after the third week, and most were
dead by the fourth week.

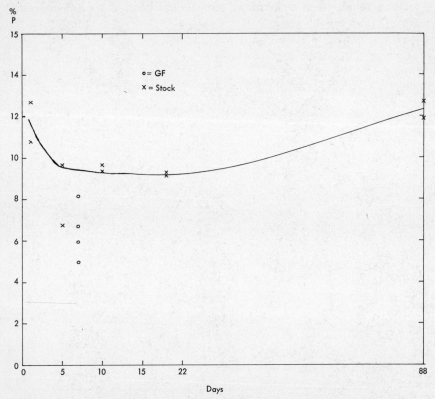

Fig. 4.22. Bone phosphorus in albino rats (dry basis). The hand-fed germfree
rats appeared to have less than dam-fed conventional rats.

A study of vitamin A deficiency in germfree rats by Beaver (1961)
indicated the simultaneous onset of many symptoms at 7 weeks. These
included a temporary squint with periorbital crusting, weight loss,
dull coat, alopecia, and a humped posture. Food and water consumption remained constant in the animals surviving as long as 15 weeks.
Gross observation in which these rats may differ from normal germfree rats appeared to be the decreased size of the pituitary gland,
variation in liver color, and renal calcification with hydronephrosis in

some of the rats. The latter syndrome appeared in older germfree animals fed adequate diets (Reyniers and Sacksteder, 1959a). Microscopic observations by Beaver indicated many abnormalities. Hepatic necrosis of isolated areas with some tubular degeneration was noted. Thin zona glomerulosa, vacuolar degeneration, and reduced lipid of the adrenal glands was sometimes seen. Of the 10 rats 2 showed cortical hemorrhagic necrosis with pigmented casts in both the convoluted and collecting tubules. Some rats had extensive tubular calcification. In the skin was found cystic atrophy of the sebaceous glands

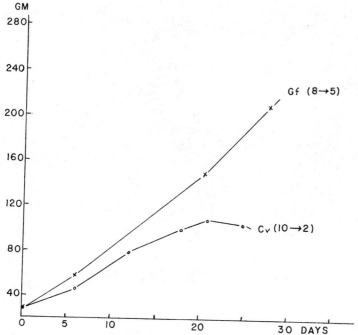

FIG. 4.23. Growth of Leghorn chicks fed vitamin A deficient diet. The growth rate of the germfree birds is comparable to those fed a complete diet (Fig. 4.16).

and hair follicles around the buccal pouch, eyelids, and the perianal region. Vacuolation was seen in sections of the mammary glands. A remarkable lack of inflammation was seen in degenerative and necrotic cells in the squamous epithelium of the salivary, lacrimal, and orbital glands. The ventricular myocardium exhibited necrosis in focal areas of the heart which had mononuclear cell infiltration. The pancreas showed minimal squamous metaplasia with slight keratinization in the pancreatic duct. Marked tubular degeneration of the sertoli cells and the germinal epithelia of testes, and absence of sperm were observed. Atrophy and degeneration were noted in the prostate glands and the epithelium of the seminal vesicles. Vaginas were found to be heavily keratinized and had no leucocytic infiltration. The ovaries showed several large corpora lutea present in each female. No major change was noted in bronchi, bronchioles, brain, nerves and nerve ganglia, gastrointestinal tract, pituitary, thyroid, and parathyroid tissue.

B Vitamins

Experiments with a B vitamin complex deficiency were performed by Balzam (1938), in which he showed the germfree birds died of a B vitamin deficiency in the same manner and time that conventional birds did. One might speculate that the primary cause of death was the lack of thiamine. It is suspected that the early workers in germfree research were plagued by B vitamin deficiency. The vitamin concept was not known at the time Nuttal and Thierfelder or Schottelius began work; an understanding of vitamins developed during the work of Cohendy. Therefore, these early workers had no idea of the need for, nor the chemical characteristics of, these micronutrients. Heat sterilization of their diets would probably have destroyed enough vitamins to make their diets deficient. Later experiments in which all the B vitamins were omitted from a syntype diet (Reyniers et al., 1960c) confirmed the observations of Balzam (1938). Both germfree and conventional Leghorns failed to grow, showed opisthotonus and leg weakness, and died within 9–12 days. This occurred whether the chicks were started at hatch or at 1 month of age. Such data would indicate that the stores of thiamine of the birds were no greater at 1 month of age than they were at birth.

Germfree and conventional White Wyandotte Bantam chickens and White Leghorn chickens fed a thiamine-deficient diet did not grow and died in 9–12 days. Opisthotonus and anorexia were regularly seen characteristics of the deficiency. The deficient birds had friable yellow adrenal glands with normal adrenal cholesterol content. The clotting time was retarded in some of these birds, and the spleen and testicles were reduced in weight. The gall bladder was enlarged in most deficient birds, a symptom characteristic of anorexic chicks. Injection of thiamine into paralyzed chicks in both environments brought a marked improvement in the disability.

TABLE 4.11

THIAMINE METABOLISM IN BANTAM CHICKS AT 11 ± 3 DAYS

(μg/gm on wet basis)

μg/100 gm Diet	Category	Liver n^a	Liver M^b	Cecum n	Cecum M	Rectal n	Rectal M
1	Germfree	8	1.2 (0.17–3.04)	7	4.9 (2.45–8.98)	1	29.1
	Conventional	4	2.2 (1.71–3.23)	3	15.5 (6.41–9.50)	3	40.3 (29.3–60.9)
200	Germfree	2	5.6 (pooled)	2	7.1 (pooled)	—	—
	Conventional	4	4.1 (2.41–8.21)	4	23.9 (9.9–53.4)	1	55.5

[a] n = number of chicks.
[b] M = mean value. The range is given in parentheses.

TABLE 4.12

ANALYSIS OF THE LIVERS OF GERMFREE AND CONVENTIONAL CHICKS[a,b]

| | Complete diet | | Diet deficient in | | | | | | | |
| | | | Thiamine | | Riboflavin | | Niacin | | Folic acid | |
Analysis	Gf	Conv.	Gf	Conv.	Gf	Conv.	Gf	Conv.	Gf	Conv.
Thiamine										
M	3.99	3.00	0.824	0.647	3.27	3.86	4.94	4.26	2.49	2.42
P_1	—		<0.01	<0.01	0.148	0.23	0.041	0.013	<0.001	0.27
P_2	0.048		0.686		0.36		0.125		0.56	
Riboflavin										
M	21.6	23.3	17.5	25.0	7.1	12.5	34.7	22.7	34.9	19.2
P_1	—		0.067	0.155	0.001	<0.001	<0.001	0.53	<0.001	0.49
P_2	0.50		0.016		0.076		0.117		0.002	
Niacin										
M	109	108	69.3	104	86	123	145	110	104	87
P_1	—		0.003	0.85	<0.001	0.53	<0.001	0.69	<0.001	0.69
P_2	0.94		0.43		0.016		<0.001		0.55	
Ca pantothenate										
M	66.4	48.0	47.6	45.0	57.7	47.3	54	51	17.6	15.3
P_1	—		0.153	0.63	0.53	0.90	0.18	0.40	<0.001	<0.001
P_2	0.001		0.82		0.63		0.12		0.38	

Biotin										
M	5.14	4.31	4.47	4.70	4.3	4.0	5.1	6.5	4.15	3.49
P_1	—		0.43	0.83	0.94	0.66	0.94	0.037	0.078	0.9+
P_2	0.215		0.87		0.64		0.27		0.41	
Folic acid										
M	4.41	3.27	3.70	2.96	5.2	2.8	2.9	2.3	3.60	2.31
P_1	—		0.49	0.16	0.38	0.45	0.079	0.032	0.24	0.016
P_2	0.021		0.53		0.127		0.044		0.022	

[a] Data of Luckey (1959c).

[b] Symbols: Gf, germfree; Conv., polycontaminated (conventional) chicks. M = average $\mu g/gm$, wet basis. P_1, probability for chicks on a complete diet, as compared to those on a deficient diet; P_2, probability for germfree chicks as compared to conventional chicks on the same diet. (5–18 chicks each except thiamine analysis in germfree chicks is only 3 chicks.)

One of the important things noted in thiamine deficiency was the quantity of thiamine being excreted in germfree chicks (see Table 4.11). The diet was very low in thiamine, but the rectal contents and the excreta had considerable quantities of thiamine in them. The tissues of the bird were losing an amount of thiamine, which, if the chicken would re-ingest its excreta, could quite possibly save his life. Knight (1960) and Wostmann and Knight (1961) studied thiamine deficiency in germfree and conventional animals using $Na_2S^{35}O_4$. They found that very little thiamine was synthesized. When they fed feces containing S^{35} thiamine, they found no thiamine absorption.

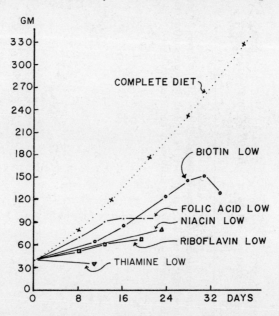

Fig. 4.24. Growth rate of germfree White Leghorn chicks fed B vitamin deficient diets compared to the germfree control fed the complete diet.

Analysis of tissues of thiamine-deficient Leghorn chicks at 10–11 days (the animals were moribund from a thiamine deficiency) indicated that the liver had much less thiamine in it than was found in chicks fed thiamine. There was no difference in the thiamine content of the livers of germfree and conventional chicks when both groups were fed the thiamine-deficient diet. Thiamine deficiency interfered with the storage of liver niacin, but not other B vitamins (Table 4.12).

Riboflavin deficiency in germfree White Wyandotte Bantam chicks resulted in a severe paralysis of the chicks; at $2\frac{1}{2}$ weeks of age they were found lying on their backs. When germfree White Leghorn chicks were fed a riboflavin-deficient diet, the chicks did not grow at a rate comparable to that of conventional birds (see Fig. 4.24) and died within 3 weeks. The conventional birds lived longer than the germfree birds in the few experiments tried. The riboflavin-deficient germfree White Leghorn chicks appeared to have enlarged hearts and bursae of Fabricius, but smaller thymus glands and spleens than were found in germfree birds fed adequate diets (Reyniers et al., 1960c).

Analysis of the livers of riboflavin-deficient chicks (Table 4.12) at 3 weeks showed few significant changes. Niacin in the livers of riboflavin-deficient germfree birds was found to be low. As expected, the riboflavin content of the livers was lower than in chicks fed the complete diet. The biotin in cecal contents of riboflavin-deficient germfree birds appeared to be much higher than in either deficient conventional birds or germfree birds fed the complete diet. A balance study conducted on complete intake and excretion of germfree rats which were fed a diet adequate in riboflavin indicated no net synthesis of riboflavin in the germfree rat tissue (Fig. 4.25).

When conventional birds were fed a syntype diet with niacin omitted, diet L-235, growth rate was not retarded in the majority of chicks. When germfree birds were fed this diet, they showed decreased growth rate and many chicks died within 3 weeks. However, in another experiment with germfree birds, growth was equal to that of conventional birds fed the same autoclaved diet. Apparently more work will be needed to settle definitely the question of the source of niacin in the conventional birds or the possible increased requirement of niacin in the germfree birds. Metabolism of B vitamins in the liver was little changed in niacin deficiency (Table 2.12). A niacin balance study in germfree rats (Fig. 4.25) indicated that no net niacin synthesis occurred in tissues.

Pantothenic acid deficiency in the germfree rat was never accompanied by adrenal necrosis (Daft, 1959). Daft (1960) found both dietary penicillin and ascorbic acid to have no effect on the deficiency of pantothenic acid in germfree rats. Either of these substances would prevent a deficiency from developing in conventional rats which had access to their feces but not in conventional rats with tail cups.

The growth rate of the chicks fed a biotin-deficient diet appeared to be only slightly depressed (Fig. 4.24). The growth of biotin-deficient germfree chicks was equal to, or better than, that of biotin-deficient conventional birds (Reyniers *et al.*, 1960c). There was a slight dermatitis noted on the legs of germfree chicks, but no clear-cut syndrome developed. The growth rate of germfree rats fed a biotin-deficient diet (low in folic acid and vitamin K) was comparable to that of rats fed the complete diet (Luckey, 1956a). After 4 months, signs of disease became increasingly apparent; diarrhea, alopecia,

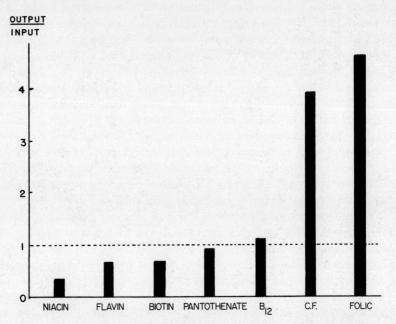

Fig. 4.25. B vitamin balance in germfree rats. Total quantity of vitamin found in excreta plus carcass is divided by the quantity in the food eaten and litter mates at the start.

spectacle eyes, and a dry dermititis developed. "Dry" spots on the skin of the shoulders developed into open sores (Fig. 4.26). When one rat died the other was given 100 μg biotin by intramuscular injection, the growth depression was quickly reversed, but 20 days later body weight began to decrease. When biotin was added to the diet, appetite was restored, the body weight increased, and after 3 weeks, new growth of fur was evidenced and the open sores began to heal. When a balance study was made, about 75% of the biotin intake was recovered (Fig. 4.25).

Germfree birds fed a diet low in folic acid appeared to grow more slowly than did germfree birds fed a complete diet (Fig. 4.24); the growth rate was equivalent to that of conventional birds fed the deficient diet. The deficient germfree birds became moribund and died, while the conventional birds, which grew no better and looked no better, continued to live. The germfree chicks exhibited slow

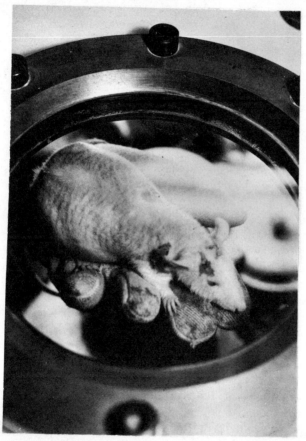

Fig. 4.26. Biotin deficient germfree rat. Note the new hair growing over the back and the open ulcers on the head and shoulders.

feather development but no gross abnormality in the feather structure. Anemia was present in the germfree birds fed a folic acid deficient diet; the red cell count was as low as 1.18 million red blood cells per cubic millimeter. Analysis of the livers of germfree birds (Table 4.12) indicated a lower concentration of thiamine, pantothenic acid, and vitamin B_{12} in folic acid deficiency than in birds fed a complete diet. No differences were noted in the liver content of niacin, biotin, or folic acid. Riboflavin was found to be higher in the liver of folic acid deficient germfree birds than in those fed in the complete diet. In comparisons of liver vitamin concentration in deficient birds, germfree chicks were found to be similar to conventional birds in thiamine, niacin, pantothenic acid, and biotin, and they had more riboflavin and folic acid and less vitamin B_{12} than deficient conventional chicks. The folic acid concentration in cecal contents was lower in both germfree and conventional deficient birds than in those fed folic acid. There was less folic acid in the cecal contents of deficient germfree birds than in deficient polybiotic birds.

Miller (1962) found that *Escherichia coli* (a folic acid producing organism) inoculation prevented a deficiency in chicks fed a folic acid low diet, while inoculation of *Streptococcus faecalis* (a folic acid requiring microorganism) decreased the growth rate when compared with germfree chicks fed the same diet. A more complete presentation of work with gnotophoric chicks is presented in Chapter 6.

When germfree rats were fed a diet containing no folic acid, biotin, or vitamin K for 5–6 months, the folic acid excretion decreased. When biotin was injected, a tremendous increase was seen in urinary folic acid (Luckey *et al.*, 1955b). A confirmatory study, (Fig. 4.26) indicated that there was a synthesis of folic acid by germfree rats. Concurrent analysis indicated that a synthesis in citrovorum factor occurred which was of the same magnitude as that for folic acid. In contrast to these results, Hayes and Luckey (1957) found no increase in the folic acid content of embryonated eggs from the beginning of incubation to hatch, and McDaniel (1960) obtained a decrease in growth rate after 8 weeks in germfree rats fed diets low in folic acid. Typical symptoms of folic acid deficiency which developed were weight loss, marked leucopenia, anemia, and excretion of large amounts of forminioglutamic acid. Folic acid would prevent or correct the deficiency. Conventional rats fed the same diet showed no signs of a folic acid deficiency. Dietary differences (the amount of ascorbic acid or biotin) may explain this discrepancy in results with germfree rats.

When Miyakawa (1960) omitted folic acid, vitamins B_{12}, and ascorbic acid from the diet of germfree guinea pigs, he found anemia accompanied by a dramatic macroblastosis or megaloblastosis in the spleen and bone marrow. This syndrome did not develop as dramatically if any one of these three vitamins were present in adequate quantities.

In an experiment designed to permit a decision on the capability of the germfree rat to synthesize biologically labile methyl groups, du Vigneaud *et al.* (1950, 1951) fed deuterium water followed by the determination of deuterium-labeled methyl groups. The deuterium content of the methyl groups in tissue choline and creatine of germfree rats was comparable to that found in conventional rats fed the same diet (Table 4.13). Prentiss *et al.* (1960) found that about 37%

TABLE 4.13
CHOLINE AND CREATINE SYNTHESIS:
DEUTERIUM CONTENT OF METHYL GROUPS OF CHOLINE AND CREATINE

| | | Atoms % excess deuterium in | | | Atoms % excess deuterium in | |
Category	Days D_2O	Body water	Methyl group of choline	Incorporation (%)	Methyl group of creatine	Incorporation (%)
Germfree	23	2.44	0.16	6.4	0.17	7.0
Germfree	10	2.99	0.10	3.3	0.12	4.0
Conventional	21	2.20	0.21	9.6	0.31	13.9
Conventional	21	2.27	0.20	8.8	0.22	9.5

of the choline fed was converted to trimethylamine in conventional rats while less than 1% of administered choline was found as urinary trimethylamine in germfree rats. Such results indicate that most of this difference was mediated by the microbial flora. The site of action and the specific action of microorganisms has not been demonstrated.

When fed a choline-free, vitamin B_{12}-free, biotin-free, 4% casein diet, germfree rats developed cirrhosis of the liver more rapidly than did conventional rats. This, plus the observation that dietary antibiotics delayed the symptoms in conventional rats led Levenson *et al.* (1960a) to suggest that interactions between the host and the microbial flora were involved.

Vitamin C

The qualitative vitamin C requirement of guinea pigs has been studied by Cohendy and Wollman (1922), Phillips *et al.* (1959b), and Miyakawa (1960). When vitamin C was removed from diet L-445 supplemented with extra thiamine and a metabolic "supplement," the germfree guinea pigs of Phillips *et al.* (1959) began losing weight at 27 days. At 28 days they were less active and walked with difficulty, and within 1 week all had assumed the scorbutic position with respiratory difficulties, had swollen and tender knee joints, and were unable to stand. Supplementation with vitamin C gave marked improvement in 48 hours and within 12 days the animals appeared to be normal. The deficiency symptoms followed the same course in conventional guinea pigs but recovery took about three times longer than it had taken in germfree guinea pigs. Miyakawa (1960) reported that changes in bones and teeth in ascorbic acid deficiency were comparable in germfree and conventional guinea pigs.

Vitamin D

When a vitamin D deficient diet was fed to germfree and conventional White Leghorn chicks (Reyniers *et al.*, 1960a) poor growth was obtained (Fig. 4.27). In both groups the bones felt soft, mild perosis was noted, the keel bones were crooked, and some chicks had beaded ribs. Feathering was extremely poor (see Fig. 4.28). Enlarged hearts

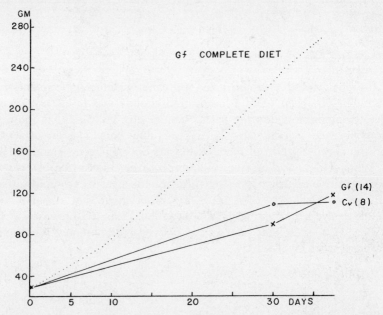

Fig. 4.27. Growth of germfree White Leghorn chicks fed a vitamin D deficient diet. The rate is considerably less than that obtained when the complete diet was fed.

were seen in some of the deficient chicks; the heart of one germfree
bird was 1.2% of the body weight. The bone ash, brain ash, and dry
weight of bones in both deficient groups were considerably below
normal (Table 4.14). Rather surprisingly, the amount of muscle ash

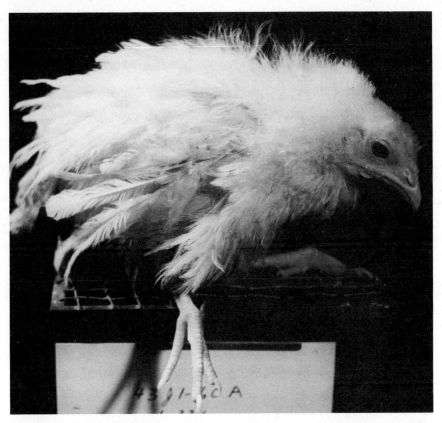

Fig. 4.28. Germfree White Leghorn fed a vitamin D deficient diet. A 48
day old male; note abnormal feather formation. The perosis makes the foot of the
chick fall to the side and the chick often walks on the tibia.

in germfree deficient chicks was considerably higher than that found
for deficient conventional birds and considerably higher than was
found in germfree birds fed a complete diet. The fat content of the
liver of both groups of birds fed the vitamin-deficient diet was much
lower than that of chicks fed a complete diet. Either directly or indirectly, the microbial fauna appears to affect vitamin D functions.

TABLE 4.14

TISSUE COMPOSITION IN VITAMIN D DEFICIENCY

Tissue	Category[a]	Vitamin D	Dry weight		Ash (% dry weight)		N_2 (% wet weight)		Fat (% wet weight)	
			M	P	M	P	M	P	M	P
Liver	Gf	−	28.9	0.53	6.05	0.62	3.34	0.91	1.85	<0.001
		+	27.1	0.71[b]	6.49	0.75[b]	3.13	0.54[b]	5.25	0.63[b]
	Cv	−	28.8	1.0	5.74	0.63	3.27	0.92	1.46	0.16
		+	28.8	—	5.39	—	3.46	—	4.07	—
Muscle	Gf	−	20.8	0.55	7.32	0.019	—	—	2.89	0.14
		+	21.7	0.67[b]	5.23	0.073[b]	—	—	2.34	0.59[b]
	Cv	−	20.0	0.046	4.82	0.45	—	—	4.55	<0.001
		+	23.2	—	4.35	—	—	—	2.25	—
Brain	Gf	−	19.3	0.076	5.17	<0.001	1.63	0.46	5.79	0.26
		+	16.0	0.65[b]	12.4	0.53[b]	1.64	0.9+[b]	6.79	—
	Cv	−	18.5	0.61	5.53	<0.001	1.55	0.041	—	—
		+	17.8	—	8.4	—	1.73	—	5.80	—
Bone	Gf	−	40.3	—	49.9	<0.001	—	—	2.08	<0.001
		+	—	0.79[b]	66.6	0.68[b]	—	—	21.2	0.50[b]
	Cv	−	41.3	—	49.0	<0.001	—	—	0.45	<0.001
		+	—	—	64.6	—	—	—	22.0	—

[a] Each group consisted of 3–4 White Leghorn chicks.
[b] Comparison of germfree and conventional chicks fed the deficient diet.

Vitamin E

When White Leghorn chicks were fed diet L-245 with vitamin E omitted, both germfree and conventional chicks could be divided by growth into two distinct groups: half of the birds had a depressed growth rate and others grew as well as did the birds fed vitamin E. The reason for this difference is not known. Some of the birds which did not grow well developed leg weakness and a small gizzard. Irrespective of size, most chicks developed a cervical tic as they approached 100 days of age. No basic differences were noted between germfree and conventional chicks when vitamin E was removed from the diet.

When germfree rats were fed the Himsworth diet (without vitamin E) and were limited in their food intake, all showed definite hemorrhagic necrosis of the liver. When allowed to eat *ad libitum,* they developed no liver necrosis (Luckey *et al.,* 1954a). It is possible that *ad libitum* feeding allowed the germfree rats to eat enough yeast to receive a supply of the antioxidant of *Torula* isolated by Forbes *et al.* (1958b).

Vitamin K

When germfree chickens were fed either the practical diet of Ansbacher or the syntype diet with the vitamin K deleted, the deficiency was seen about 1 week earlier than it was seen in conventional birds (Fig. 4.29). The vitamin K content of the diet must have been almost high enough to meet the needs of the birds since the germfree birds apparently recovered spontaneously from a vitamin K deficiency. A similar experience has been reported by Barnes *et al.* (1959) with conventional rats, using cups to prevent coprophagy.

Surprisingly, vitamin K deficiency was found to markedly influence the metabolism of B vitamins (Table 4.15). The liver concentrations of thiamine, riboflavin, pantothenic acid, and probably niacin were lower in germfree chicks fed the deficient diet than in those fed the complete diet. Biotin, folic acid, and vitamin B_{12} were similar in both groups. Livers from germfree deficient chicks had less niacin than was found in polybiotic deficient chicks. The concentration of pantothenic acid in cecal contents of germfree chicks fed the vitamin K deficient diet was greater than that of chicks in either control group. In the cecal contents, the concentration of folic acid and riboflavin was lower and niacin was greater in germfree chicks fed the diet low in vitamin K than that of germfree chicks fed the complete diet.

When germfree rats were fed a similar diet with vitamin K, folic acid, and biotin omitted (diet L-283) for 1 year, they exhibited no vitamin K deficiency (Luckey, 1955b). Apparently, rats fed this diet

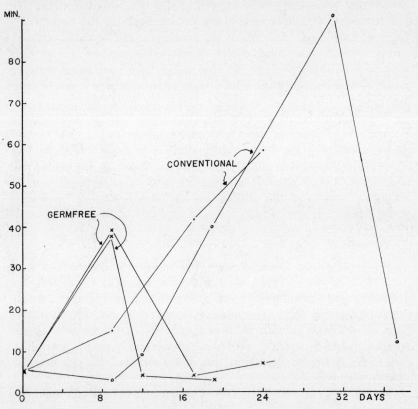

FIG. 4.29. Whole blood clotting in White Leghorn chicks fed the Ansbacher diet. Note that in each experiment the whole blood clotting time returned to normal without supplementation.

had a requirement less than the amount present in the diet. When this experiment was repeated by Gustafsson (1959d) with a diet in which the ingredients had been ether extracted, more than 50% of the germfree rats exhibited a vitamin K deficiency: whole blood clotting time and prothrombin clotting times were prolonged. Conventional rats fed the same diet showed no symptoms of vitamin K deficiency.

TABLE 4.15

EFFECT OF VITAMIN K UPON B VITAMIN METABOLISM

Vitamin	Category[a]	Vitamin K	Liver		Cecal contents	
			M	P	M	P
Thiamine	Gf	−	4.52	<0.001	—	—
		+	3.99	0.86[b]	—	—
	Cv	−	4.48	0.24	—	—
		+	3.00	—	—	—
Riboflavin	Gf	−	16.1	<0.001	3.6	0.011
		+	21.6	0.07	10.9	0.26[b]
	Cv	−	10.9	<0.001	2.6	0.001
		+	23.3	—	1.38	—
Niacin	Gf	−	130	0.023	25.0	<0.001
		+	109	0.50[b]	12.1	0.11[b]
	Cv	−	141	0.110	19.1	0.041
		+	108	—	37.2	—
Pantothenate	Gf	−	19.6	<0.001	16.2	<0.001
		+	66.4	0.9+[b]	5.47	0.016[b]
	Cv	−	17.9	<0.001	3.88	0.046
		+	48.0	—	7.74	—
Biotin	Gf	−	4.7	0.47	0.35	0.36
		+	5.14	0.88[b]	0.241	0.20[b]
	Cv	−	3.7	0.52	0.49	0.9+
		+	4.31	—	0.488	—
Folic acid	Gf	−	5.0	0.39	1.05	0.001
		+	4.41	0.52[b]	2.29	0.10[b]
	Cv	−	3.4	0.84	0.67	0.020
		+	3.27	—	1.83	—
Vitamin B$_{12}$	Gf	−	0.266	0.34	—	—
		+	0.323	0.28[b]	—	—
	Cv	−	0.252	0.32	—	—
		+	0.171	—	—	—

[a] Each group consisted of 4–5 birds. Data given in terms of μg/gm fresh weight.
[b] Comparison of germfree and conventional fed deficient diets.

When germfree rats with prolonged prothrombin clotting times were transferred to a conventional environment, or inoculated with micro-organisms, normal prothrombin clotting times were noted within 48 hours. In further experiments supplements of vitamin K gave normal prothrombin clotting times at 16 hours, while menadione sulfate and the fat-soluble menadione showed no change. Further studies by Gustafsson (1960) indicated that male germfree rats developed a vitamin K deficiency earlier than germfree female rats. The vitamin K deficiency in germfree rats fed an extracted protein (Brambel, 1960) was complicated as shown by abnormal hematology and bone erythrocyte indices. The appreciable number of germfree rats which showed no deficiency of vitamin K in the Gustafsson experiments is to be noted.

Unknown Factors

One of the first uses proposed for animals with no intestinal bac-teria was to determine how many, if any, new vitamins might be required. The results of a search for new vitamins with germfree chicks fed diet 56227 are given in Table 4.16 (Reyniers *et al.*, 1950).

TABLE 4.16
GROWTH OF GERMFREE WHITE LEGHORN CHICKS FED SOURCES
OF UNIDENTIFIED COMPOUNDS

Supplement to diet PD56227	No. chicks	Weight at 4 weeks	
		Average	Range
None[a]	5	306	270–365
Yeast extract, liver powder, and fermentation residue (2% each)	6	256	208–298
Fresh liver extract	5	264	213–295

[a] Three chicks received 50 μg thiamine per day *per os*.

Growth on the unsupplemented syntype diet was as good as that obtained when it was supplemented with 2% of any or all of the following sources of unidentified factors: dried yeast extract, liver powder, bacterial fermentation residue powder, and fresh liver extract. Combining groups fed different basal diets, these investigators re-ported sixteen chicks fed fresh liver extract weighed an average of 265 gm and thirteen germfree chicks fed the same diet without liver weighed 267 gm at 4 weeks. Thus, the intestinal microorganisms contributed little, if any, important unidentified nutrients not present in the diet under the conditions described. It is possible that the diets carried significant quantities of an unknown factor or that newly hatched chicks possessed a reserve of some factor adequate for the first few weeks of life. The work presented thus delineated the problem but did not treat it exhaustively. This work could be repeated with other sources of unknown vitamins, a chemically defined diet, or parameters other than growth, hemoglobin formation, and general appearance.

Horton and Hickey (1961) suggested that the germfree guinea pigs needed some growth factor not present in their syntype diet No. 17 after electron beam sterilization (2×10^6 rads). Conventional guinea pigs grew 5.6 gm per day, while germfree guinea pigs grew only 4.2 gm per day.

The growth of male germfree rats (see Fig. 4.18) indicated the possibility that an unknown nutrient might be required. However, the germfree rats of Gustafsson (1959a) grew as well as the conventional control rats. Wostmann (1959a) found male germfree rats grew at a rate comparable to 80% of that of conventional rats and female rats grew at a less acceptable rate. And Gordon (1959b) has shown that the decreased growth rate was statistically significant in both male and female rats. Wostmann (1959a) suggested the growth rate of germfree mice was not as great as that of conventional mice. The data of Gordon (1959b) also suggested this, but he pointed out that the differences were not statistically significant. Thus, no definitive studies have been made on the possible requirement of germfree mammals for unknown vitamins. Gordon suggested overcrowding may be a factor in the germfree experiments.

Until the factors required for the reduction of the ceca of germfree rodents are identified, this must be considered an unknown nutritional factor in mammals. The addition of fiber to the diet helped, but even practical diets, which carried a variety of fibers, did not eliminate the condition. Food restriction at the beginning of solid food intake was helpful but was not the complete solution. The enlarged cecum is presently the greatest problem in rearing germfree rabbits (Wostmann, 1959a) and seems to be the limiting factor in the production of germfree guinea pig colonies. Bausor et al. (1960) found germfree guinea pigs had grossly enlarged ceca when fed sterile live plants. They suggest that enteric microorganisms were producing an unknown growth factor. Since the addition of bacteria to the germfree rat reduced the cecum size within 3 days (Gustafsson, 1959a and Gordon, 1960b), the physical or metabolic activities of certain microorganisms may be implicated. The presence of microorganisms such as *Lactobacillus acidophilus* did not materially reduce the size of the rat cecum.

Effect of Antibiotics

When Moore *et al.* (1946) discovered the growth stimulation of dietary antibiotics, they proposed that the action of these substances could be directly upon the tissues of the chick. They also suggested that antibiotics could act indirectly via the intestinal microorganisms which might depress growth either by producing toxins or by robbing the host of essential nutrients. The germfree animal presented an ideal test system to resolve this dilemma. Preliminary results on the growth of germfree chicks fed antibiotics released in symposium were negative. Subsequent work with lower levels of antibiotics gave an entirely different picture; Table 4.17 summarizes the data obtained (Luckey, 1958). Growth stimulation in germfree chicks was noted with statistical significance when low levels of antibiotics were fed. The negative results obtained with relatively high levels of antibiotics have been confirmed by Forbes *et al.* (1959b) and Forbes and Park (1959) and Gordon *et al.* (1958b), although the data of Forbes and Park (1959) indicated that antibiotics might be active in male germfree chicks fed suboptimum diets. Details of the effect of dietary antibiotics upon germfree chick organ weight, tissue composition (Gordon, 1959b), and vitamin metabolism (Luckey, 1959a,b) have been presented. Greater differences were found in conventional chicks than were found in germfree chicks.

When antibiotics were fed to germfree Beltsville White turkey poults, a growth stimulus was noted in males and no increase was seen in the females (Luckey, 1958). When data on both sexes were combined the growth rate of those fed antibiotics was statistically greater ($p = 0.003$) than the growth rate of those fed no antibiotics. Forbes *et al.* (1958c) found no consistent increased growth rate in germfree poults fed either penicillin or oleandomycin. Work with inoculated chicks is reviewed in Chapter 6.

The stimulatory action of subharmful concentrations of antibiotics fitted the pattern of other germicidal drugs and many harmful agents. The generalized action, called *hormoligosis,* has been reviewed by Luckey (1959a). The action of antibiotics in the total replacement of certain B vitamins in the diet was also reviewed (Luckey, 1959a). When 50 mg procaine penicillin was fed to germfree rats with no thiamine added to the diet, Wostmann *et al.* (1958) found no effect.

TABLE 4.17
EFFECT OF ANTIBIOTICS ON GERMFREE CHICKS

Drug	High level				Low level				P
	Expt. no.	ppm[a]	No. birds	GI[b]	Expt. no.	ppm[a]	No. birds	GI[b]	
Streptomycin	1	50	8	97	2[e]	8	6	117	0.31
Chloramphenicol	5	50	6	103	—	—	—	—	—
Oxytetracycline	7	50	5	83	4	25	7	112	0.001
	8	50	6	88	20	25	10	108	0.011
	13	50	6	114[c]	22	25	9	134	0.001
	15	50	6	79	—	—	—	—	—
	16	50	8	106[d]	—	—	—	—	—
	19	50	9	94	—	—	—	—	—
Procaine penicillin	9	50	12	98	24	10	8	106	0.026
	14	50	5	90	—	—	—	—	—
Bacitracin	10	50	12	97	—	—	—	—	—
Sulfasuxadine	11	2(%)	8	79	—	—	—	—	—

[a] The amounts added are given: the amount destroyed by sterilization, mixing into the diet, and storage was not well examined (see Table 4.3).

[b] GI = growth index.

[c] All chicks fed the basal diet were females and all fed the drug were males.

[d] Data taken at 21 days (due to a glove break on the 22nd day).

[e] These chicks were sick for 1 week. The chicks in experiment No. 23 died the first week and experiments No. 6, 12, 17, 18, and 21 were contaminated during the first 10 days.

That quantity of penicillin allowed no increased body weight nor did the liver weights change in the germfree rats (liver weights increased when conventional rats were fed penicillin). Thiamine stores of rats fed the deficient diet plus procaine penicillin were aligned with those fed the thiamine-deficient diet. Since no record was made of coprophagy in this experiment, it is difficult to compare results in conventional rats with those from germfree rats. Daft (1960) found penicillin would partially "replace" pantothenic acid in the diet of conventional rats but not in germfree rats.

Summary

Failure of early investigators to produce germfree animals was attributed primarily to poor understanding of principles of nutrition. Germfree animals could be readily procured, but acceptable growth rates and reproduction were not obtained during the first half-century of germfree research. When germfree animals became available, problems in nutrition were the first experiments performed. A major problem in theoretical nutrition is an evaluation of the role of the intestinal microflora in meeting the nutritional requirements of the host without coprophagy or rumination.

In order to evaluate the importance of the myriad reactions which occur during diet sterilization, much effort was directed to determine the chemistry of those changes. Emphasis was placed upon the vitamin losses during different methods of sterilization. The results indicate that sterilization by radiation was the preferred method for dry diets, although with certain precautions, steam or chemicals (ethylene oxide) were satisfactory.

Examples are presented of nutritional problems met in obtaining the first germfree colony. Different methods were examined to assure maturity of young at the Cesarean operation. The colostrum factor was shown to be dispensable. Rat milk was analyzed in an effort to determine what mother rats fed their young. On the basis of this knowledge, the use of high fat diets increased the half-life of hand-fed rats from 3 to 10 days. Then an "over-feeding technique" was inaugurated which prolonged the half-life of the young animals well passed weaning. As soon as the young rats were weaned they ate too much solid food, the abdomen became distended, the cecum became enlarged, and spontaneous fractures ensued. Analyses of muscle and bone ash indicated a phosphorus deficiency; however, it was found that simply restricting the diet during the transition to solid food would alleviate or prevent this syndrome. The difficulty with the cecum enlargement was never entirely solved; restricted feeding and the addition of a small amount of fiber to the diet reduced the size of the cecum enough to allow survival and reproduction. Finally, a lactation problem was overcome and the first germfree colony was established. Once germfree rat colonies were started, problems in the hand-feeding of rats were abandoned. Germfree weanling rats may be fed a variety of syntype or practical diets. The growth rate appears to be approximately the same in germfree and conventional rats according to the later reports.

No serious attempts have been made to raise germfree amphibia or fish in the recent past, therefore dietary needs of these animals have not been studied. Most of the work with germfree chickens has been done with steam-sterilized diets. It was found that steam-sterilized practical diets needed extra protein as well as vitamins in order to meet the nutrient requirement of chicks. Attempts to rear guinea pigs were made by most investigators in germfree research. Although present-day investigators raise guinea pigs which look good, all are plagued with the problem of the enlarged cecum, and reproduction is considerably slowed by this malformation. However, germfree guinea pigs grow satisfactorily and they have reproduced on a variety of diets. Germfree mice have been reared by hand with some difficulty. The success was adequate to start colonies of mice for an indefinite period; foster suckling has allowed the introduction of different strains of mice. Difficulties have been encountered in raising germfree rabbits. A good percentage of hand-fed, Cesarean born rabbits can be weaned in the germfree state, but these all have enlarged ceca and reproduction is poor. Since food restriction and dietary fiber do not decrease the size of the cecum to reasonable proportions, early ligation of part of the cecum has been used to prevent it from becoming too large. Reproduction has occurred although no colonies have been established. No major problem was encountered in raising germfree monkeys and pigs for a short period of time. Germfree ruminants may become most useful germfree animals for nutrition research. Both syntype diets and natural milk have been used in attempts to rear goats and lambs.

The nutritional requirements of germfree animals have been approached systematically. They appear to require the same amount of food and water as do conventional animals, and metabolic studies indicate they excrete a similar quantity per gram body weight. Germfree animals withstand starvation as well as do conventional animals and their food efficiency for growth is equal to that of conventional animals. Few studies are reported on the protein, energy, mineral, or roughage requirement of germfree animals. The vitamin requirements of germfree animals have been studied in some detail. They appear to require all of the known vitamins normally required by conventional animals of the same species. Vitamin A deficiency has been studied in germfree chicks and rats. When all the B-vitamins were left out of the diet, chicks died within 10 to 12 days. The symptoms shown were those of thiamine deficiency. When thiamine was withheld from the diet the chicks did not grow, exhibited anorexia, and died at 10 to 12 days. Riboflavin deficiency in germfree chicks elicited decreased growth rate and sometimes enlarged hearts. Niacin metabolism appeared to be upset in riboflavin deficiency. When niacin was omitted from the diet, germfree birds grew less well than do the conventional birds. Biotin-deficient germfree chicks showed the same dermatitis and lack of growth found in conventional birds. Germfree chicks fed folic acid low diets grew slowly and exhibited poor feather development and became anemic. Riboflavin metabolism may be changed in a folic acid deficiency. The chicks died in each deficiency reviewed. Germfree rats required pantothenic acid and biotin. Germfree rats were found to synthesize folic acid and citrovorum factor when fed high vitamin diets, but they became deficient when fed oridnary diets low in folic acid. Germfree rats can apparently synthesize methyl groups as shown by the deuterium labeling of choline when deuterium water was fed. Guinea pigs have been shown to require vitamin C and germfree chicks required vitamin D. Vitamin E deficiency was also obtained in some of the chicks. Growth was very poor in half of the chicks and the other half grew satisfactorily. Vitamin K deficiency has been obtained in both germfree chicks and rats. Spontaneous recovery of vitamin K deficiency in germfree chicks was reported. Vitamin K deficiency changed the metabolism of B vitamins. There is no good evidence that unidentified vitamins were required for germfree birds, however germfree mammals may require an unknown nutrient to maintain normal cecal size.

Finally, work with antibiotics in germfree animals was reviewed. It is obvious that the high levels of antibiotics are not effective in stimulating growth in germfree chicks while low levels of antibiotics have been found to stimulate growth of germfree chicks. The data from germfree turkeys is controversial. Further work may clarify the role of antibiotics in germfree animals.

CHAPTER 5

Characteristics of Germfree Animals

Introduction

The characteristics of the germfree animal are important because the germfree animal is uncomplicated by the stimulus of living microbial forms, has fewer variables as a biological unit, and thus forms the baseline or control for animals harboring microorganisms. This is reflected mathematically in the mean variation of those organs which come into contact with microorganisms—namely, intestinal tract, lungs, lymph nodules, liver, and blood. Where comparisons are made it is appropriate that the germfree animal should serve as the base while conventional (polycontaminated) or gnotobiotic animals which contain one or more microorganisms should be considered as the variable or experimental group. This logical approach is sometimes difficult because there is little data for the characteristics of germfree animals.

Throughout this work, unless stated otherwise, groups are compared when the animals are the same strain, are fed sterilized diet of the same composition, and are provided with food and water *ad libitum*. Since most of the conventional animals were maintained in stock colony or laboratory rooms, their environment differed from that of the germfree animal in more ways than the presence of a microbial flora. Other factors included slightly lower air pressure; air with a wider variety of dust and odors, humidity, temperature (no heat cycles during autoclave procedures), differences in lighting cycles, intensity and direction of light; greater variety of visual stimuli; less variety in sounds; differences in cage space and arrangement; different number of animals per unit area; ingestion of nonsterile water and food (although it had undergone sterilization treatment); different ions in water; and differences in the relationship to the caretaker. Since many such details were not given in the published literature, it is not possible to be sure of all of the differences which existed between the

283

germfree animal and the conventional animal. Most of these unwanted variables could be eliminated by rearing the contaminated animals in a germfree cage, and inoculating with one or more known organisms as the experimental variable. A normal flora could not be maintained when a conventional animal was fed sterile food and maintained in a sterile environment (Kijanizin, 1895; Nelson, 1941; and Reback, 1942). A "cage control" animal with conventional flora was obtained by having a daily visitor from the conventional stock colony. Each day a new visitor was exchanged for the visitor of the previous day. Thus continuous "normal flora" inoculum was provided without bringing any of the cage control animals out of the contaminated cage. Data taken from these animals clearly identified them with the conventional animals and indicated they were quite distinct from germfree animals. Apparently none of the uncontrolled variables were as important as the microbial vector. Experiments with precise control of the qualitative microbial component are presented in the last chapter.

Microorganisms contribute to the characteristics of the conventional laboratory animal; unfortunately this contribution is not well defined. So few direct experiments have been performed that it is best to simply provide comparisons between the germfree animals and those containing microorganisms without necessarily delineating cause–effect relationships. The effect of the microorganisms is greatest where the contact is the most intimate. Each of these contacts affects the cellular and chemical composition of the blood which reflects the conditions of the tissues it services. The difference between germfree animals and animals with a microbial flora of undefined composition provides a key to the study of defense mechanisms, the role of intestinal microflora in nutrition, the study of infectious diseases, and the many facets of the microorganisms' contribution to the host. These problems can be studied best by the inoculation of germfree animals with one or more microorganisms. While much work has been done with invertebrates, the major part of that work has been concerned with diet, methods, and apparatus useful for obtaining and maintaining different species in the axenic state, or with the basic nutritional problems required to rear invertebrates from one stage to another. No basic studies are known wherein the morphological, biochemical, physiological, serological, and immunological characteristics of a germfree invertebrate are compared with those of a contaminated or inoculated counterpart.

Far less work has been done with germfree fish than with invertebrates. Germfree platyfish have been reared by Baker and Ferguson (1942), and germfree guppies have been obtained by Shaw (1957). In both cases, the prime attempt was to obtain germfree young and observe the growth and development over a short period of time. Neither experiment was carried through reproduction, and in neither case was there a systematic attempt to evaluate the animal *per se* or to carry experiments with them. Our state of knowledge with respect to germfree amphibia is comparable to that of germfree fish. Most of the workers who have used amphibia have only tried to obtain germfree eggs and to determine whether or not the tadpole would grow and develop in the absence of bacteria. Except for the material presented in Chapter 2 on the conditions of rearing, the diet, growth rate, general morphology, and mortality of amphibia, little is available in the reports by O. Metchnikoff (1903), Wollman and Wollman (1915), and Moro (1905). None of these authors investigated the animal *per se* in a systematic fashion.

While Küster (1912) conceived of germfree experimentation in broad terms, it remained for the workers who are presently active to do work in more than one or two aspects of germfree life. Except for the morphological survey of the germfree guinea pig by Glimstedt (1936a) and bits of information gleaned from other workers prior to 1950, the major work presented in this chapter on the morphological, biochemical, physiological, and serological characterization of germfree animals was published in the past dozen years. Future work will increase the significance of the basic survey of germfree chicks and rats; however enough is known at present to warrant a compilation of data into a ready reference. It is hoped that such a background of information will accrue for germfree mice, rabbits, dogs, and other laboratory mammals.

The early experiments with each species contributed important historical material. For this reason Chapter 2 contained not only accounts of the first efforts to obtain and rear such species, but also presented, where possible for each species, the characteristics of growth, general appearance, obvious signs of disease, and success in reproduction. In Chapter 4 may be found the main nutritional characteristics known for each germfree animal species. Here may be found growth rates of animals fed different diets, vitamin requirements, characteristics of specific vitamin deficiencies, syndromes with disease-producing diets, and a review of the work with antibiotic feeding in germfree animals. Reference must be made to both of these chapters in order to learn all that is available regarding the characteristics of any one species.

Details of most methods used for examination of chicks and rats and statistical treatment of the data (and much of the data without specific citation) were given by Reyniers *et al.* (1960a), and methods for the morphological survey of guinea pigs were given by Glimstedt (1936a). Methods used for other species are similar but have not been collected in one place. Animals were sacrificed by electronarcosis, decapitation, ether, or severing of the cervical vertebrae; and animals used only for serological work were usually sacrificed by exsanguination via cardiac puncture. The method of sacrifice had no apparent effect upon the gross morphological or biochemical data. Theoretically, animals with abnormal morphology of function (i.e., enlarged cecum) are not acceptable as experimental material: in practice, most methods of inquiry are not sensitive enough to distinguish the nonintestinal tissue of a normal animal from one with enlarged cecum. Animals having a *greatly* distended cecum or any other symptoms of pathology were not used in the survey.

The presentation of the characteristics of germfree animals begins with a description of the total animal and details of growth and reproduction which were not presented as a part of history or nutrition. Morphological and biochemical characteristics of organs and tissues are arranged according to the major systems: integument, skeletal, musculature, circulatory, respiratory, digestive with accessory organs, nervous, sensory, lymphatic, and endocrine. The chick, guinea pig, and rat data presented under the above systems are compiled in separate tables as an aid to those interested in results from a single species. This approach brings chemical similarities and differences into focus from a different point of view and gives a more concise presentation of the biochemical character of each species. Metabolism and physiology, histology and cytology form a small portion of the total chapter because little information is available. The material on body defense mechanisms forms a skeleton of needed knowledge. The last part of the chapter presents abnormalities in form and function seen in germfree animals.

General Characteristics

The gross appearance and over-all development of germfree birds were quite comparable to those of conventional birds (Fig. 5.1). The main difference one sometimes saw was that the germfree birds were less clean than conventional birds. This was attributed to the some-

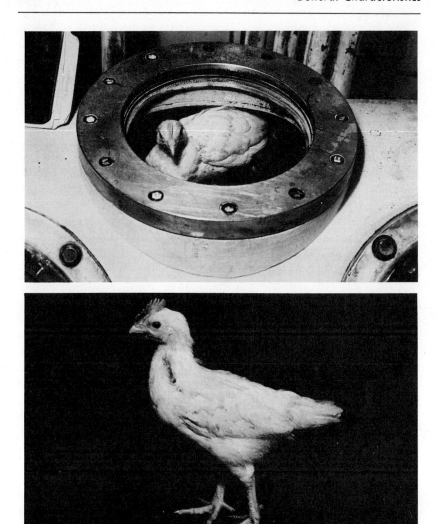

FIG. 5.1. Germfree pullet (*top*) and cockerel (*bottom*) at 4 weeks of age fed a syntype diet. (Reyniers *et al.*, 1950.)

what higher humidity in the germfree cage. When the humidity was high, diet, fecal matter, and other waste material tended to stick to the feathers, and the birds did not keep clean (see Fig. 2.6). When fewer birds were maintained in one cage and the air flow was adequate and dry, the germfree birds would clean themselves. The other difference which could be readily noted was in the odor of the germ-free bird. While conventional birds had the odor of the fecal flora, the germfree bird had no strong odor distinct to itself. The main odor associated with the germfree birds was that of the autoclaved diet. The unfed germfree bird had the pungent aroma of newly let blood. Neither germfree nor conventional chicks fed synthetic-type diet had distinctive taste. The meat may have been more tender, but the author had insufficient evidence to assert this point. The detailed presentation of the growth of germfree single comb White Leghorn, and the rose comb White Wyandotte chickens (Reyniers *et al.*, 1949b,d, 1960a) indicated that germfree chicks might grow at a somewhat faster rate than did conventional chicks. This has been confirmed by Forbes *et al.* (1959), Wostmann *et al.* (1958–1960), and A. W. Phillips *et al.* (1959). Reproduction was obtained in germfree White Wyandotte Bantam chickens (Reyniers *et al.*, 1949a).

Nuttall and Thierfelder (1895–1896) found the general appearance of their 8 day old, germfree guinea pig to be perfectly normal accord-ing to "expert witness." Both it and the control weighed 83 gm at age 1 week. The germfree animal had eaten 330 ml of milk in 8 days and was judged to have grown, without the actual weight at birth being known. Their other two guinea pigs were obviously not normal and had not gained as much as the controls in the 10 day experiment. The distended abdomen was found to be caused by a greatly enlarged cecum. Gradual improvement in the health, nurture, and general ap-pearance of germfree guinea pigs may be traced through the experi-ments of Cohendy and Wollman (1914) and Glimstedt (1936a) to the excellent guinea pigs reared by Phillips *et al.* (1959b). This group re-ported on 4 guinea pigs over 1 year of age: "The animals were alert and active throughout their lives. On external examination the guinea pigs appeared well developed and in good state of nutrition." These animals had the ever present "greatly distended ceca." Abrams *et al.* (1960) found germfree guinea pigs grew as well as conventional ani-mals, had excellent external appearance, and showed no signs of nutri-tional deficiencies in the tissues. Reproduction was first obtained in germfree guinea pigs by Teah in 1959 (personal communication) and Newton in 1960. The general appearance of these animals is shown in Fig. 2.8.

The morphologic ideas of weanling germfree rats was colored in the early literature by the swollen abdomen caused by the distended cecum (Gustafsson, 1947). Except for the full abdomen and slight lethargy, germfree and conventional rats give the same general appearance by gross observation. Gordon (1960b) suggested that the decreased growth rate found in germfree rats (Luckey, 1956a) might have been caused by overcrowding. Gustafsson (1959a) finds no difference in growth. All recent work with germfree rats has been done with albino rats, *Rattus norvegicus*. The Lobund strain was developed from Wistar and Sprague Dawley stock.

The author recently examined 5 male albino mice of the Swiss strain donated by the University of Notre Dame Department of Biology. They were 6 months of age from the fifth generation in germfree environment. Four were fed diet No. 462 and one was fed a practical diet. All were sacrificed by separation of the cervical vertebrae. The gross appearance of these germfree mice (Fig. 2.12) was comparable to that of conventional mice. Several differences could be noted upon close observation. The enlarged cecum causes in every germfree mouse abnormal fullness of the abdomen which is particularly noticeable from the dorsal view. The sides appear more distended than does the ventral surface of the abdomen. Other differences were in the fur (as detailed in the section on integument), and in the integrity of the skin. The conventional mice had various minor skin infections, particularly on the ears. The preliminary observation indicated the possibility that the ratio of body length to tail length was greater in germfree mice than in conventional mice. The tail length appeared to be the same in both groups (9.4–9.8 cm) but the body length seemed to be longer in germfree mice (11.1–11.5 cm) than in conventional mice (10.3–10.5 cm).

From the few reports and from limited personal observation, it might be stated that the general appearance of germfree and conventional monkeys and pups was comparable. Rabbits in the germfree state began to show somewhat distended abdomens shortly after weaning. This general view is presented in Fig. 2.13.

There is little published data on the chemical analysis of total carcass of animals, although much is available on the chicken embryo, and a considerable body of evidence was available for different organs and tissues. Table 5.1 summarizes the limited data in which germfree and conventional birds are compared on a total organism basis. At 4 weeks of age there was an apparent difference in the dry weight of the birds: the germfree birds appeared to have a somewhat greater amount of moisture than had conventional birds. This difference was not reflected in the ash content of the birds. The riboflavin, biotin, and folic acid concentrations in the total carcass of the germfree and conventional birds were almost identical. Conventional birds had a slightly, but significantly, higher concentration of niacin and pantothenic acid than had the germfree birds. The concentration of biotin (0.24 μg/gm at hatch) and riboflavin (2.29 μg/gm at hatch) of a

TABLE 5.1
WHOLE BODY COMPOSITION OF 6 WEEK-OLD LEGHORN CHICKS

	Category	No.[a]	Mean	Min—Max	σ[d]	P[e]
Dry wgt (%)	Gf[b]	3	29.6	28.4—30.9	1.63	0.018
	Cv[c]	3	33.7	33.1—34.1	0.462	
Ash (%)	Gf	3	11.8	4.4—12.1	0.286	0.89
	Cv	3	10.0	9.25—11.6	1.13	
Riboflavin (μg/gm)	Gf	3	4.25	3.84—4.51	0.294	0.96
	Cv	3	4.62	3.68—5.28	0.678	
Niacin (μg/gm)	Gf	3	45.2	44.0—46.1	1.10	0.001
	Cv	3	54.6	52.9—56.6	1.66	
Pantothenic acid (μg/gm)	Gf	3	26.0	25.1—26.9	0.848	0.001
	Cv	3	22.2	20.9—23.5	0.119	
Biotin (μg/gm)	Gf	3	0.070	0.052—0.085	0.0438	0.93
	Cv	3	0.064	0.045—0.088	0.0567	
Folic acid (μg/gm)	Gf	3	6.95	5.45—8.25	1.17	0.94
	Cv	3	6.02	5.65—6.10	0.192	

[a] Number of observations (this applies to all tables).
[b] Gf = Germfree chicks.
[c] Cv = Conventional chicks.
[d] σ = Standard deviation.
[e] P = Probability.

chick doubled from 0 to 30 days. Pantothenic acid (3.6 μg/gm at hatch) increased almost 8-fold during this time. The niacin concentration (3.9 μg/gm at hatch) increased more than 10-fold, while the concentration of folic acid (0.21 μg/gm at hatch) increased approximately thirty times.

Comparable data are not available on the composition of the total body of other germfree animals, excepting B-vitamin content of germfree rats (Luckey et al., 1955b). Gustafsson et al. (1957b) found 6.9–7.8 μg histidine per gram fresh tissue in whole germfree rats; this concentration was comparable to that for conventional rats.

Systems, Organs, and Tissues

Integument

The skin of germfree White Leghorn chicks 5 weeks of age comprised 9.4% of the total body weight while that of conventional chicks was 10.8% (Table 5.2). The feathers of well fed germfree birds were well formed and equal in quantity (about 6.6% of the body weight), quality, and appearance (Fig. 5.1) to that of conventional birds. Distribution, color, and fine structure of the feathers of germfree birds were comparable to those of conventional chicks. The physical state of the scales on the leg, the claws, the beak, the wattles, comb, and skin in the germfree chicken were equivalent to those of conventional birds fed the same amount of pigment, vitamin D, and mineral in the diet. The skin, scales, and claws of the germfree birds and the diet control birds had less color than was seen in farm-reared birds or birds fed commercial diets, owing to the low quantity of carotenoid pigment in the syntype diets. Details of microscopic examination of skin and accessory structures have not yet been reported.

The snood of germfree turkeys at 1 month of age was less well developed than that of conventional turkey poults (Luckey et al., 1960). This difference was more pronounced in male than in female turkeys. Except for this observation, germfree and conventional poults appeared to be identical from the gross viewpoint.

The four guinea pigs over 1 year of age of Phillips et al. (1959b) had exceptionally clean skin and the fur had normal texture. Germfree guinea pigs in present colonies seen by the author were equal to those of the best conventional stock animals in general appearance. They were alert with quick movement; their eyes were bright, and the fur was lustrous. However, upon close examination a swollen abdomen was seen in many individuals.

Abnormalities in the skin and hair development of hand-fed, preweaned, germfree rats was presented in the nutrition chapter. No gross pathology of the skin was seen in germfree rats which were cared for by their mother. The ears were opened by the 3rd day of life; the eyes opened at the 12th to 14th day; and teeth erupted on schedule. Hair growth began at 1 week and the young were covered with a white hair coat by the age of 12–14 days. The adult fur was thick and of typical ivory-white color as long as the humidity was not too high. When humidity rose excessively, the fur was not kept clean

TABLE 5.2
BODY WEIGHT AND RELATIVE ORGAN WEIGHT[a] IN GERMFREE
AND CONVENTIONAL WHITE LEGHORN CHICKENS[b]
AND WHITE WYANDOTTE BANTAM CHICKENS[c]

	Category	Leghorn Mean (%)	Wyandotte Mean (%)
Body weight (gm)	Gf	340	289
	Cv	399	241
Feathers	Gf	6.763	—
	Cv	6.292	—
Skin	Gf	9.368	—
	Cv	10.78	—
Skeleton	Gf	11.10	—
	Cv	10.25	—
Musculature	Gf	47.15	—
	Cv	47.29	—
Trachea	Gf	0.207	—
	Cv	0.178	—
Lungs	Gf	0.613	0.408
	Cv	0.573	0.496
Heart	Gf	0.601	0.487
	Cv	0.548	0.612
Mediastinum	Gf	0.542	—
	Cv	0.614	—
Esophagus	Gf	0.322	—
	Cv	0.294	—
Crop	Gf	0.680	—
	Cv	0.610	—
Proventriculus	Gf	0.419	1.850
	Cv	0.452	3.060
Gizzard	Gf	2.255	0.343
	Cv	2.092	0.522
Small intestine	Gf	1.400	1.650
	Cv	1.925	3.210
Ceca, both	Gf	0.191	0.173
	Cv	0.294	0.288
Large intestine (mg/100 gm)	Gf	91.0	—
	Cv	67.0	—
Cloaca (mg/100 gm)	Gf	70.9	—
	Cv	78.0	—
Intestinal contents	Gf	1.791	—
	Cv	1.787	—
Cecal content	Gf	0.343	—
	Cv	0.347	—

TABLE 5.2 (Continued)

	Category	Leghorn Mean (%)	Wyandotte Mean (%)
Liver	Gf	2.880	2.90
	Cv	2.579	4.33
Bile	Gf	0.130	—
	Cv	0.127	—
Pancreas	Gf	0.333	0.225
	Cv	0.244	0.311
Gonads (testes) (mg/100 gm)	Gf	23.6	—
	Cv	79.3	—
Kidney	Gf	0.901	—
	Cv	0.919	—
Brain	Gf	0.701	0.760
	Cv	0.611	0.940
Eyeballs, two	Gf	0.924	0.726
	Cv	0.823	0.768
Spleen	Gf	0.093	0.196
	Cv	0.165	0.209
Trident (mg/100 gm)	Gf	25.5	26
	Cv	43.2	90
Bursa of Fabricius	Gf	0.274	0.231
	Cv	0.362	0.221
Thymus	Gf	0.314	0.500
	Cv	0.455	0.394
Pituitary (mg/100 gm)	Gf	0.83	—
	Cv	0.78	—
Thyroid	Gf	3.86	4.4
	Cv	8.39	5.9
Adrenals (mg/100 gm)	Gf	11.8	11.9
	Cv	10.9	12.4
Blood	Gf	5.149	—
	Cv	5.269	—
Fat	Gf	0.216	—
	Cv	0.772	—
Evaporation	Gf	4.104	—
	Cv	3.076	—

[a] Organ weight in gm per 100 gm corrected live weight. Corrected weight obtained by deducting from the live body weight the somewhat variable contents of the oral cavity, esophagus, crop, proventriculus, and gizzard. The rest of the gastrointestinal contents were left to form a part of "body weight" as to permit an appraisal of their relative participation. Data of Gordon (1960a).

[b] Age 30-35 days, 3 chickens in each group.

[c] Age 46-64 days, 3 chickens in each group.

and the predominant color became a light reddish brown from the diet and waste material which clings to the fur. Occasionally a streak of reddish pigment was seen in the hair of the neck and shoulders. It was not clear whether this was simply unclean fur or the red, non-hemin pigment seen occasionally in conventional rats.

The fur of germfree mice appeared smooth and of ivory-white color as compared to the more fuzzy, chalk-white fur of conventional mice. Possibly the difference was caused by the cleaning activity of the conventional mice which were constantly ridding themselves of infestations. The skin was clear and supple in both groups. The vibrissae were of variable length in all mice; some had hairs no longer than 0.5 cm while the vibrissae of some approached 2.5 cm.

Gustafsson et al. (1957b) found 10.6–15.8 μg of histidine per gram of back skin in germfree rats 120 days of age. The abdominal skin was found to contain 17.5–22.7 μg/gm. These ranges were comparable to those found for conventional rats of the same age.

Skeletal System

The development of the osseous system was comparable in germfree birds to that of conventional birds. The osseous material of germfree White Leghorns was 11.1% of the body weight and that of conventional birds was 10.2% (Table 5.2). Gordon (1959b) suggested that the skeleton is always heavier in germfree animals. No systematic quantitative study of the morphology of the skeletal sysetm has been

TABLE 5.3

COMPARISON OF SKULL DEVELOPMENT IN RATS FROM CEPHALOROENTGENOGRAMS[a]

Category	No.	Age	Weight	Skull measurement (mm)[b]		
				O-N	C-M	D-L
Conventional	16	160	338	45.8	21.4	13.4
Germfree, hand-fed	13	168	281	40.9	19.3	11.8
Coventional	23	195	328	45.9	22.2	13.2
Germfree, dam-fed	9	214	250	44.7	21.5	12.3

[a]Orland et al. (1954).
[b]See fig. 5.2 for measurements used.

reported except that done on morphological and histological aspects of the teeth of the germfree rat in connection with dental caries by Orland et al. (1954). These workers found that the growth of the skull (Fig. 5.2 and Table 5.3) and femur of germfree rats was comparable to that of conventional rats. Correlation of bone growth to body weight is similar in germfree and conventional rats (Fig. 5.3). Germfree guinea pigs were reported to have well developed teeth (Phillips *et al.* 1959). Bones and teeth of germfree and conventional mice were comparable in size, color, and breaking strength. The upper incisors of mice were pigmented (old ivory color) but the lower incisors were chalky white.

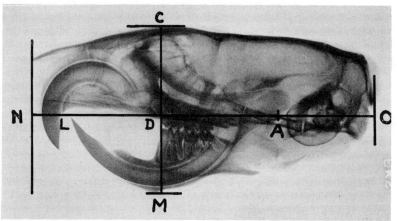

FIG. 5.2. Measurement of rat skull. Craniometric planes for the determination of the rat skull growth pattern. (Point A is at the comparable site of sella turcica in man, this landmark being absent in the rat.) (Orland *et al.*, 1954.)

The chemical composition of bones, using total femurs, has been studied in some detail (Table 5.4). On the dry weight basis, the percent ash of bones of germfree Leghorn chicks at 10 weeks of age was equal to that of conventional birds; the apparent difference was not statistically significant. The percent of fat in the bones of the two groups of birds was very similar. The nitrogen content of the bones of germfree birds was 3.07%; this would indicate the crude protein to be about 19%. The riboflavin, niacin, pantothenic acid, biotin, and vitamin B_{12} content of the bones of conventional birds was very similar to that of germfree birds. The mean folic acid content of bones of conventional birds was approximately one-half that of germfree birds. However, the variability was too great for statistical validity to be reached.

The dry weight of bones of the germfree rats was not noted. The bone ash of newly weaned germfree first generation rats was considerably less than that dam-fed conventional rats (see Table 5.5).

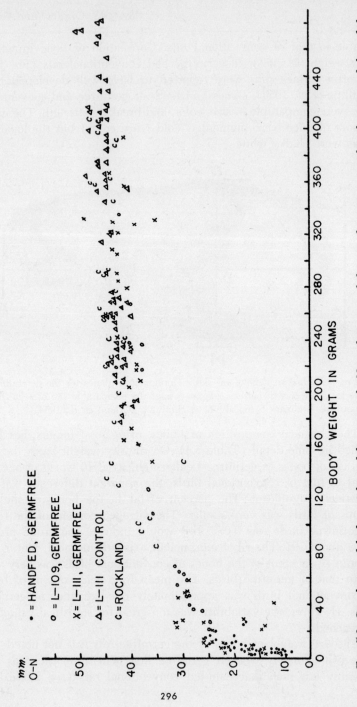

Fig. 5.3. Correlation of body weight and bone growth. Note that most of the germfree rats are within the range of those fed Rockland Stock Diet (from Arcady Mills, Inc., Chicago, Illinois). O–N equals the skull length.

TABLE 5.4
COMPOSITION OF TISSUES OF GERMFREE AND CONVENTIONAL WHITE
LEGHORN CHICKS FED SYNTYPE DIET L-245

| | | Composition of Bone | | | | | | | | | |
| | | Age 4 – 7 weeks | | | | | Age 10 – 11 weeks | | | | |
	Category	No.	Mean	Limits	σ	P	No.	Mean	Limits	σ	P
Dry weight, (%)	Gf	—	—	—	—	—	—	—	—	—	—
	Cv	—	—	—	—	—	—	—	—	—	—
Ash (%, dry basis)	Gf	—	—	—	—	—	4	66.6	65.3 67.6	2.72	—
	Cv	—	—	—	—	—	4	64.4	61.0 67.1	2.95	0.38
Fat (%)	Gf	—	—	—	—	—	3	21.2	20.3 22.7	1.06	—
	Cv	—	—	—	—	—	3	22.0	21.5 22.5	1.28	0.53
Nitrogen (%, total)	Gf	—	—	—	—	—	4	3.07	3.32 3.95	—	—
	Cv	—	—	—	—	—	—	—	—	—	—
Riboflavin (μg/gm)	Gf	3	14.3	6.7 25.0	7.86	—	—	—	—	—	—
	Cv	3	12.8	9.5 14.6	2.23	0.80	—	—	—	—	—
Niacin (μg/gm)	Gf	3	32.0	22.4 42.7	8.46	—	—	—	—	—	—
	Cv	3	20.5	19.4 21.2	0.88	0.52	—	—	—	—	—
Pantothenic acid (μg/gm)	Gf	3	5.93	4.7 8.1	1.55	—	—	—	—	—	—
	Cv	4	5.23	4.2 6.3	1.00	0.58	—	—	—	—	—
Biotin (μg/gm)	Gf	3	1.69	1.01 2.94	0.89	—	—	—	—	—	—
	Cv	4	0.92	0.57 1.25	0.25	0.23	—	—	—	—	—
Folic acid (μg/gm)	Gf	2	3.7	2.8 4.6	0.9	—	—	—	—	—	—
	Cv	3	1.8	1.6 2.1	0.2	—	—	—	—	—	—
Vitamin B$_{12}$ (μg/gm)	Gf	3	5.99	3.6 8.5	2.00	—	—	—	—	—	—
	Cv	3	3.43	3.4 3.5	0.06	0.61	—	—	—	—	—
Vitamin C (μg/gm)	Gf	—	—	—	—	—	—	—	—	—	—
	Cv	—	—	—	—	—	—	—	—	—	—

TABLE 5.4 (Continued)

		Composition of Muscle									
		Age 4 – 7 weeks					Age 10 – 11 weeks				
	Category	No.	Mean	Limits	σ	P	No.	Mean	Limits	σ	P
Dry weight (%)	Gf	3	22.8	22.5 23.2	0.48	—	4	21.7	20.9 22.5	0.87	—
	Cv	4	22.6	21.5 24.5	1.04	0.74	4	23.2	22.2 23.8	0.73	0.08
Ash (%, dry basis)	Gf	3	5.23	4.93 5.51	0.26	—	4	7.26	6.32 8.17	0.86	—
	Cv	4	4.35	3.24 5.89	0.96	0.26	4	6.39	5.74 7.16	0.54	0.17
Fat (%)	Gf	3	2.43	2.40 2.50	0.14	—	4	2.47	2.01 2.86	0.32	—
	Cv	4	2.25	2.10 2.50	0.17	0.27	3	1.69	1.60 1.74	0.10	0.02
Nitrogen (%, total)	Gf	—	—	—	—	—	4	2.96	2.75 3.11	0.19	—
	Cv	—	—	—	—	—	4	2.98	2.73 3.25	0.25	0.94
Riboflavin (μg/gm)	Gf	3	8.1	5.7 9.8	1.8	—	—	—	—	—	—
	Cv	4	10.9	9.0 13.6	1.7	0.59	—	—	—	—	—
Niacin (μg/gm)	Gf	3	33.5	23.6 43.4	8.10	—	—	—	—	—	—
	Cv	4	46.5	37.0 58.0	7.65	0.89	—	—	—	—	—
Pantothenic acid (μg/gm)	Gf	3	17.5	16.5 18.3	1.32	—	—	—	—	—	—
	Cv	4	14.3	12.4 16.5	1.44	0.86	—	—	—	—	—
Biotin (μg/gm)	Gf	3	3.00	2.42 3.32	0.41	—	—	—	—	—	—
	Cv	3	2.83	2.27 3.30	0.41	0.69	—	—	—	—	—
Folic acid (μg/gm)	Gf	3	0.86	0.75 0.94	0.11	—	—	—	—	—	—
	Cv	4	1.06	0.72 1.46	0.25	0.33	—	—	—	—	—
Vitamin B_{12} (μg/gm)	Gf	3	15.1	11.9 17.7	2.50	—	—	—	—	—	—
	Cv	3	15.6	12.8 17.4	2.01	0.83	—	—	—	—	—
Vitamic C (μg/gm)	Gf	3	16.6	16.0 17.1	0.46	—	—	—	—	—	—
	Cv	3	24.7	22.1 28.4	2.69	<0.01	—	—	—	—	—

TABLE 5.4 (Continued)

	Category	Composition of Lungs Age 10 – 11 weeks					Composition of Small Intestine Age 10 – 11 weeks				
		No.	Mean	Limits	δ	P	No.	Mean	Limits	δ	P
Dry weight (%)	Gf	3	21.2	20.7 22.1	1.34	—	4	25.3	22.7 27.0	1.74	—
	Cv	4	21.8	20.9 22.7	0.78	0.59	4	23.4	21.6 24.9	1.60	0.20
Ash (%, dry basis)	Gf	4	7.50	7.05 7.76	0.39	—	4	6.50	5.04 7.87	0.98	—
	Cv	4	6.29	5.99 6.52	0.28	<0.01	4	6.09	5.24 7.04	0.60	0.56
Fat (%)	Gf	3	4.76	4.61 4.89	0.20	—	3	5.24	4.87 5.64	0.25	—
	Cv	4	3.40	2.74 3.81	0.55	0.02	4	4.15	3.43 5.00	0.66	0.06
Nitrogen (%, total)	Gf	4	2.64	2.40 2.75	0.14	—	4	2.74	2.64 2.90	0.10	—
	Cv	3	2.46	2.36 2.54	0.10	0.15	3	2.41	2.37 2.45	0.02	0.01
Riboflavin (μg/gm)	Gf										
	Cv										
Niacin (μg/gm)	Gf										
	Cv										
Pantothenic acid (μg/gm)	Gf										
	Cv										
Biotin (μg/gm)	Gf										
	Cv										
Folic acid (μg/gm)	Gf										
	Cv										
Vitamin B_{12} (μg/gm)	Gf										
	Cv										
Vitamin C (μg/gm)	Gf										
	Cv										

TABLE 5.4 (Continued)

	Category	Composition of Cecal Contents									
		Age 4 – 7 weeks					Age 10 – 11 weeks				
		No.	Mean	Limits	δ	P	No.	Mean	Limits	δ	P
Dry weight (%)	Gf	10	13.5	12.3 16.4	1.97	—	4	11.1	9.6 12.6	1.1	—
	Cv	8	21.4	17.2 25.1	2.86	<0.01	3	16.2	13.3 17.7	2.0	<0.01
Ash (%, dry basis)	Gf	10	20.3	15.7 25.4	3.52	—	4	18.4	12.8 24.3	4.19	—
	Cv	8	24.3	16.1 30.9	4.56	0.070	4	22.3	20.4 24.1	1.23	0.19
Fat (%)	Gf	—	—	—	—	—	—	—	—	—	—
	Cv	—	—	—	—	—	—	—	—	—	—
Nitrogen (%, total)	Gf	—	—	—	—	—	3	0.817	0.748 0.900	0.053	—
	Cv	—	—	—	—	—	3	1.150	0.870 1.350	0.204	0.10
Riboflavin (μg/gm)	Gf	3	10.9	1.3 19.6	7.57	—	—	—	—	—	—
	Cv	10	7.3	2.4 11.0	2.38	0.09	—	—	—	—	—
Niacin (μg/gm)	Gf	9	12.1	5.6 25.0	6.67	—	—	—	—	—	—
	Cv	13	28.9	9.1 51.0	14.10	<0.01	—	—	—	—	—
Pantothenic. acid (μg/gm)	Gf	9	5.47	2.1 7.7	2.40	—	—	—	—	—	—
	Cv	12	7.74	4.0 15.3	3.72	0.68	—	—	—	—	—
Biotin (μg/gm)	Gf	9	0.24	0.06 0.62	0.18	—	—	—	—	—	—
	Cv	13	0.49	0.14 0.81	0.20	0.01	—	—	—	—	—
Folic acid (μg/gm)	Gf	7	2.29	1.60 3.10	0.46	—	—	—	—	—	—
	Cv	13	1.82	0.61 3.10	0.94	0.26	—	—	—	—	—
Vitamin B_{12} (μg/gm)	Gf	7	14.5	3.6 32.1	—	—	—	—	—	—	—
	Cv	2	18.4	4.7 31.7	—	—	—	—	—	—	—
Vitamin C (μg/gm)	Gf										
	Cv										

TABLE 5.4 (Continued)

	Category	Composition of Rectal Contents Age 10 - 11 weeks					Composition of Kidney Age 10 - 11 weeks				
		No.	Mean	Limits	σ	P	No.	Mean	Limits	σ	P
Dry weight (%)	Gf	3	15.5	11.4 18.5	3.0	—	3	21.3	20.9 21.7	0.33	—
	Cv	4	18.7	17.3 21.8	2.9	0.27	3	21.4	21.3 21.5	0.17	0.72
Ash (%, dry basis)	Gf	3	17.53	12.34 20.70	3.74	—	4	7.22	6.42 8.41	0.72	—
	Cv	3	8.09	6.80 9.33	1.06	0.02	4	6.23	5.78 6.74	0.30	0.08
Fat (%)	Gf	—	—	—	—	—	4	4.62	3.62 5.64	0.72	—
	Cv	—	—	—	—	—	3	5.02	4.81 5.20	0.14	0.46
Nitrogen (%, total)	Gf	—	—	—	—	—	4	2.22	1.91 2.52	0.18	—
	Cv	3	2.25	2.20 2.33	0.14	—	3	2.32	2.23 2.43	0.15	0.55
Riboflavin (μg/gm)	Gf										
	Cv										
Niacin (μg/gm)	Gf										
	Cv										
Pantothenic acid (μg/gm)	Gf										
	Cv										
Biotin (μg/gm)	Gf										
	Cv										
Folic acid (μg/gm)	Gf										
	Cv										
Vitamin B_{12} (μg/gm)	Gf										
	Cv										
Vitamin C (μg/gm)	Gf										
	Cv										

TABLE 5.4 (Continued)

	Category	Composition of Brain									
		Age 4 – 7 weeks					Age 10 – 11 weeks				
		No.	Mean	Limits	σ	P	No.	Mean	Limits	σ	P
Dry weight (%)	Gf	3	22.0	19.3 23.8	1.89	—	4	16.0	14.4 17.9	1.53	—
	Cv	4	22.0	20.8 23.4	0.95	1.00	4	17.8	16.7 19.1	1.61	0.20
Ash (%, dry basis)	Gf	3	8.40	7.9 9.0	0.46	—	4	12.4	11.5 13.0	1.21	—
	Cv	4	7.08	6.5 7.7	0.51	0.03	4	8.01	7.27 8.72	0.48	<0.01
Fat (%)	Gf	3	5.50	4.7 6.7	0.87	—	4	6.79	5.34 8.28	1.23	—
	Cv	4	6.85	5.3 9.1	0.46	0.27	3	5.80	5.68 5.97	0.22	0.29
Nitrogen (%, total)	Gf	—	—	—	—	—	4	1.64	1.51 1.74	0.14	—
	Cv	—	—	—	—	—	3	1.73	1.64 1.85	0.05	0.34
Riboflavin (μg/gm)	Gf	3	2.33	1.1 3.4	0.96	—	—	—	—	—	—
	Cv	4	2.10	2.0 2.3	0.14	0.70	—	—	—	—	—
Niacin (μg/gm)	Gf	3	25.4	20.6 30.2	3.92	—	—	—	—	—	—
	Cv	4	21.8	21.1 22.4	1.67	0.19	—	—	—	—	—
Pantothenic acid (μg/gm)	Gf	3	55.3	49 59	1.55	—	—	—	—	—	—
	Cv	4	64.8	59 70	0.95	<0.01	—	—	—	—	—
Biotin (μg/gm)	Gf	3	0.88	0.59 1.10	0.21	—	—	—	—	—	—
	Cv	4	1.11	1.05 1.18	0.89	0.16	—	—	—	—	—
Folic acid (μg/gm)	Gf	3	0.53	0.48 0.56	0.04	—	—	—	—	—	—
	Cv	4	0.55	0.53 0.61	0.11	0.80	—	—	—	—	—
Vitamin B$_{12}$ (μg/gm)	Gf	3	15.1	9.8 18.7	5.12	—	—	—	—	—	—
	Cv	4	16.3	14.1 20.1	2.36	0.74	—	—	—	—	—
Vitamin C (μg/gm)	Gf	3	401	371 454	42.0	—	—	—	—	—	—
	Cv	4	361	306 407	35.5	0.18	—	—	—	—	—

TABLE 5.4 (Continued)

| | | Composition of Bile | | | | | | | | | |
| | | Age 4 – 7 weeks | | | | | Age 10 – 11 weeks | | | | |
	Category	No.	Mean	Limits	δ	P	No.	Mean	Limits	δ	P
Dry weight (%)	Gf	—	—	—	—	—	3	22.9	21.0 24.0	0.49	—
	Cv	—	—	—	—	—	3	24.9	23.5 26.8	0.57	0.01
Ash (%, dry basis)	Gf	—	—	—	—	—	3	11.6	11.2 12.2	0.43	—
	Cv	—	—	—	—	—	3	12.5	10.3 14.3	1.37	0.41
Fat (%)	Gf	—	—	—	—	—	—	—	—	—	—
	Cv	—	—	—	—	—	—	—	—	—	—
Nitrogen (%, total)	Gf	—	—	—	—	—	3	0.716	0.701 0.724	0.01	—
	Cv	—	—	—	—	—	3	0.703	0.506 0.914	0.17	0.93
Riboflavin, (μg/gm)	Gf	3	48.2	40.7 56.7	6.56	—	—	—	—	—	—
	Cv	3	12.7	2.2 20.1	8.00	<0.01	—	—	—	—	—
Niacin (μg/gm)	Gf	3	7.60	4.1 11.3	2.94	—	—	—	—	—	—
	Cv	3	8.77	2.9 20.1	7.90	0.85	—	—	—	—	—
Pantothenic acid (μg/gm)	Gf	4	3.05	1.8 4.0	0.87	—	—	—	—	—	—
	Cv	3	2.27	1.8 2.8	0.14	0.27	—	—	—	—	—
Biotin (μg/gm)	Gf	3	0.24	0.23 0.24	0.01	—	—	—	—	—	—
	Cv	3	0.07	0.02 0.13	0.05	<0.01	—	—	—	—	—
Folic acid (μg/gm)	Gf	4	0.36	0.20 0.53	0.10	—	—	—	—	—	—
	Cv	3	0.40	0.28 0.62	0.11	0.94	—	—	—	—	—
Vitamin B$_{12}$ (μg/gm)	Gf	3	6.00	3.06 9.35	—	—	—	—	—	—	—
	Cv	2	3.86	3.06 4.66	—	—	—	—	—	—	—
Vitamin C (μg/gm)	Gf										
	Cv										

TABLE 5.4 (Continued)

| | | Composition of Liver | | | | | | | | | |
| | | Age 4 – 7 weeks | | | | | Age 10 – 11 weeks | | | | |
	Category	No.	Mean	Limits	σ	P	No.	Mean	Limits	σ	P
Dry weight (%)	Gf	10	25.9	23.9 28.5	1.55	—	4	27.1	22.6 31.3	3.20	—
	Cv	8	29.5	28.1 31.6	1.32	<0.01	4	28.8	28.3 29.4	1.27	0.41
Ash (%, dry basis)	Gf	9	5.80	5.00 6.33	0.44	—	4	6.49	6.22 7.05	0.30	—
	Cv	7	4.25	3.71 5.60	0.90	0.02	4	5.39	4.92 5.75	0.34	0.01
Fat (%)	Gf	5	4.02	3.0 4.8	0.73	—	4	5.25	4.48 5.82	0.27	—
	Cv	4	7.45	5.4 9.8	1.57	0.01	4	4.07	2.45 5.77	1.22	0.24
Nitrogen (%, total)	Gf	—	—	—	—	—	3	3.13	2.94 3.23	0.198	—
	Cv	—	—	—	—	—	4	3.46	3.27 3.68	0.158	0.10
Riboflavin, (μg/gm)	Gf	10	21.6	18.2 24.0	2.06	—	—	—	—	—	—
	Cv	13	23.3	16.7 36.0	7.25	0.50	—	—	—	—	—
Niacin (μg/gm)	Gf	8	199	90.0 129	9.9	—	—	—	—	—	—
	Cv	14	108	31.8 174	45.1	>0.90	—	—	—	—	—
Pantothenic acid (μg/gm)	Gf	5	66.4	49 79	10.4	—	—	—	—	—	—
	Cv	10	48.0	28 57	9.9	<0.01	—	—	—	—	—
Biotin (μg/gm)	Gf	13	5.1	3.4 6.7	1.00	—	—	—	—	—	—
	Cv	18	4.3	1.1 7.9	2.10	0.22	—	—	—	—	—
Folic acid (μg/gm)	Gf	12	4.4	2.8 5.9	1.26	—	—	—	—	—	—
	Cv	18	3.3	2.1 4.7	1.15	0.02	—	—	—	—	—
Vitamin B_{12} (μg/gm)	Gf	13	323	109 402	145.6	—	—	—	—	—	—
	Cv	18	171	40 430	168.5	<0.02	—	—	—	—	—
Vitamin C (μg/gm)	Gf	4	23.8	14.5 38.7	9.0	—	—	—	—	—	—
	Cv	4	104.0	59.0 151.0	44.3	<0.01	—	—	—	—	—

This difference was not seen in subsequent age groups up to 2 months of age. The fat content of bones of weanling rats showed a tremendous difference. The hand-fed first generation germfree rats were found to have approximately ten times more fat in the bone than the dam-fed conventional rats. This difference was seen in rats up to 160 days of age. Presumably diet and the hand-feeding difficulty accounted for part of the differences noted. By 256 days, no real difference was seen between the fat content of the bone of germfree and conventional rats. The phosphorus content of bone of rat at 67 days of age was similar in germfree and conventional rats; however, at 160 and 256 days of age the germfree bones contained significantly more phosphorus than did the conventional bones. The average fluorine content of the femur of germfree rats at 143 ± 2 days of age was 67.6 ppm. The value for conventional rats fed the same fluorine low diet was 48.8 ppm. No data are available for the composition of bone in other species.

Musculature

By gross observation, the musculature of germfree birds and mammals was entirely comparable to that of farmyard birds and conventional mammals. The notable exception is the muscle tonus in the cecal walls of germfree mammals. Histological studies of muscle have not been reported. An evaluation of the percentage of muscle in germfree birds (Table 5.2) showed it to be present in the same quantity as was found in conventional White Leghorn chicks. Muscle tonus and control of germfree birds was good (Fig. 5.1).

The composition of the muscle of germfree chickens is presented in Tables 5.4 and 5.6. As can be seen, there was no difference in the dry weight of the muscle of White Wyandotte Bantam chicks between the conventional and the germfree category from 10 days up to 1 year of age. Likewise, the sparse data for germfree White Leghorn chickens confirmed this identity. The percentage of ash (dry weight basis) of the muscle of Leghorn germfree chicks was the same as that for conventional chicks from 4 to 10 weeks. The fat content of muscle of conventional chicks was similar to that of germfree birds at 4–7 weeks of age. However, there was a tendency for the fat of the muscle in conventional birds to be somewhat less prominent than that of the germfree birds. The phosphorus content of muscle of birds at 4–7 weeks of age was similar with a possibility existing that conventional birds had somewhat more muscle phosphorus than had germfree birds.

	Category	Age 29 Days					Age 67 Days					Age	
		No.	Mean	Min./Max.	σ	P	No.	Mean	Min./Max.	σ	P	No.	Mean
Body (gm)	Gf	4	37.0	32/41	4.0625	<0.001	5	156	134/191	23.313	<0.01	4	259
	Cv	5	77.3	70.9/85.3	6.663	—	5	198	135/225	32.50	—	10	342
												Composition	
Dry weight	Gf	3	26.03	25.1/27.2	0.9316	0.163	4	28.0	26.3/29.2	0.150	<0.01	4	26.275
	Cv	5	24.0	21.9/26.8	1.8607	—	5	25.0	24.6/25.7	1.0761	—	4	24.5
Ash	Gf	4	4.96	4.32/5.45	0.3944	0.22	5	6.00	4.97/7.42	1.0488	0.0485	4	4.75
	Cv	5	5.27	5.04/5.49	0.1736	—	4	4.58	4.35/4.93	0.2666	—	4	5.73
Fat	Gf	4	4.39	3.98/4.63	0.2453	0.014	5	3.34	2.91/3.67	0.3611	0.02	3	3.95
	Cv	5	2.96	1.75/3.76	0.7752	—	4	4.00	3.72/4.33	0.2085	—	—	—
Nitrogen	Gf	3	2.76	1.16/3.95	0.9767	0.712	4	3.74	3.46/3.79	0.0187	0.01	4	4.06
	Cv	5	2.96	2.75/3.20	0.1849	—	5	2.90	2.50/3.15	0.2297	—	5	3.386
												Composition	
Dry weight	Gf												
	Cv	5	55.42	54.6/56.4	9.7500	—	5	62.26	60.2/64.9	1.7465	—	5	75.9
Ash	Gf	4	54.1	52.2/55.6	2.05	0.01	5	64.46	60.8/67.0	2.1648	0.470	4	68.5
	Cv	5	60.92	60.0/61.8	0.640	—	5	65.28	65.0/65.7	0.2786	—	5	69.6
Fat	Gf	3	9.9	7.4/13.2	2.1645	0.01	4	1.95	1.8/2.2	3.8730	—	3	3.5
	Cv	5	1.02	0.456/1.84	0.4926	—	—	—	—	—	—	3	2.0
Phosphorus	Gf	5	210.6	197/225	10.2394	—	3	209	197/217	8.6410	0.335	4	204.75
	Cv	—	—	—	—	—	4	194.75	191/203	4.8153	—	5	191.8
												Composition	
Dry weight	Gf	4	20.5	17.7/25.3	2.7486	0.2	4	23.7	21.9/25.3	0.7399	0.655	4	24.375
	Cv	5	22.6	21.2/23.5	1.3077	—	4	25.1	24.5/25.6	1.1906	—	—	—
Ash	Gf	4	7.47	7.25/7.89	0.2499	<0.01	5	7.27	6.84/7.64	0.2587	0.50	3	6.54
	Cv	5	9.18	7.76/10.12	0.5853	—	4	5.79	5.50/6.59	1.5549	—	—	—
Nitrogen	Gf	—	—	—	—	—	—	—	—	—	—	—	—
	Cv	5	3.03	2.93/3.15	0.0907	—	—	—	—	—	—	—	—

5.5
OF RAT TISSUE
weight)

	162 Days			Age 256 Days					All				
	Min./Max.	σ	P	No.	Mean	Min./Max.	σ	P	No.	Mean	Min./Max.	σ	P
	192 / 323	55.340	0.23	5	247	220 / 322	37.811	6.167	—	—	—	—	—
	217 / 530	107.878	—	3	316	250 / 418	73.16	—	—	—	—	—	—
of Muscle													
	25.3 / 27.5	0.8261	0.095	5	28.2	26.2 / 29.6	0.4775	0.027	13	27.5	25.3 / 30.4	7.374	0.282
	23.5 / 25.5	1.3370	—	3	25.7	24.5 / 26.5	1.5780	—	12	25.0	23.5 / 26.5	1.524	—
	4.63 / 4.92	0.1937	0.115	4	5.65	5.40 / 6.06	0.1168	0.64	13	5.51	4.63 / 7.42	0.8304	0.653
	4.36 / 6.93	0.8968	—	3	5.85	5.17 / 6.26	0.5247	—	11	5.35	4.35 / 6.93	0.8193	—
	3.61 / 4.13	0.2921	—	5	4.45	3.62 / 5.32	0.5434	0.269	13	3.909	2.91 / 5.32	0.6508	0.525
	—	—	—	3	3.40	3.3 / 3.5	1.530	—	7	3.70	3.3 / 4.33	1.8915	—
	3.97 / 4.20	0.08573	0.345	3	3.65	3.07 / 3.96	0.3638	0.193	11	3.83	3.07 / 4.20	0.2942	0.590
	3.26 / 3.52	0.0900	—	3	3.283	3.27 / 3.30	0.4842	—	13	3.175	2.50 / 3.52	0.2735	—
of Bone													
	71.7 / 78.8	1.9458	—	3	70.87	69.4 / 72.2	0.9182	—	13	69.5	60.2 / 78.8	6.1814	—
	68.4 / 68.6	1.8527	0.45	5	71.0	70.5 / 71.6	2.4274	0.50	14	68.0	60.8 / 71.6	2.3910	0.99
	68.8 / 70.6	1.7939	—	3	69.6	69.4 / 69.8	2.1610	—	13	67.95	65.0 / 70.6	2.2791	—
	3.3 / 3.7	0.1633	0.010	3	3.43	3.4 / 3.5	0.1584	0.575	9	2.9	1.8 / 3.7	0.6438	0.355
	1.8 / 2.2	0.1633	—	3	2.9	1.7 / 4.6	1.2359	—	6	2.5	1.7 / 4.6	0.8554	—
	194 / 217	8.8987	0.025	5	199	178 / 219	3.3467	<0.01	12	203	178 / 219	15.3487	0.068
	189 / 195	2.3152	—	2	183.5	180 / 187	3.5	—	11	191	180 / 203	12.9474	—
of Spleen													
	23.5 / 25.4	0.7628	—	4	24.975	23.3 / 25.8	1.0419	0.99	12	24.3	23.0 / 25.8	1.8514	0.99
	—	—	—	3	27.2	23.6 / 29.7	2.6090	—	7	26.0	23.6 / 29.7	2.1925	—
	6.40 / 6.74	0.2536	—	5	6.66	6.24 / 7.16	0.2979	0.640	13	6.87	6.24 / 7.64	0.3689	0.45
	—	—	—	3	9.23	6.28 / 11.0	2.0832	—	7	7.37	5.50 / 11.0	2.1431	—
	—	—	—	—	—	—	—	—	—	—	—	—	—
	—	—	—	—	—	—	—	—	—	—	—	—	—

TABLE 5.5

	Category	Age 29 Days					Age 67 Days					Composition Age	
		No.	Mean	Min./Max.	σ	P	No.	Mean	Min./Max.	σ	P	No.	Mean
Dry weight	Gf	5	28.8	28.0/29.4	0.5678	0.445	4	29.0	27.8/30.2	1.650	0.415	4	29.4
	Cv	5	28.1	27.2/29.3	1.656	—	4	28.07	27.5/29.2	0.8589	—	5	28.38
Ash	Gf	5	5.31	5.07/5.47	0.2504	0.99	5	5.01	4.44/5.39	0.3313	0.855	4	4.765
	Cv	5	5.30	4.44/6.17	0.6279	—	4	5.05	4.89/5.18	0.1905	—	4	4.30
Fat	Gf	4	6.65	5.28/8.88	1.2744	0.830	5	6.80	5.69/7.36	0.6374	0.432	4	6.76
	Cv	5	6.83	5.80/8.38	0.8541	—	5	6.43	5.23/7.17	0.6285	—	—	—
Nitrogen	Gf	4	3.38	3.06/3.50	0.2272	0.026	5	3.52	2.61/4.50	0.6153	0.0155	4	3.55
	Cv	5	2.98	2.93/3.02	0.1588	—	5	2.51	2.21/2.73	0.2449	—	5	3.34

	Category	No.	Mean	Min./Max.	σ	P	No.	Mean	Min./Max.	σ	P	Composition No.	Mean
Dry weight	Gf	4	20.5	18.2/23.1	1.4327	<0.01	5	16.9	15.0/19.2	1.921	<0.01	2	25.1
	Cv	5	25.8	24.2/28.6	1.2207	—	4	22.5	21.5/23.6	1.4133	—	5	27.88
Ash	Gf	5	11.8	8.11/13.7	1.8677	<0.01	4	14.4	12.9/16.6	0.7314	0.094	2	15.85
	Cv	5	15.6	14.4/17.3	0.8843	—	4	21.1	19.5/23.3	5.8764	—	4	23.15
Nitrogen	Gf	—	—	—	—	—	—	—	—	—	—	—	—
	Cv	5	1.594	1.49/1.71	0.0889	—	5	1.37	1.05/1.61	0.1922	—	5	1.39

	Category	No.	Mean	Min./Max.	σ	P	No.	Mean	Min./Max.	σ	P	Composition No.	Mean
Dry weight	Gf	4	23.1	22.4/24.2	2.9449	0.645	4	24.9	23.0/26.7	1.3874	0.9	4	25.1
	Cv	5	24.22	22.0/27.6	1.8605	—	5	25.1	22.9/27.7	2.3495	—	5	25.5
Ash	Gf	5	5.83	5.56/6.00	0.160	0.01	4	6.22	4.86/7.80	1.0601	0.837	4	7.15
	Cv	4	7.21	6.37/8.27	0.7521	—	5	6.08	5.21/7.25	0.6918	—	5	7.07
Fat	Gf	3	5.60	5.31/5.83	0.2909	0.7	4	5.74	5.06/6.02	0.1601	0.99	4	4.93
	Cv	5	7.15	5.74/9.91	5.8635	—	4	5.48	5.26/6.00	0.3017	—	—	—
Nitrogen	Gf	4	2.96	2.52/3.29	0.3350	0.478	5	2.90	2.41/3.45	0.3230	0.10	4	2.52
	Cv	5	2.85	2.70/3.11	0.1579	—	5	2.52	2.06/2.77	0.2629	—	5	2.77

(Continued)

of Liver

162 Days			Age 256 Days					All				
Min./Max.	σ	P	No.	Mean	Min./Max.	σ	P	No.	Mean	Min./Max.	σ	P
27.9 / 31.5	1.375	0.265	5	30.5	29.0 / 32.8	2.0407	0.750	13	29.7	27.8 / 32.8	1.8562	0.093
27.5 / 29.3	0.8450	—	3	29.0	29.0 / 29.1	1.3917	—	12	28.4	27.5 / 29.3	1.6963	—
4.51 / 5.04	0.2045	0.081	5	4.81	4.46 / 5.30	0.3433	<0.01	14	4.87	4.44 / 5.37	0.3013	0.385
4.00 / 4.69	0.3176	—	3	6.16	5.73 / 6.56	0.2721	—	11	5.08	4.00 / 6.56	0.7809	—
6.32 / 7.70	0.5307	—	4	9.89	8.82 / 11.2	0.9027	0.01	13	7.74	5.69 / 11.2	1.5672	0.084
—	—	—	3	6.9	6.6 / 7.3	0.7681	—	8	6.61	5.23 / 7.3	0.6730	—
3.26 / 3.76	0.08247	0.08	5	3.27	2.85 / 3.72	0.3777	0.805	14	3.44	2.85 / 4.50	0.4464	<0.01
3.13 / 3.54	0.1626	—	3	3.03	2.71 / 4.66	1.7239	—	13	3.03	2.21 / 4.66	0.6087	—

of Cecal Contents

162 Days			Age 256 Days					All				
Min./Max.	σ	P	No.	Mean	Min./Max.	σ	P	No.	Mean	Min./Max.	σ	P
21.3 / 28.9	3.8012	0.2	5	16.8	15.3 / 19.0	1.7082	<0.01	12	18.2	15.0 / 28.9	3.9403	<0.01
26.3 / 28.9	0.8588	—	3	24.8	24.5 / 25.1	0.2450	—	12	25.3	21.5 / 28.9	2.6985	—
15.8 / 15.9	0.050	<0.001	5	15.9	14.6 / 17.6	1.3602	<0.01	11	15.3	12.9 / 17.6	1.7147	<0.01
21.6 / 25.0	1.3086	—	3	24.0	23.5 / 24.3	1.3204	—	11	22.6	19.5 / 25.0	2.1558	—
—	—	—			—					—		
1.32 / 1.51	0.1276	—	3	1.35	1.21 / 1.44	0.0277	—	13	1.374	1.05 / 1.61	0.1354	—

of Kidney

162 Days			Age 256 Days					All				
Min./Max.	σ	P	No.	Mean	Min./Max.	σ	P	No.	Mean	Min./Max.	σ	P
23.5 / 26.9	0.3039	0.580	5	25.76	24.2 / 27.0	0.9178	0.645	13	25.3	23.0 / 27.0	1.092	0.775
23.9 / 27.3	0.502	—	3	26.2	25.8 / 26.9	1.4059	—	13	25.5	22.9 / 27.7	2.097	—
4.70 / 10.1	0.4327	0.99	4	5.97	4.54 / 7.70	1.1286	0.675	12	6.45	4.54 / 10.1	1.7240	0.390
5.10 / 10.1	1.7561	—	3	8.91	6.10 / 12.1	2.4642	—	13	7.12	5.10 / 12.1	1.9596	—
4.48 / 5.44	0.5926	—	5	6.00	4.61 / 7.17	3.1244	0.0135	16	5.59	4.48 / 7.17	0.7300	0.0340
—	—	—	3	6.70	6.40 / 6.90	0.2160	—	12	6.48	5.26 / 9.91	1.2566	—
2.33 / 2.72	0.1678	0.0565	4	2.98	2.82 / 3.32	0.0945	0.01	13	2.806	2.33 / 3.45	0.2856	0.08
2.60 / 3.07	0.1277	—	3	2.49	2.39 / 2.60	0.0860	—	13	2.61	2.06 / 3.07	0.2353	—

TABLE 5.5

		Age 29 Days					Age 67 Days					Composition Age	
	Category	No.	Mean	Min./Max.	σ	P	No.	Mean	Min./Max.	σ	P	No.	Mean
Dry weight	Gf	4	18.9	18.1/19.3	0.4062	0.021	3	20.66	20.1/21.6	0.8472	0.265	3	21.7
	Cv	5	19.6	18.0/20.4	0.2324	—	5	19.3	17.2/20.8	1.5697	—	5	19.2
Ash	Gf	5	8.40	6.97/10.7	2.2731	0.99	4	7.82	6.82/8.80	0.8896	0.031	3	6.98
	Cv	5	8.30	7.39/9.17	0.6009	—	5	6.61	6.19/7.10	0.2002	—	5	7.61
Fat	Gf	4	10.5	8.9/12.7	1.6553	<0.01	3	9.30	8.23/11.6	2.4489	0.705	3	8.54
	Cv	5	7.50	7.29/7.78	0.3093	—	5	8.79	8.26/9.70	0.4975	—	—	—
Nitrogen	Gf	—	—	—	—	—	—	—	—	—	—	—	—
	Cv	5	1.96	1.91/2.12	0.0808		4	1.78	1.56/1.95	0.0612	—	5	1.65

There was almost complete identity between the total nitrogen in the muscle of conventional birds and that of germfree birds at 10 weeks of age. At 4–7 weeks of age, it was seen that there was no difference between the riboflavin, niacin, pantothenic acid, biotin, folic acid, or vitamin B_{12} content of muscle from Leghorn chicks in the conventional or contaminated state. The vitamin C content of muscle of conventional birds was considerably greater than that of germfree birds. This interesting observation should bring to mind the suggestion of Reyniers et al. (1946) that germfree suckling rats may require vitamin C. Fraenkel (1954) found the carnitine content of the muscle of germfree chicks (175–350 μg/gm, dry tissue) to be comparable to that of conventional chicks.

The dry weight of the muscle of conventional rats at 67 and at 256 days was somewhat less than that of germfree rats (Table 5.5). Statistical significance was not reached by the data in other age groups. The muscle ash was almost identical in germfree and conventional rats, although there was a tendency at 67 days for the germfree rats to have higher muscle ash than the conventional rat. The conventional rats had a lower percentage of fat in the muscle than did the germfree rats at 29 days, a greater percentage at 67 days, and no difference at 256 days. The nitrogen and crude protein content of muscle was equivalent in germfree and conventional rats at 29, 162,

(Continued)

of Brain 162 Days			Age 256 Days					All				
Min. Max.	σ	P	No.	Mean	Min. Max.	σ	P	No.	Mean	Min. Max.	σ	P
20.1 23.4	0.6191	0.187	5	20.9	19.5 22.0	1.2830	0.535	11	21.05	19.5 23.4	1.1534	0.555
16.2 21.8	2.5413	—	3	20.3	18.3 21.3	0.7638	—	13	19.5	16.2 21.8	8.1147	—
6.69 7.56	0.7496	0.399	4	7.55	7.06 8.14	0.4988	0.645	11	7.49	6.69 8.80	0.7675	0.99
6.31 8.89	0.8698	—	3	8.97	8.0 10.1	0.8301	—	13	7.45	6.19 8.89	1.1236	—
4.41 12.5	0.9902	—	3	11.5	9.5 12.8	1.4353	0.99	9	9.85	4.41 12.8	2.5588	0.54
—	—	—	3	9.93	9.3 10.6	0.5903	—	8	9.22	8.26 10.6	0.7375	—
—	—	—	—	—	—	—	—	—	—	—	—	—
1.44 1.85	0.1623	—	3	1.64	1.42 1.83	0.1687	—	12	1.69	1.42 1.95	0.1617	—

and 256 days. However, at 67 days the conventional rats had less nitrogen in their muscle than did the germfree rats. The riboflavin, pantothenic acid, and folic acid content of muscle (Table 5.7) was similar in conventional and germfree rats. Conventional rats had only one-third as much biotin in their muscle as was present in germfree rats. No differences were noted (Gustafsson et al. 1957b) in the histamine content of muscle of germfree (1.7–4.9 µg/gm) and conventional (2.7–4.3 µg/gm) rats at 120 days of age.

The muscle of 2 germfree pups was found to average 21.3% (20.8–21.7%) dry weight and 3.7% (3.66–3.86) fat. Data from a single germfree rabbit is presented in Table 5.8. Küster (1914) found the water content of muscle in one germfree goat to be comparable to that of the naturally reared twin.

Circulatory System

The hearts of conventional birds and germfree chickens were similar in size, shape, relative weight, dry weight, color, and position by gross examination (Table 5.2). The values for relative weight of heart are lower than those obtained by Latimer (1924). This may be caused by the increased growth rate and/or the restricted movement of the individual. The blood vessels of germfree birds were grossly comparable to those of conventional birds.

TISSUE COMPOSITION IN GERMFREE AND CONVENTIONAL WHITE

		Age 2 weeks			Age 5 weeks					
	Gf Cv	Average wgt. 43 gm Average wgt. 50 gm			Average wgt. 143 gm Average wgt. 123 gm					
		No.	Mean	Limits	No.	Mean	Limits	σ	P	No.
Dry weight (%)	Gf	3	27.6	23.4 30.3	12	23.8	19.2 33.2	4.1	—	13
	Cv	2	23.5	23.0 24.0	11	22.9	18.3 34.2	4.2	0.63	13
										Composition
Dry weight (%)	Gf	3	23.2	22.6 24.0	12	22.0	16.8 26.5	2.6	—	13
	Cv	2	21.6	21.5 21.8	12	21.2	19.1 23.9	1.5	0.41	14
										Composition
Dry weight (%)	Gf	3	23.9	22.5 25.9	12	21.5	15.7 29.5	4.0	—	13
	Cv	2	19.9	17.6 22.2	11	22.0	18.6 28.6	3.2	0.77	14
										Composition
Dry weight (%)	Gf	3	22.3	21.1 23.8	12	24.1	19.7 30.9	3.0	—	13
	Cv	2	22.6	22.2 23.0	12	22.3	17.1 25.8	3.0	0.15	14
										Composition
Dry weight (%)	Gf	3	25.3	23.7 27.3	12	25.3	20.9 32.9	3.5	—	13
	Cv	2	24.2	22.0 26.5	11	24.5	22.1 27.6	1.9	0.49	14
										Composition
Dry weight (%)	Gf	3	28.8	24.4 34.2	12	24.1	19.8 33.3	3.3	—	13
	Cv	2	23.0	20.1 26.0	12	23.4	17.2 27.2	2.7	0.63	14
										Composition
Dry weight (%)	Gf	3	26.3	21.3 32.0	10	21.1	18.6 24.1	1.5	—	13
	Cv	2	23.7	22.4 25.1	12	22.0	15.5 26.9	3.2	0.43	14
										Composition
Dry weight (%)	Gf	—	—	—	8	15.2	9.7 19.8	—	—	4
	Cv	—	—	—	1	24.8	—	—	—	3
Ash (%, dry basis)	Gf	—	—	—	7	12.7	6.1 17.3	—	—	4
	Cv	—	—	—	1	11.6	—	—	—	3

5.6
WYANDOTTE BANTAM CHICKENS FED SYNTYPE DIET L-137

| | Age 8 weeks | | | | Age 23 weeks | | | | | Age 32-52 weeks | | |
| | Average wgt. 273 gm / Average wgt. 237 gm | | | | Average wgt. 847 gm / Average wgt. 667 gm | | | | | Average wgt. 813 gm / Average wgt. 944 gm | | |
Organ	Mean	Limits	σ	P	No.	Mean	Limits	σ	P	No.	Mean	Limits
	22.6	19.7–24.6	1.4	—	5	25.5	20.6–28.6	2.6	—	3	25.8	25.2–26.2
	23.1	19.4–26.6	2.0	0.53	6	25.4	23.1–31.2	2.7	1.00	3	24.6	23.1–26.4
of Heart	21.5	20.1–24.2	1.2	—	5	23.2	21.1–25.8	1.8	—	3	23.0	22.7–23.4
	21.1	19.4–27.4	1.7	0.40	7	23.0	20.3–26.0	2.0	0.80	3	22.6	21.5–23.8
of Lungs	22.8	20.1–25.5	3.3	—	5	25.7	24.8–28.6	1.4	—	3	27.3	26.1–29.4
	21.9	17.6–26.1	3.1	0.48	7	25.3	23.2–28.0	1.9	0.73	3	21.5	17.8–23.7
of Proventriculus	24.3	22.6–27.0	1.3	—	5	25.6	23.6–28.7	1.7	—	3	24.5	23.3–25.4
	23.9	19.9–27.3	1.7	0.44	7	25.4	23.5–28.1	1.7	0.86	3	23.5	22.6–24.1
of Gizzard	23.6	21.0–25.7	1.7	—	5	26.5	23.4–29.7	1.4	—	3	26.9	24.9–29.5
	23.7	18.6–27.9	2.4	0.98	6	27.4	23.7–30.0	2.3	0.54	3	25.0	23.4–27.0
of Small Intestine	25.7	20.3–30.4	2.7	—	5	27.6	25.4–29.8	1.4	—	3	30.2	25.9–32.4
	24.7	21.4–30.1	2.3	0.30	7	25.5	22.6–28.8	1.8	0.07	3	28.2	27.5–28.8
of Ceca	24.3	21.6–27.6	1.8	—	5	28.3	26.2–30.4	1.6	—	3	23.4	19.4–25.5
	23.4	17.5–27.6	2.7	0.29	7	23.3	19.8–27.2	2.9	0.01	3	21.1	18.6–23.2
of Cecal Contents	13.2	12.2–14.5	0.83	—	5	15.2	11.9–20.9	—	—	—	—	—
	25.6	21.8–27.8	2.72	<0.01	1	26.9	—	—	—	—	—	—
	12.9	9.2–19.5	4.0	—	5	13.6	10.7–18.3	—	—	—	—	—
	12.9	10.8–15.6	2.2	1.00	1	18.6	—	—	—	—	—	—

TABLE 5.6

		Age 2 weeks			Age 5 weeks					
	Gf	Average wgt. 43 gm			Average wgt. 143 gm					
	Cv	Average wgt. 50 gm			Average wgt. 123 gm					
		No.	Mean	Limits	No.	Mean	Limits	σ	P	No.
										Composition
Fat (%)	Gf	—	—	—	3	2.68	2.29 3.34	—	—	—
	Cv	—	—	—	2	3.33	2.23 4.43	—	—	—
Nitrogen (%, total)	Gf	—	—	—	—	—	—	—	—	—
	Cv	—	—	—	—	—	—	—	—	—
Thiamine (μg/gm)	Gf	—	—	—	—	—	—	—	—	2
	Cv	—	—	—	—	—	—	—	—	—
Riboflavin (μg/gm)	Gf	—	—	—	4	44.8	6.6 88.4	31.59	—	3
	Cv	—	—	—	3	16.5	6.3 24.9	7.72	0.25	1
Niacin (μg/gm)	Gf	—	—	—	2	3.9	2.7 5.1	—	—	3
	Cv	—	—	—	3	82.8	24.1 166.0	—	—	2
Pantothenic acid (μg/gm)	Gf	—	—	—	2	55.7	37.6 73.8	—	—	3
	Cv	—	—	—	2	28.4	26.0 30.8	—	—	1
Pyridoxine (μg/gm)	Gf	—	—	—	—	—	—	—	—	3
	Cv	—	—	—	—	—	—	—	—	1
Biotin (μg/gm)	Gf	—	—	—	—	—	—	—	—	3
	Cv	—	—	—	—	—	—	—	—	2
Folic acid (μg/gm)	Gf	—	—	—	2	2.19	2.16 2.22	—	—	1
	Cv	—	—	—	—	—	—	—	—	—
										Composition
Dry weight (%)	Gf	3	28.3	26.3 32.3	12	28.4	23.3 39.0	4.8	—	13
	Cv	2	28.7	28.5 28.8	12	26.4	22.4 30.2	2.4	0.23	14
Ash (%, dry basis)	Gf	—	—	—	13	5.50	4.67 6.31	0.641	—	10
	Cv	—	—	—	7	5.28	4.61 6.11	0.438	0.45	8
Fat (%)	Gf	—	—	—	11	5.32	4.31 6.81	0.705	—	10
	Cv	—	—	—	8	6.06	4.82 7.29	0.852	0.07	6
Phosphorus (%)	Gf	—	—	—	—	—	—	—	—	5
	Cv	—	—	—	4	0.626	0.464 0.816	—	—	5

(Continued)

	Age 8 weeks Average wgt. 273 gm Average wgt. 237 gm				Age 23 weeks Average wgt. 847 gm Average wgt. 667 gm					Age 32-52 weeks Average wgt. 813 gm Average wgt. 944 gm		
	Mean	Limits	σ	P	No.	Mean	Limits	σ	P	No.	Mean	Limits
of Cecal Contents (continued)												
	—	—	—	—	1	3.19	—	—	—	—	—	—
	—	—	—	—	—	—	—	—	—	—	—	—
	—	—	—	—	3	1.26	1.16 / 1.39	—	—	—	—	—
	—	—	—	—	1	2.38	—	—	—	—	—	—
	8.75	5.2 / 12.3	—	—	4	4.16	2.12 / 6.45	1.66	—	2	8.77	5.84 / 11.70
	—	—	—	—	3	8.68	5.78 / 12.00	2.56	0.05	2	11.30	9.31 / 13.30
	17.0	15.7 / 18.7	—	—	2	5.51	4.98 / 6.04	—	—	3	4.43	2.37 / 7.00
	5.3	—	—	—	—	—	—	—	—	2	8.90	5.32 / 12.40
	14.6	10.2 / 23.3	—	—	—	—	—	—	—	3	19.1	11.4 / 25.1
	48.3	38.5 / 58.0	—	—	—	—	—	—	—	2	56.6	45.8 / 67.3
	37.7	33.6 / 42.8	—	—	—	—	—	—	—	3	20.6	6.7 / 32.5
	11.6	—	—	—	—	—	—	—	—	2	20.9	16.3 / 25.5
	1.8	1.2 / 2.5	—	—	4	0.89	0.72 / 1.12	—	—	2	2.0	1.5 / 2.5
	2.4	—	—	—	—	—	—	—	—	1	5.9	—
	0.766	0.705 / 0.821	—	—	—	—	—	—	—	2	0.749	0.595 / 0.904
	2.050	0.703 / 3.410	—	—	—	—	—	—	—	2	4.900	0.640 / 9.160
	2.13	—	—	—	—	—	—	—	—	2	0.527	0.372 / 0.687
	—	—	—	—	—	—	—	—	—	2	2.24	1.71 / 2.77
of Liver												
	27.6	23.1 / 33.2	2.3	—	5	29.9	29.2 / 31.8	1.0	—	3	28.1	26.6 / 29.7
	29.3	26.2 / 34.7	2.1	0.06	7	31.2	27.2 / 34.0	2.7	0.37	3	27.9	25.5 / 30.8
	5.23	4.47 / 6.14	0.558	—	5	4.26	3.97 / 4.54	0.22	—	3	5.19	5.01 / 5.53
	5.68	4.34 / 6.82	0.619	0.14	3	5.17	3.92 / 6.68	1.14	0.17	2	5.04	4.35 / 5.85
	5.41	3.95 / 7.17	0.893	—	5	6.07	5.78 / 6.71	0.328	—	3	4.58	3.20 / 5.60
	5.71	4.71 / 6.60	0.725	0.52	2	6.13	5.16 / 7.10	—	—	2	7.09	5.33 / 8.85
	0.818	0.341 / 1.28	0.397	—	1	0.882	—	—	—	3	0.545	0.340 / 0.882
	1.06	0.702 / 1.49	0.277	0.07	—	—	—	—	—	2	1.09	0.92 / 1.26

TABLE 5.6

	Gf Cv	Age 2 weeks Average wgt. 43 gm Average wgt. 50 gm			Age 5 weeks Average wgt. 143 gm Average wgt. 123 gm					
		No.	Mean	Limits	No.	Mean	Limits	σ	P	No.
										Composition
Nitrogen (%, total)	Gf	—	—	—	—	—	—	—	—	5
	Cv	—	—	—	4	3.16	2.50 3.72	—	—	1
N P N (%)	Gf	—	—	—	—	—	—	—	—	2
	Cv	—	—	—	2	0.054	0.047 0.06	—	—	—
Thiamine (µg/gm)	Gf	—	—	—	11	2.99	1.57 4.77	1.12	—	4
	Cv	—	—	—	3	6.19	4.73 7.43	1.11	<0.01	3
Riboflavin (µg/gm)	Gf	—	—	—	10	13.7	12.2 17.0	1.57	—	5
	Cv	—	—	—	5	12.4	9.9 14.9	1.84	0.20	3
Niacin (µg/gm)	Gf	—	—	—	7	103	61 147	28.4	—	7
	Cv	—	—	—	3	124	108 152	19.9	0.35	3
Pantothenic acid (µg/gm)	Gf	—	—	—	7	98.1	60.0 142.0	29.6	—	6
	Cv	—	—	—	3	37.4	26.4 57.4	14.7	0.02	3
Pyridoxine (µg/gm)	Gf	—	—	—	7	8.97	6.1 11.5	2.28	—	7
	Cv	—	—	—	4	8.74	7.5 9.8	0.91	0.86	2
Biotin (µg/gm)	Gf	—	—	—	3	18.9	15.8 21.8	2.46	—	5
	Cv	—	—	—	3	21.6	17.8 24.6	2.82	0.35	3
Folic acid (µg/gm)	Gf	—	—	—	4	7.65	6.51 9.66	1.09	—	7
	Cv	—	—	—	3	4.15	1.63 5.68	1.92	0.04	2
										Composition
Dry weight (%)	Gf	3	28.6	22.9 35.4	12	26.1	20.5 32.8	3.7	—	12
	Cv	2	21.5	17.4 25.4	12	26.6	19.8 31.2	2.7	0.69	14
										Composition
Dry weight (%)	Gf	—	—	—	6	18.7	10.8 25.9	—	—	3
	Cv	—	—	—	4	17.0	13.9 19.1	—	—	2
										Composition
Dry weight (%)	Gf	—	—	—	5	19.6	13.9 26.6	5.1	—	9
	Cv	—	—	—	7	20.6	14.0 30.4	6.1	0.79	9

	Age 8 weeks					Age 23 weeks					Age 32-52 weeks	
	Average wgt. 273 gm Average wgt. 237 gm					Average wgt. 847 gm Average wgt. 667 gm					Average wgt. 813 gm Average wgt. 944 gm	
Mean	Limits	σ	P	No.	Mean	Limits	σ	P	No.	Mean	Limits
of Liver (Continued)											
3.11	2.94 3.35	—	—	4	3.03	2.88 3.12	—	—	2	3.19	3.16 3.21
2.46	—	—	—	—	—	—	—	—	2	2.77	2.39 3.14
0.16	0.10 0.22	—	—	—	—	—	—	—	2	0.23	0.22 0.23
—	—	—	—	—	—	—	—	—	1	0.10	—
3.76	2.31 4.08	1.03	—	4	8.04	7.00 8.71	0.40	—	2	7.22	5.92 8.52
3.40	2.92 3.64	0.34	0.71	3	7.43	5.85 10.3	1.89	0.60	2	13.18	7.96 18.4
8.08	6.16 10.1	1.63	—	5	7.71	4.40 10.4	2.52	—	3	17.8	11.5 23.5
15.50	8.75 19.9	4.85	0.03	3	12.10	7.66 18.0	4.37	0.16	2	22.9	16.2 29.6
131	83 185	32.2	—	5	133	99 169	23.2	—	3	149	138 163
88	65 100	16.5	0.09	3	169	135 236	45.5	0.23	2	126	119 133
65.9	57.2 77.5	6.7	—	5	80.2	57.8 99.6	18.8	—	—	—	—
84.1	62.6 101.0	16.1	0.07	3	73.7	65.3 87.1	9.6	0.63	—	—	—
8.58	7.1 9.5	—	—	5	11.6	7.7 14.1	2.31	—	2	8.8	7.5 10.0
9.97	8.8 11.1	—	—	3	10.4	9.3 11.7	1.00	0.15	2	8.0	7.4 8.5
13.1	12.0 16.7	1.36	—	5	13.2	10.8 15.8	2.06	—	3	12.7	5.2 19.1
11.9	8.8 15.8	2.91	0.52	3	12.6	9.2 25.3	7.83	0.89	2	17.7	15.1 20.2
2.61	1.90 3.76	—	—	5	2.81	1.78 4.12	0.92	—	2	4.21	4.02 4.49
5.90	4.29 7.40	—	—	3	2.42	1.21 3.95	1.14	0.65	2	7.85	6.18 9.62
of Pancreas											
29.3	25.7 32.7	2.3	—	5	32.0	28.8 36.6	3.4	—	3	30.7	28.7 32.6
26.6	22.8 30.7	1.9	0.01	7	28.1	22.9 34.0	3.5	0.18	3	26.3	22.0 28.6
of Testicles											
14.4	12.8 16.2	—	—	3	14.7	14.5 14.9	—	—	1	13.1	—
19.9	19.3 20.5	—	—	2	14.2	13.3 15.2	—	—	2	13.7	13.3 14.2
of Ovary											
18.0	15.1 21.2	2.0	—	—	—	—	—	—	—	—	—
17.4	13.5 21.4	2.5	0.62	—	—	—	—	—	—	—	—

TABLE 5.6

	Gf / Cv	Age 2 weeks Average wgt. Gf 43 gm / Cv 50 gm			Age 5 weeks Average wgt. Gf 143 gm / Cv 123 gm					
		No.	Mean	Limits	No.	Mean	Limits	σ	P	No.
										Composition
Dry weight (%)	Gf	3	24.3	20.1 28.0	12	23.0	17.7 30.2	3.4	—	12
	Cv	2	21.3	20.4 22.2	12	23.0	18.1 32.8	3.5	1.00	13
										Composition
Dry weight (%)	Gf	3	18.0	16.3 19.0	12	17.4	13.4 22.8	2.9	—	13
	Cv	2	20.3	19.7 21.0	12	17.2	13.2 22.3	2.4	0.85	11
										Composition
Dry weight (%)	Gf	1	26.1	—	10	22.3	17.1 28.0	3.8	—	13
	Cv	2	25.6	25.6 25.6	11	21.0	17.2 29.3	3.3	0.42	14
Lymphocyte concentration ($\times 10^6$ per mm^3 fresh tissue)	Gf	—	—	—	10	1.0	0.7 1.6	0.3	—	13
	Cv	—	—	—	11	1.0	0.7 1.4	0.2	0.90	11
										Composition
Dry weight (%)	Gf	3	20.9	20.0 22.5	12	18.9	14.7 22.9	2.4	—	13
	Cv	2	17.5	17.0 18.1	12	18.2	13.1 21.3	1.2	0.36	14
										Composition
Dry weight (%)	Gf	3	22.0	15.6 27.2	12	20.9	13.0 24.6	3.6	—	13
	Cv	2	19.9	16.2 23.6	12	21.6	18.1 28.3	3.3	0.70	14
Thymocyte concentration ($\times 10^6$ per mm^3 fresh tissue)	Gf	—	—	—	11	3.8	2.7 5.2	0.8	—	13
	Cv	—	—	—	10	4.0	2.6 5.8	1.0	0.56	11

(Continued)

	Age 8 Weeks				Age 23 weeks				Age 32-52 weeks		
	Average wgt. 273 gm Average wgt. 237 gm				Average wgt. 847 gm Average wgt. 667 gm				Average wgt. 813 gm Average wgt. 944 gm		
Mean	Limits	σ	P	No.	Mean	Limits	σ	P	No.	Mean	Limits
of Kidney											
22.4	19.1–26.5	2.3	—	5	23.1	21.1–26.2	1.7	—	3	22.9	19.8–25.3
21.7	17.6–25.2	1.8	0.44	7	24.2	21.0–28.2	2.7	0.46	2	21.6	20.5–22.8
of Brain											
18.7	17.1–20.8	1.1	—	5	19.6	18.3–21.6	1.3	—	3	20.6	19.3–21.8
18.7	17.1–20.6	1.1	1.00	7	19.1	18.0–20.4	1.0	0.47	2	19.7	19.2–20.2
of Spleen											
21.6	18.6–26.0	2.0	—	5	25.3	23.6–27.4	1.3	—	3	24.8	23.5–25.8
21.9	20.2–27.0	1.6	—	7	23.0	20.7–25.8	1.7	0.04	3	22.5	21.9–22.9
1.7	1.1–2.3	0.4	—	5	2.0	1.3–2.7	0.5	—	—	—	—
1.4	1.1–2.0	0.3	0.12	6	1.4	1.0–1.8	0.3	0.05	—	—	—
of Bursa											
19.6	16.3–23.8	1.8	—	—	—	—	—	—	—	—	—
18.8	14.6–22.7	1.7	0.29	—	—	—	—	—	—	—	—
of Thymus											
21.0	18.6–23.1	1.5	—	5	22.7	21.4–24.9	1.3	—	3	22.4	18.9–25.2
19.8	18.0–20.9	0.8	0.02	6	23.8	20.4–28.4	3.1	0.55	3	23.7	21.0–26.9
4.3	3.4–5.0	0.5	—	5	3.6	2.0–4.9	1.1	—	—	—	—
3.9	3.3–5.0	0.6	0.11	6	3.6	2.0–5.5	1.6	1.00	—	—	—

TABLE 5.7
VITAMINS IN RAT MUSCLE

	Germfree rats[a]		Conventional rats[a]	
	Mean	Min - Max	Mean	Min - Max
Weight (gm)	268	205 - 368	376	268 - 484
Riboflavin (μg/gm)[b]	1.89	1.61 - 2.11	1.99	1.28 - 2.95
Pantothenic acid (μg/gm)	19.2	15.9 - 21.2	21.3	10.8 - 43.0
Biotin (μg/gm)	0.455	0.412 - 0.537	0.158	0.142 - 0.201
Folic acid (μg/gm)	0.779	0.252 - 2.49	0.620[c]	0.469 - 772

[a]Age, 162 ± 17 days; 3 males, 3 females.
[b]All vitamin concentrations are given in μg/gm on a fresh weight basis.
[c]Only 2 rats in this group; all other groups have 6.

Phillips *et al.* (1959) found the circulatory system of adult germfree quinea pigs to be in normal condition, and Glimstedt (1936a) found the hearts of germfree and conventional guinea pigs to have the same relative weight (Table 5.9). Gordon (1960b) found no difference between the heart size of germfree and conventional rats. The circulatory system of germfree and conventional mice are comparable by gross observation at autopsy.

TABLE 5.8
ANALYSIS OF GERMFREE RABBIT[a]

	Liver	Muscle	Cecum	Bone	Brain
Dry wt (%)	29.9	23.8	16.0	75.2	25.4
Ash (dry basis, %)	4.7	14.0	9.9	66.2	5.4
Niacin (μg/gm)	92	92	50.	—	—
Riboflavin (μg/gm)	10.3	2.4	1.7	—	—
Pantothenate (μg/gm)	22.0	5.3	6.5	—	—
Biotin (μg/gm)	4.3	0.083	0.028	—	—
Folic acid (μg/gm)	1.94	0.084	0.44	—	—

[a]Female, 9 months old.

Blood Morphology

Blood samples taken from germfree White Leghorn chicks have the same gross appearance as those taken from conventional birds. In

TABLE 5.9
ORGAN WEIGHT IN GUINEA PIGS[a]

Organ	Age 30 days				Age 61 days			
	Conventional (7)[b]		Germfree (5)[b]		Conventional (12)[b]		Germfree (3)[b]	
	Mean	Percent of body[c]	Mean	Percent of body[c]	Mean	Percent of body[c]	Mean	Percent of body[c]
Body weight	—	—	170	—	—	—	298	—
Body weight without ingesta	176	100	141	100	308	100	238	100
Lymph nodes	0.654	0.372	0.147	0.104	0.880	0.286	0.237	0.0995
Lymph nodes, cervical	0.144	0.0818	0.024	0.017	0.190	0.0617	0.050	0.021
Lymph nodes, scapular	0.050	0.0284	0.018	0.013	0.068	0.221	0.029	0.012
Lymph nodes, inguinal	0.045	0.0256	0.016	0.011	0.76	0.0247	0.033	0.014
Lymph nodes, mesenteric	0.349	0.198	0.066	0.0468	0.390	0.127	0.093	0.0391
Lymph nodes, pancreatic	0.024	0.0137	0.011	0.0078	0.064	0.0208	0.018	0.0076
Lymph nodes, bronchial	0.027	0.0153	0.007	0.0050	0.076	0.0247	0.014	0.0059
Spleen	0.301	0.171	0.160	0.114	0.483	0.0157	0.291	0.122
White pulp	0.039	0.0222	0.016	0.0114	0.085	0.0276	0.039	0.0163
Total lymph	0.693	0.394	0.164	0.116	0.958	0.318	0.276	0.116
Thymus	0.240	0.136	0.122	0.0864	0.304	0.0986	0.131	0.055
Liver	8.243	4.68	5.9	4.19	14.94	4.85	10.2	4.3
Kidney	1.80	1.02	1.17	0.830	3.36	1.082	2.13	0.894
Adrenal	0.072	0.0409	0.056	0.0397	0.204	0.0662	0.131	0.055
Heart	0.613	0.348	0.47	0.333	1.25	0.406	0.86	0.361
Lung	1.38	0.786	0.91	0.645	2.609	0.847	1.74	0.732
Gastrointestinal tract without ingesta	18.43	9.80	11.3	8.02	22.73	7.37	13.5	5.67
Gastrointestinal tract with ingesta	27.3	—	44	—	48.6	—	60	—

[a] From Glimstedt (1936a).
[b] Numbers in parentheses indicate number of animals.
[c] Percent body weight taken without ingesta.

TABLE 5.10
HEMATOLOGY OF GERMFREE AND CONVENTIONAL ANIMALS

White Wyandotte Bantam chick (Gordon)

	Category	Age 2 weeks (2/2)[a]		Age 5 weeks (10-12/11-12)[a]				Age 8 weeks (14/13)[a]				Age 23 weeks (7/5)[a]			
		Mean	Limits	Mean	Limits	σ	P	Mean	Limits	σ	P	Mean	Limits	σ	P
Hemoglobin (%)	Gf	9.53	9.41 9.65	9.20	7.66 13.56	1.68	—	8.82	7.59 11.37	1.02	—	12.04	10.35 13.97	1.52	—
	Cv	9.38	8.26 10.50	8.53	6.08 13.11	1.89	0.42	8.99	6.26 11.21	1.19	0.71	10.92	8.70 13.00	1.50	0.28
Red blood cells x 10[3]	Gf	3.50	3.17 3.83	3.47	2.83 4.20	0.38	—	3.18	2.11 4.10	0.57	0.97	3.41	3.03 4.05	0.38	—
	Cv	2.84	2.74 2.93	2.96	2.46 3.67	0.35	<0.01	3.17	2.50 4.28	0.50	—	3.47	2.42 4.49	0.71	0.87
White blood cells[b]	Gf	10.42	8.14 12.70	14.17	5.10 31.60	6.76	—	18.14	9.63 26.50	5.65	—	19.72	12.80 25.60	4.48	—
	Cv	15.95	13.90 18.00	21.54	6.90 44.50	9.58	0.05	31.55	9.35 79.00	16.47	0.01	35.17	19.00 51.80	11.45	0.03
Heterophils[b] (chick) or Neutrophils[b] (mammal)	Gf	4.29	2.36 6.22	3.42	0.71 7.90	1.86	—	5.87	2.52 10.34	2.65	—	4.11	1.22 6.91	2.27	—
	Cv	3.37	3.34 3.40	3.53	1.45 6.00	1.41	0.88	5.00	1.68 15.00	3.61	0.50	4.57	1.04 8.88	2.21	0.76
Eosinophils[b]	Gf	0.08	0 0.16	0.04	0 0.32	0.10	—	0.15	0 0.58	0.16	—	0.12	0 0.23	0.10	—
	Cv	0.14	0 0.28	0.06	0 0.27	—	0.90	0.07	0 0.44	0.14	0.90	0.10	0 0.46	0.17	1.00
Basophils[b]	Gf	0.72	0.63 0.81	0.41	0 0.71	0.21	—	0.62	0.12 1.23	0.32	—	0.60	0.17 1.02	0.34	—
	Cv	0.60	0.36 0.83	0.81	0.20 1.86	0.48	0.02	0.74	0.20 2.00	0.61	0.50	0.76	0 2.07	0.62	0.65
Lymphocytes[b]	Gf	5.07	4.64 5.50	9.46	3.90 21.50	4.78	—	10.67	5.20 18.60	4.16	—	13.81	9.86 17.01	2.90	—
	Cv	10.71	8.62 12.80	16.23	5.00 36.00	7.99	0.03	24.42	6.45 61.60	13.05	<0.01	27.93	13.90 45.60	10.77	0.07

		White Leghorn chick (Gordon)								Guinea pig					Rat (Gordon)		
		Age 4-7 weeks (7/6)[a]				Age 10-1/2 weeks (4/4)[a]				Miyakawa Age 4 weeks (5/3)[a]		Phillips Age 4 weeks (10)[a]			Age 12-14 weeks (9/6)[a]		
		Mean	Limits	σ	P	Mean	Limits	σ	P	Mean	Limits	Mean	Limits	P	Mean	Limits	P
Monocytes[b]	Gf	0.27	0.16–0.38	0.73	—	0.55	0.10–1.90	0.82	—	0.26	0.35–1.23	1.09	0.51–1.63	—	0.37	—	—
	Cv	1.14	0.83–1.44		—	0.59	0–1.78	0.72	—	0.96	0.31–3.55	1.81	1.14–3.11	0.69	—	—	0.09
Whole blood clotting (sec)	Gf	900	840–960	231	—	207	61–685	327	—	207	93–755	184	115–252	—	47	—	—
	Cv	96	90–103	155	—	133	27–433	294	—	171	90–640	335	232–475	—	82	—	<0.01
Hemoglobin (%)	Gf	—	—			10.27	8.36–11.71	1.25	—	—	—	14.9	11.7–17.1	—	—	—	—
	Cv	—	—			8.72	8.13–9.57	0.59	0.10	—	—	—	—	—	—	—	—
Red blood cells x10³	Gf	2.79	2.44–3.24	0.32	—	3.05	2.54–3.55	0.40	—	—	—	5.73	3.54–7.52	0.01	10.2	—	0.01
	Cv	2.77	2.48–3.32	0.67	1.00	3.05	2.68–3.41	0.33	1.00	—	—	—	—	—	8.1	—	—
White blood cells[b]	Gf	8.45	3.58–12.67	2.96	—	13.03	9.30–17.46	3.27	—	2.07	1.80–2.50	1.90	0.80–5.75	—	4.91	—	0.23
	Cv	24.28	9.88–44.40	12.06	0.02	26.86	10.00–44.40	13.36	0.13	2.84	2.40–3.50	—	—	—	6.71	—	—
Heterophils[b] (chick) or Neutrophils[b] (mammal)	Gf	2.34	0.90–3.09	0.76	—	2.82	1.40–3.60	0.85	—	0.568	0.560–0.575	1.05	0.30–1.56	—	0.69	—	0.01
	Cv	2.80	0.78–6.66	2.01	0.65	2.69	1.90–4.00	0.83	0.84	1.020	0.820–1.540	—	—	—	1.36	—	—
Eosinophils[b]	Gf	0.10	0–0.33	0.11	—	0.23	0–0.35	0.14	—	0	0–0.02	0	0–0.02	—	0.048	—	0.14
	Cv	0	0	0	—	0.02	0–0.10	0.04	—	0.04	0–0.08	—	—	—	0.099	—	—

TABLE 5.10 (Continued)

		White Leghorn chick (Gordon)								Guinea pig				Rat (Gordon)		
		Age 4-7 weeks (7/6)[a]				Age 10-1/2 weeks (4/4)[a]				Miyakawa Age 4 weeks (5/3)[a]		Phillips Age 4 weeks (10)[a]		Age 12-14 weeks (9/6)[a]		
		Mean	Limits	σ	P	Mean	Limits	σ	P	Mean	Limits	Mean	Limits	Mean	Limits	P
Basophils[b]	Gf	0.41	0.22 0.76	0.17	—	1.11	0.85 1.20	0.15	—	0.014	0 0.02	0.01	0 0.04	0	—	—
	Cv	0.77	0 1.78	0.59	0.20	0.70	0 1.72	0.64	0.33	0.025	0 0.03	—	—	0	—	—
Lymphocytes[b]	Gf	5.32	2.40 8.50	2.07	—	8.32	5.77 11.91	2.56	—	1.40	1.18 1.81	0.80	0.32 1.56	3.86	—	0.40
	Cv	19.99	7.71 39.52	10.64	<0.01	22.81	7.40 39.5	12.50	0.09	1.61	0.70 2.95	—	—	4.61	—	—
Monocytes[b]	Gf	0.29	0.07 0.44	0.14	—	0.55	0.10 0.74	0.26	—	0.052	0.028 0.070	0.049	0 0.133	0.14	—	0.45
	Cv	0.72	0 3.38	1.10	0.40	0.66	0.30 1.03	0.31	0.65	0.084	0.032 0.129	—	—	0.09	—	—
Whole blood clotting (sec)	Gf	260	42 600	206	—	313	15 483	183	—	—	—	—	—	—	—	—
	Cv	243	40 408	122	0.98	321	115 463	131	1.00	—	—	—	—	—	—	—

[a] Numbers in parentheses indicate number conventional/number germfree.
[b] $\times 10^3$ per mm³.

324

the younger germfree White Wyandotte Bantam birds, the red blood cell count was somewhat higher than in conventional chickens. In the older groups and in all groups of the White Leghorn birds, the morphologic similarity of the circulating red blood cells was confirmed by microscopic observation. Nor were differences seen in hemoglobin or hematocrit values in any category when germfree and conventional chicks of the same age group were compared (Table 5.10).

The white blood cells of the conventional birds were generally 2–5 times more numerous than those of germfree birds. The lymphocytes presented the same picture as the total white blood count. Despite the high variability, the differences were great enough that it might be said with statistical confidence that the presence of living microorganisms and/or their products had an effect on the numbers of circulating lymphocytes. In both germfree and conventional birds, there was a preponderance of the small lymphocytes which usually amounted to about 65% of the total. The morphology of the lymphocytes originating from the germfree or conventional birds were comparable by microscopic observation.

The expressed blood volume of germfree and conventional Leghorn chicks was 5.2% of the body weight. Total circulating blood volumes have not been reported for any germfree animal. Zweifach *et al.* (1958) reported the blood pressure for pentobarbital anesthetized germfree rats ranged between 145 and 165 mm Hg, while the blood pressure of similarily treated conventional rats was only 100–120 mm Hg.

The morphologic characteristics of the cells in peripheral blood of germfree guinea pigs as presented by Tajima (1955) and Miyakawa *et al.* (1958c) and Phillips *et al.* (1959b) are summarized in Table 5.10. The red cells of germfree and conventional guinea pigs were morphologically comparable according to Tajima (1955). Phillips *et al.* (1959) and Horton and Hickey (1961) found that the hemoglobin, hematocrit, and red blood cell counts of germfree guinea pigs were not significantly different from the values of conventional guinea pigs. The data indicated increased white cell count, eosinophil population, granulocyte count, and lymphocyte count in the blood of conventional guinea pigs when compared to germfree animals. The decreased proportion of lymphocytes of total blood leucocytes, from 88% to 54%, seen during the first 20 days of life in a conventional guinea pig was not seen (Miyakawa *et al.*, 1957a) in germfree guinea pigs until a much later age. The number of mitochondria per lymphocyte increased from 10.1 in late embryos to 13.5 in conventional guinea pigs at one month, while no change was seen in the number (9.5) seen in germfree guinea pigs (Tajima, 1955). The percentage of neutrophils in germfree guinea pigs (82%) was much higher than the 8–23% found in conventional guinea pigs; in contrast to this, the lymphocytes constitute a lower percentage in germfree guinea pigs (42%) than the 76–90% usually encountered in conventional guinea pigs.

The cellular components of the blood of germfree rats did not follow entirely the pattern seen in chicks and guinea pigs as shown by the data of Gordon (1959a,b). The germfree male rats 85–95 days of age showed a statistically significant greater quantity of red blood cells than was found in the conventional rats. The total white blood cell count was lower in the germfree rats than in the conventional rats but the difference was not as striking as seen for other species, nor was the difference of statistical significance ($p = 0.23$), nor did the lymphocyte count show a difference ($p = 0.40$). Apparent contradictions found when different species are compared may reflect differences in antigenicity of diets.

Heterophils and Neutrophils

In both White Leghorn and White Wyandotte Bantam chickens, the conventional birds had the same number of circulating heterophils in both young and old birds. Although differences were indicated, they were never statistically significant. Females in both environments were found to have somewhat higher values than the males. No morphological difference was seen in the heterophils, most of which were mature forms.

The neutrophil count was only ½ as great in germfree rats as in conventional rats according to Gordon (1959b). Tajima (1955) and Miyakawa (1958a) found this same relationship in guinea pigs.

Eosinophils and Basophils

Generally, there was no difference in the number or morphology of circulating eosinophils and basophils found in either Wyandotte Bantam or Leghorn chickens, irrespective of their germfree or conventional status. Several animals in both groups were found which had no heterophils of the basophilic type. Among conventional birds twice as many were found to be free of eosinophil cells as were found among the germfree birds.

No eosinophils were seen and basophilic cells were rare in the blood of germfree guinea pigs 22–70 days old examined by Phillips *et al.* (1959). They saw no Kurloff cells in germfree guinea pigs, while Tajima (1955) found almost as many Kurloff cells in the blood of germfree guinea pigs as he found in conventional animals, and cited this as evidence that Kurloff cells are not parasites. Gordon (1959b) found no basophil cells in the blood of germfree or conventional rats. The increased number of eosinophils seen in conventional rat blood above those found in germfree rat blood was not significant.

Monocytes

In White Wyandotte Bantam chicks, the absolute monocyte count in the blood of conventional birds was 2 times greater than that seen in germfree birds after six weeks of age. Microscopically, no differences were seen in the morphology of the monocyte whether its origin was from germfree or conventional birds. No clear picture was seen from monocyte counts in White Leghorn chicks where great variability masked any possibility for statistical difference. Miyakawa (1958a) found more monocytes in conventional guinea pigs than in germfree animals. No difference was seen between germfree and conventional rats in the monocyte count of the blood (Gordon, 1959b).

Blood Clotting

In White Wyandotte Bantam chicks fed a complete diet, L-137, there was an apparent prolonged whole blood clotting time in the young chick 2 weeks old. This decreased by the 5th week from 900 to 251 seconds. At 23 weeks of age the clotting time in germfree chicks was statistically less than was found for the conventional birds. The whole blood clotting time of germfree and conventional White Leghorn chicks were almost identical at 4 to 10 weeks of age. Details of the requirement of germfree chicks and rats for vitamin K are presented in the nutrition chapter.

Biochemistry of Blood

No riboflavin could be found in the whole blood of either germfree or conventional White Leghorn chicks fed diet L-245. No niacin could be found by microbiological assay in the blood of conventional chicks fed this diet while niacin was present (2.62 μg/gm) in the blood of germfree birds. This phenomenon should be investigated further to look for a bacterial inhibitor. The whole blood of germfree White Leghorn chicks contained pantothenic acid (0.89 μg/gm), folic acid (0.72 μg/gm), and vitamin B_{12} (2.86 mμg/gm) in concentrations similar to those found in conventional birds fed the same diets.

Melville and Horner (1953) reported 5.8 mg ergothionine per 100 ml of red blood cells in germfree chicks at 5 weeks of age. Conventional chicks erythrocytes contained 3.8 mg per 100 ml. This finding indicated that ergothionine comes from sources other than the intestinal microflora.

Forbes *et al.* (1958a) found no difference between the serum concentration of cholesterol in germfree and conventional chicks fed a cholesterol free diet. This was verified by Wostmann and Wiech (1960) for chicks at 70 days of age, but they found that at 1 month of age the serum cholesterol level was considerably higher in germfree chicks than it was in conventional chicks. The data of Kritchevsky *et al.* (1959), summarized in Table 5.11, indicated the cholesterol

TABLE 5.11
SERUM CHOLESTEROL IN CHICKS (28 days old)
FED 3.0% CHOLESTEROL AND 5% CORN OIL

Diet		Germfree			Conventional		
		No.	Mean	Range	No.	Mean	Range
Protein 25%	Carbohydrate 54%						
Casein	Glucose	11	888	492-1482	10	742	208-1530
Casein	Sucrose	10	1155	720-1452	10	1352	458-2575
Casein	Starch	10	627	262-1052	10	539	300-1062
Promine (soya protein)	Starch	10	521	233-1328	10	365	245-587

Data of Kritchevsky *et al.* (1959).

found in both germfree and conventional chicks varied with other dietary constituents. The high values obtained with sucrose diets would be most meaningful if they could be confirmed in mammalian species. Germfree rats were found to have significantly higher serum cholesterol levels than those found in conventional rats fed the same diet (Gustafsson, 1959a; Danielsson and Gustafsson, 1959). Wostmann and Wiech (1960) reported that the serum cholesterol level for germfree rats fed fortified commercial diets averaged 127 ± 7 mg per 100 ml while those for conventional rats averaged 77 ± 2 mg per 100 ml. Further work should help explain the species differences noted.

Blood glucose was found to be present in the same concentration in conventional lambs as it was in germfree lambs (Smith and Trexler, 1960). In germfree lambs the value found was 51 mg per 100 ml of blood during fasting and 70 mg per 100 ml of blood 3 hours after fasting.

Wright *et al.* (1959) found ammonia in the portal blood of germfree guinea pigs. The quantity present was much less than in the portal blood of classic guinea pigs (Warren *et al.*, 1959). No consistent difference was found in peripheral blood.

Serum Proteins

The globulin fraction of the blood of germfree animals is usually lower than that of conventional animals. Wostmann (1959b) presented the electrophoretic patterns of several species of germfree animals compared to conventional animals (Fig. 5.4). The major serum globulin deficiency in germfree chicks was in the γ-2 fraction. The γ-1- and β-fractions were also low. The difference in γ-globulin in germfree and conventional chicks was found to increase with age: little change was found in serum γ-globulin of germfree chicks as they matured, while serum γ-globulin increased markedly with age in conventional chicks.

Tajima (1955) found the total serum protein of germfree guinea pigs to be as high as that of conventional guinea pigs (Table 5.12). He noted that the γ-globulin serum proteins were low in germfree guinea pigs while the α- and β-fractions were present in serum at levels comparable to those of conventional guinea pigs. Miyakawa (1958a) reported germfree guinea pigs have a high serum albumin and low γ-globulin content when compared to conventional guinea pigs. Neither observation could be verified by Newton *et al.* (1960a). Wostmann (1961a) found no serum γ-globulin in germfree guinea pigs fed no milk; but when fed milk, they had about one-half as much serum γ-globulin as was found in classic animals.

The α-2, β-, and γ-globulins in the serum of 90 day old germfree male rats were statistically lower than the same fractions in classic rats (Wagner and Wostmann, 1961). Wostmann (1959b) found this difference in globulins was compensated by the presence of a higher serum albumin content in germfree rats. This, and the lack of euglobulins found by Sacquet *et al.* (1961) for germfree rats and mice, confirmed the observation of Gustafsson and Laurell (1958), who studied the serum protein pattern in 5 generations of germfree rats.

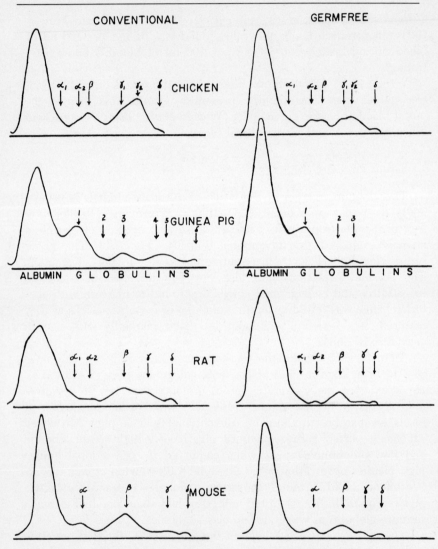

FIG. 5.4. Electrophoretic patterns of serum proteins in germfree and conventional animals. (B. Wostmann, 1959b, 1961a and unpublished.)

They suggested that the production of γ-globulins in classic rats was 3 times greater than that of germfree rats.

Preliminary information regarding the electrophoretic pattern of serum proteins in Swiss mice (Fig. 5.4) indicated that the differences seen in rats were similar in mice; lowered serum globulin fractions

TABLE 5.12
SERUM PROTEINS IN GUINEA PIGS[a]

Category	Age (days)	No.	Protein (gm/100ml)	Albumin	Composition of Protein (%, range)		
					α-Globulin	β-Globulin	γ-Globulin
Naturally reared	30	4	4.5(4.2-4.8)	62.8(56.5-67.5)	9.9(8.0-12.1)	10.9(9.6-12.1)	16.4(13.9-21.1)
Artificially reared	30	3	5.2(4.8-5.8)	54.9(51.8-56.8)	14.8(14.3-16.6)	13.0(12.2-14.3)	17.0(15.3-19.4)
	90	1	5.2	61.2	13.8	11.9	13.1
	102	1	5.6	43.7	20.7	10.3	25.3
Germ-free	20	3	5.5(4.6-6.7)	59.9(54.5-67.0)	13.3(9.2-17.1)	15.1(11.9-16.9)	11.8(11.5-11.9)
	40	1	5.9	67.0	10.0	12.0	11.0
	82	1	6.0	63.4	15.0	10.0	11.6
	150	1	6.0	58.6	18.5	8.9	13.9

[a]Data of Tajima (1955).

compensated by an increased serum albumin (Wostmann, 1959b). Germfree rabbits, sheep and a goat had very low amounts of serum γ-globulin (Wostmann, 1961a). No difference was found in β-globulins while the α-globulins were in somewhat higher concentrations in classic than germfree sheep and goat.

Sacquet *et al.* (1961) report less heparin in the serum of germfree rats than in classic rats (the ratio was 6:10).

Respiratory System

The nostrils and beaks of germfree chicks appeared to be very similar to those of classic birds. The trachea, bronchii, and lungs of conventional birds showed no conspicuous differences from those seen in germfree birds (Table 5.13). There was a tendency for the relative wet weight of the lungs of older classic birds to be somewhat higher than that of germfree birds irrespective of body weight or sex in both White Wyandotte Bantam and White Leghorn chicks, but it never reached statistical significance. As Latimer (1924) pointed out, male birds show a higher proportion of lung tissue in their body than do females, particularly in older age groups. The lungs of White Wyandotte Bantam chicks is similar in both categories (Table 5.14). Since most lung tissue beyond the secondary bronchii in classic animals is normally bacteria free, one would expect no changes from direct contact of microorganisms in the finer structures and none are reported. Surprisingly, the trachea of germfree White Leghorn chicks may be heavier than that of conventional chicks (Table 5.13).

The relative weight of the lungs of guinea pigs at 30 and 60 days of age appeared somewhat smaller in germfree than in conventional environments (Glimstedt, 1936a; Table 5.9). The respiratory system of germfree guinea pigs was reported to be normal by Phillips *et al.* (1959). The nose and paranasal cavities of germfree rats were found to be free of inflammation by Kelemen (1960). The lungs of germfree and conventional rats usually appeared to be normal. However newborn germfree rats and mice were susceptible to extensive lung consolidation. A virus has been suspected but never found.

No differences were seen in the percentage dry weight of lungs of conventional and germfree White Wyandotte Bantam chicks in all age groups (Table 5.6). Nor were differences seen in the dry weight of lungs of White Leghorn chicks at 10 weeks of age (Table 5.4). The percentage of ash and fat in lungs on a dry basis was somewhat less in conventional Leghorn chicks than was found for germfree

TABLE 5.13
ORGAN WEIGHTS (gm) IN GERMFREE AND CONVENTIONAL
WHITE LEGHORN CHICKS   FED SYNTYPE DIET L-245

	Category	No.[a]	Mean[a]	Min—Max[a]	No.[b]	Mean[b]	Min—Max[b]
Heart	Gf	—	—	—	4	3.79	3.20 - 4.54
	Cv	—	—	=	4	4.53	2.58 - 5.70
Lungs	Gf	—	—	—	4	5.43	5.07 - 5.81
	Cv	—	—	—	4	6.56	4.88 - 8.36
Proventriculus	Gf	6	1.54	1.31 - 1.88	4	2.70	2.34 - 3.06
	Cv	8	1.65	1.42 - 2.08	4	3.57	3.07 - 4.39
Gizzard	Gf	6	7.67	6.87 - 8.29	3	12.72	12.11 - 13.10
	Cv	8	7.79	6.10 - 8.91	4	15.28	11.71 - 18.55
Small intestine	Gf	6	6.22	5.58 - 7.01	4	12.20	10.55 - 13.80
	Cv	8	8.40	6.83 - 10.83	4	17.35	15.36 - 13.80
Ceca, empty	Gf	6	0.51	0.42 - 0.61	4	1.33	1.04 - 1.78
	Cv	8	0.98	0.70 - 1.16	4	2.14	1.36 - 2.51
Cecal contents	Gf	6	1.42	0.47 - 2.66	4	2.69	0.84 - 5.35
	Cv	8	0.80	0.17 - 1.96	4	2.40	0.91 - 3.67
Liver	Gf	6	7.22	5.16 - 9.27	4	16.36	14.39 - 18.89
	Cv	8	7.16	5.51 - 8.83	4	20.10	14.75 - 26.60
Pancreas	Gf	5	1.03	0.90 - 1.20	4	1.38	1.07 - 1.66
	Cv	8	1.07	0.72 - 1.44	4	1.82	1.48 - 2.43
Kidney	Gf	—	—	—	3	21.3	20.9 - 21.7
	Cv	—	—	—	3	21.4	21.3 - 21.5
Spleen	Gf	6	0.36	0.28 - 0.53	—	—	—
	Cv	8	0.45	0.23 - 0.61	—	—	—
Trident	Gf	6	0.11	0.10 - 0.15	4	0.16	0.14 - 0.18
	Cv	8	0.18	0.13 - 0.23	4	0.25	0.22 - 0.31
Bursa Fabricius	Gf	6	1.48	0.93 - 2.07	4	3.21	2.20 - 4.50
	Cv	8	1.38	0.82 - 2.02	4	4.49	2.42 - 7.91
Thymus	Gf	6	1.11	0.59 - 1.58	4	3.02	2.86 - 3.25
	Cv	8	0.75	0.33 - 1.00	4	4.15	2.99 - 6.24
Adrenal glands	Gf	6	0.042	0.023 - 0.070	3	0.10	0.08 - 0.12
	Cv	8	0.037	0.025 - 0.047	3	0.11	0.09 - 0.13
Ovary	Gf	6	0.056	0.029 - 0.087	—	—	—
	Cv	8	0.052	0.066 -	—	—	—
Testicles	Gf	2	0.093	0.080 - 0.106	2	3.82	3.60 - 4.04
	Cv	4	0.071	0.053 - 0.088	3	3.23	1.92 - 5.24

[a]Age 4 – 7 weeks; average weight of germfree chicks 268 gm.; average weight of conventional chicks 248 gm.

[b]Age 10 weeks; average weight of germfree chicks 1075 gm.; average weight of conventional chicks 1171 gm. Data of Gordon (Reyniers   ., 1960a).

birds. The amount of nitrogen in lungs of conventional Leghorn chickens was similar to that of germfree Leghorn chickens. The histamine content of lungs in 4 month old germfree rats was 5.1–13.8 μg/gm and that in conventional rats was 2.1–8.2 μg/gm (Gustafsson et al. 1957b). The dry weight and fat in the lungs of germfree pups was found to be 19.5% (19.1–20.2%) and 4.9% (4.69–5.08%) respectively.

TABLE 5.14

ORGAN WEIGHTS (IN GRAMS) IN GERMFREE AND CONVENTIONAL WHITE WYANDOTTE BANTAM CHICKS FED SYNTYPE DIET L-137

	Gf / Cv Category	Age 2 weeks Average wgt. 43 gm / 50 gm			Age 5 weeks Average wgt. 143 gm / 123 gm			Age 8 weeks Average wgt. 273 gm / 237 gm			Age 23 weeks Average wgt. 847 gm / 667 gm			Age 32–52 weeks Average wgt. 813 gm / 944 gm		
		No.	Mean	Limits	No.	Mean	Limits	No.	Mean	Limits	No.	Mean	Limits	No.	Mean	Limits
Heart	Gf	3	0.258	0.235 / 0.270	12	0.841	0.690 / 1.150	13	1.27	0.77 / 2.23	5	2.87	1.66 / 4.13	3	3.98	2.80 / 4.81
	Cv	2	0.401	0.333 / 0.470	12	0.715	0.410 / 1.010	14	1.04	0.47 / 1.68	7	2.08	1.55 / 3.26	3	4.48	3.15 / 5.74
Lungs	Gf	3	0.267	0.240 / 0.300	12	0.751	0.510 / 0.950	13	1.26	0.72 / 1.85	5	2.59	1.96 / 3.14	3	2.95	2.38 / 3.91
	Cv	2	0.320	0.270 / 0.370	9	0.694	0.500 / 0.970	14	1.11	0.54 / 1.67	7	2.79	1.75 / 4.13	3	4.19	2.75 / 6.23
Proventriculus	Gf	3	0.260	0.220 / 0.310	10	0.682	0.430 / 0.900	13	0.98	0.68 / 1.43	5	1.37	1.17 / 1.74	3	1.37	1.11 / 1.65
	Cv	2	0.404	0.369 / 0.440	12	0.704	0.580 / 0.970	13	0.94	0.69 / 1.30	7	1.77	1.06 / 2.29	3	1.56	1.45 / 1.70
Gizzard	Gf	3	1.59	1.60 / 1.96	11	2.97	1.78 / 4.63	11	5.88	2.76 / 7.87	5	14.95	9.40 / 21.21	3	10.41	6.73 / 16.60
	Cv	2	1.77	1.51 / 2.04	11	3.14	2.16 / 4.42	13	6.15	3.51 / 11.80	7	10.36	8.06 / 17.11	3	14.05	8.90 / 24.20
Small intestine	Gf	3	1.80	1.35 / 2.12	12	3.63	1.74 / 5.31	13	4.24	2.20 / 6.32	4	6.40	5.72 / 7.98	3	6.30	4.35 / 7.75
	Cv	2	2.63	2.45 / 2.81	12	4.43	2.36 / 7.60	13	6.12	4.39 / 9.45	7	9.24	5.92 / 12.43	3	12.03	9.35 / 17.40
Ceca, empty	Gf	3	0.130	0.110 / 0.160	12	0.369	0.220 / 0.560	13	0.558	0.350 / 1.250	5	1.04	0.72 / 1.22	3	1.32	0.89 / 1.70
	Cv	2	0.168	0.163 / 0.174	12	0.445	0.300 / 0.670	13	0.742	0.450 / 1.100	7	1.70	1.03 / 2.11	3	2.52	1.68 / 3.55
Cecal contents	Gf	3	0.160	0.040 / 0.291	12	0.681	0.300 / 1.290	13	1.93	0.80 / 3.82	5	3.33	1.43 / 7.98	3	1.40	0.30 / 2.51
	Cv	2	0.087	0.080 / 0.095	12	0.407	0.150 / 0.870	14	1.15	0.18 / 3.41	7	3.02	0.87 / 4.84	3	4.28	3.86 / 4.65

Organ		n	mean	min	max	n	mean	min	max	n	mean	min	max	n	mean	min	max	n	mean	min	max
Liver	Gf	3	1.91	1.24	2.86	11	4.99	3.10	5.84	13	7.76	6.00	10.34	5	14.96	12.31	16.10	3	12.59	10.51	14.04
	Cv	2	3.09	2.96	3.22	12	5.01	3.78	9.10	14	8.03	4.88	12.61	7	17.39	10.50	22.39	3	18.65	13.40	26.60
Pancreas	Gf	3	0.142	0.135	0.150	11	0.419	0.250	0.520	13	0.646	0.390	1.180	5	1.15	0.93	1.24	3	1.04	0.82	1.36
	Cv	2	0.245	0.233	0.256	11	0.457	0.290	0.750	14	0.629	0.167	0.840	7	1.32	0.83	1.66	3	1.24	0.90	1.60
Spleen	Gf	3	0.037	0.030	0.045	12	0.190	0.090	0.370	13	0.486	0.220	1.140	5	1.101	0.470	1.520	3	1.07	0.580	1.500
	Cv	2	0.060	0.052	0.067	12	0.264	0.140	0.450	14	0.493	0.162	0.870	7	1.07	0.540	1.990	3	1.42	1.250	1.720
Trident	Gf	3	0.026	0.021	0.031	12	0.058	0.037	0.083	13	0.080	0.039	0.131	4	0.176	0.161	0.184	3	0.128	0.083	0.156
	Cv	2	0.033	0.032	0.034	12	0.077	0.040	0.126	13	0.167	0.055	0.420	7	0.256	0.169	0.340	3	0.202	0.161	0.272
Bursa of Fabricius	Gf	3	0.083	0.050	0.109	12	0.252	0.070	0.470	13	0.568	0.210	1.250	—				—			
	Cv	2	0.144	0.140	0.149	12	0.328	0.140	0.550	14	0.700	0.176	1.390	—				—			
Thymus	Gf	3	0.131	0.102	0.179	12	0.534	0.250	0.810	13	1.38	0.72	2.02	4	1.67	0.89	2.45	3	0.938	0.215	1.850
	Cv	2	0.151	0.111	0.119	12	0.385	0.117	0.800	14	1.00	0.30	1.88	6	1.93	0.91	2.85	3	0.783	0.298	1.140
Adrenal glands	Gf	3	008	0.005	0.012	12	0.023	0.018	0.034	12	0.028	0.018	0.052	5	0.047	0.033	0.065	3	0.057	0.050	0.063
	Cv	2	0.009	0.009	0.010	11	0.016	0.009	0.027	14	0.024	0.014	0.034	7	0.037	0.019	0.051	3	0.060	0.051	0.065
Ovary	Gf	—				6	0.037	0.019	0.054	10	0.092	0.072	0.133	—				—			
	Cv	—				8	0.042	0.028	0.057	10	0.073	0.046	0.108	—				—			
Testicles	Gf	3	0.012	0.010	0.015	6	0.066	0.040	0.094	3	0.65	0.25	0.90	3	5.72	4.80	7.03	2	3.79	3.25	4.33
	Cv	2	0.013	0.012	0.015	4	0.058	0.022	0.093	3	0.24	0.05	0.45	2	3.90	1.80	6.00	2	4.82	4.19	5.45

TABLE 5.14

Category	Gf/Cv	Age 2 weeks Gf Average wgt. 43 gm / Cv Average wgt. 50 gm No.	Mean	Limits	Age 5 weeks Gf Average wgt. 143 gm / Cv Average wgt. 123 gm No.	Mean	Limits	Age 8 weeks Gf Average wgt. 273 gm / Cv Average wgt. 237 gm No.	Mean	Limits	Age 23 weeks Gf Average wgt. 847 gm / Cv Average wgt. 667 gm No.	Mean	Limits	Age 32–52 weeks Gf Average wgt. 813 gm / Cv Average wgt. 944 gm No.	Mean	Limits
Eye, left	Gf	3	0.457	0.420 / 0.500	12	0.723	0.650 / 0.850	13	0.992	0.800 / 1.220	5	1.65	1.53 / 1.83	3	1.74	1.50 / 1.94
	Cv	2	0.430	0.410 / 0.450	12	0.732	0.600 / 0.860	14	0.961	0.690 / 1.170	7	1.48	1.37 / 1.72	2	1.89	1.87 / 1.90
Thyroid	Gf	—	—	—	11	0.0100	0.0056 / 0.0140	11	0.0157	0.0069 / 0.0267	4	0.055	0.046 / 0.062	3	0.040	0.032 / 0.047
	Cv	—	—	—	11	0.0071	0.0034 / 0.0128	12	0.0118	0.0073 / 0.0171	6	0.049	0.027 / 0.064	2	0.049	0.043 / 0.055
Brain	Gf	3	1.03	1.00 / 1.05	12	1.69	1.45 / 1.99	13	2.05	1.79 / 2.36	5	2.68	2.59 / 2.83	3	2.73	2.51 / 2.95
	Cv	2	1.09	1.01 / 1.16	12	1.65	1.40 / 1.88	14	2.00	1.62 / 2.21	7	2.45	1.59 / 3.04	2	2.93	2.80 / 3.06

Taken from data of Gordon (Reyniers, *et al.*, 1960a).

Digestive System

The oral cavity, crop and the esophagus of germfree White Wyandotte Bantam and White Leghorn chicks in gross appearance seemed to be identical with that of conventional birds. The empty crop and esophagus of germfree chicks were slightly heavier (Table 5.2) than those of conventional birds. Under 2–3 times magnification Gordon (in Reyniers et al., 1960a) found the mucosal surfaces of the esophagus and crop in older conventional birds were more rough than those found in germfree birds.

The oral cavities of germfree guinea pigs were clean and the perioral glands were pale and insignificant (Phillips et al., 1959). Miyakawa (1959b) presented pictures of the oral and nasal cavities at different cross-sectional planes. As summarized in the discussion of the lymphatic system, development of elements of defense (i.e., stratified ciliated epithelium and lymphatic tissue) was greatly retarded in germfree guinea pigs.

The mouth and pharynx of germfree and conventional rats and mice were very similar in gross appearance and development. The first teeth erupted in germfree rats at 11 days (Gustafsson, 1948). Germfree teeth may become abraded—the incisors are normally kept in the proper condition and size by abrasion—or broken, but dental caries did not occur in germfree rats (Orland et al., 1954; Fitzgerald et al., 1960b). The incidence of carious lesions in monoflora rats will be presented in the final chapter.

The gross appearance, texture, and color of the proventriculus were the same in germfree and conventional chicks. Older conventional chicks were found to have somewhat higher relative weight of the proventriculus than was found in germfree chicks. Diet also had a definite effect upon the proventriculus weight: this organ had a greater mass when practical diets were fed than when syntype diets were fed. The larynx and esophagus of germfree animals were grossly identical to those of conventional animals. One exception to this statement was the white pestules (ureate deposits?) lining the esophagus of the only second generation chick hatched *inside* the germfree cage. Since other chicks hatched from the same clutch of eggs appeared to be normal, this one exception may not be important.

The stomach and small intestine of germfree guinea pigs were "normal" (Phillips et al., 1959). The stomach of germfree mice usually had more food than was found in the stomach of conventional mice.

The histamine in the gastric mucosa of rats was 16.2–56.4 μg/gm in the germfree state and 40.7–68.7 μg/gm in conventional controls (Gustafsson *et al.*, 1957b).

The gizzards of conventional chicks appeared similar in gross morphology to that of germfree chicks. Minute erosions were seen in the epithelial lining in chicks of both groups. It was noted (Reyniers *et al.*, 1960a) that feeding crude diets encouraged the development of larger gizzards more often than did syntype diets. Apparently some dietary material had more effect on the gizzard size than the presence of microorganisms. No differences were noted in the percentage of dry weight of the gizzard when the germfree and conventional chicks were compared.

Pancreas

Gross observation of the pancreas of germfree and conventional chicks indicated they were similar. The conventional chicks consistently had higher relative wet weight of pancreas than did germfree birds in all age groups in both Leghorn and Bantam chicks (Table 5.2); however this difference never reached statistical significance. Once again, the type of diet appeared to be an important factor in determining the relative size: practical diets were correlated to heavier pancreas weights.

The dry weight of the pancreas of Bantam chickens showed no difference in the young birds. At 46–54 days of age, the pancreas of conventional birds had significantly less dry weight than that of germfree birds.

Small Intestine

The over-all length of the small intestine was approximately 10% greater in conventional chicks than in germfree chicks fed the same diet. This difference was less striking in older birds than in rapidly growing chicks. The relative weight of small intestine was greater in conventional birds than in germfree birds. This development increased with respect to the age in both Leghorn and Wyandotte Bantam chicks (Table 5.2). Chicks fed a crude diet had larger small intestines than had chicks fed a syntype diet.

Nuttall and Thierfelder (1896b) found the small intestines of guinea pigs to be empty and acid in pH. Glimstedt (1936a) found that the weight of the stomach and intestine without ingesta were about the same in germfree and conventional guinea pigs (Table 5.9). The

TABLE 5.15[a]

ORGAN WEIGHTS[b] OF GERMFREE AND CONVENTIONAL ALBINO RATS[c,d]

	Category	No. of observations	Mean	Standard deviation
Small intestine, upper 50% of length	Gf	15	513	94
	Cv	19	679	105
Small intestine, lower 50% of length	Gf	15	425	63
	Cv	19	592	112
Small intestine, total	Gf	15	939	133
	Cv	19	1270	202
Cecal sac	Gf	19	538	90
	Cv	28	210	56
Cecal contents	Gf	12	5300	665
	Cv	19	797	100
Adrenal gland	Gf	14	14.5	1.6
	Cv	19	10.9	1.5
Thymus gland	Gf	14	147	31
	Cv	17	186	45
Submandibular lymph nodes	Gf	15	27.4	6.3
	Cv	25	101.5	32.2
Cecal lymph nodes	Gf	15	3.2	1.0
	Cv	17	7.8	2.1
Peyer's patches (no.)	Gf	4	12	2
	Cv	9	16	2
Peyer's patches (wgt.)	Gf	4	34.6	8.6
	Cv	9	89.9	14.2
Spleen	Gf	15	254	34
	Cv	18	465	86

[a]From Gordon and Wostmann (1960).
[b]Organ weights in mg/100 gm body weight (live weight minus weight of cecal contents).
[c]All male rats, age 89—98 days.
[d]$P = 0.01$ or less for all comparative data; P calculated from students' tables (Fisher and Yates, 1943).

weight of the gastrointestinal tract with ingesta was about 50% greater in the germfree guinea pigs than that of the conventional animals.

The relative weight of the small intestine was found to be greater in conventional rats and mice than in germfree rats and mice respectively (Gordon, 1960b). This difference was equally valid when the upper and lower portions were compared (Table 5.15). The length of the small intestine was comparable in germfree and conventional animals. More partially digested food was seen in the intestinal canal of germfree rats (Gustafsson, 1958) and mice than was seen in conventional mammals. This might suggest the reduced muscle tonus seen so dramatically in the cecum is actually typical of the total intestinal tract.

Stenquist (1934) presented photomicrographs and discussion of the morphology of the intestinal mucosa of the germfree guinea pigs reared by Glimstedt. Microscopic examination of the intestinal mucosa

TABLE 5.16

PERCENT DISTRIBUTION OF TISSUE IN THE LOWER ILEUM[a]

Species	Age (days)	Category	Muscle	Connective tissue	Epithelium	Total
Chicken (White Leghorn)	30	Gf	46.9	20.3	32.8	100.0
		Cv	45.8	23.8	30.4	100.0
Rat (Albino)	242	Gf	17.1	29.3	53.6	100.0
		Cv	17.3	34.2	48.5	100.0

[a]Data of Gordon (1960b).

showed a greater regularity in cell structure and arrangement in germfree animals than was found in conventional animals. This tissue had less lymphatic development and less connective tissue in chickens in the germfree state (Gordon, 1960b). The general picture presented in intestinal mucosa was that the germfree animal had a relatively greater proportion of essential absorptive elements and fewer and less well developed elements of defense. Gordon (1960b) found about three times greater numbers of reticuloendothelial cells in the mucosa and submucosa of the ileum of young conventional chicks than in germfree chicks. This difference was noted also for "Schollen" or globule leucocytes found within the epithelium and in the number of plasma cells and lymphocytes in the submucosa and lamina propria of the lower ileum. The counts for other R-E cells (monocytes, heterophils, eosinophils, and basophils) was practically the same in both categories.

When Gordon (1960b) examined tissue distribution in the wall of the lower ileum of chicks and rats, he found the muscle mass of the conventional animal was almost identical in both categories for each species (Table 5.16). The amount of connective tissue in the ileum of the conventional animals of both species was greater than that in the germfree animals. The reciprocal was noted for the epithelial content: the amount of epithelium was greater in the germfree category. Gordon *et al.* (1960a) suggested that the decreased lamina propria tissue and cellular tissue associated with defense leave the mucosal surface more efficient for absorption. More recently Gordon (1961, personal communication) found that the total mucosal surface area of the small intestine of the 3–4 month old germfree rat was significantly lower than that of conventional rats (Table 5.17). This

TABLE 5.17
MUCOSAL SURFACE AREA OF SMALL INTESTINE
AND MEAN BODY WEIGHT IN RATS[a,b]

		Germfree		Conventional		P
		Mean	S. D.	Mean	S. D.	
Mucosal surface area of small intestine (sq. cm.)	Upper third	249	29	296	20	0.01
	Mid third	144	23	263	24	0.01
	Lower third	73	14	112	16	0.01
	Total	466	37	671	35	0.01
Body weight (gm.)		312	22	320	22	0.57

[a]Data of H. A. Gordon (1961).
[b]No. of rats: 7 germfree, 7 conventional; all males.
[c]S. D. = standard deviation.

was established from surface tracings of both cross and longitudinal sections of different parts of the small intestine. This method accounts for variables such as total length, cross section diameter, and the size and numbers of the villi. In preliminary studies on the tissue renewal rate, Gordon found that the number of ileal epithelial cells undergoing mitosis was 1.1% in germfree rats and 1.0% in conventional rats. The epithelium of the Lieberkuhn crypts had all the mitotic activity; none was found in the villi. The amount of lamina propria in the total area was $25.6 \pm 0.9\%$ in germfree chicks and $36.8 \pm 1.4\%$ in conventional chicks. The increased amount of lamina propria is seen in the cross sectional view of intestinal villi (Fig. 5.5).

The small intestine of conventional and germfree White Leghorn and White Wyandotte Bantam chickens had the same percentage of dry weight (Tables 5.4 and 5.6), while that of conventional rats at 3

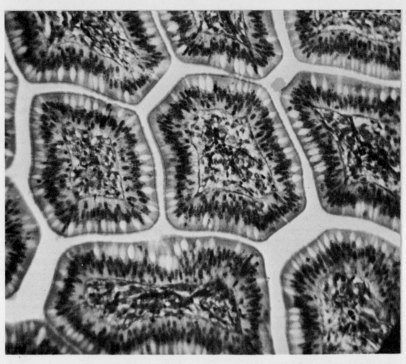
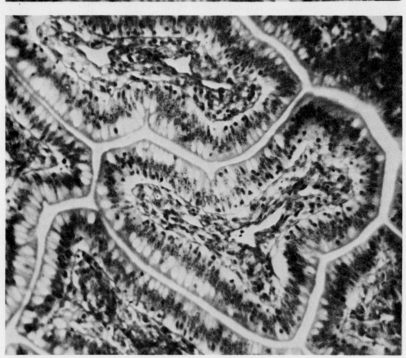

Fig. 5.5. Intestinal villi of conventional (*left*) and germfree (*right*) chicks. The cross sections were taken at mid-height of the villus, in 9 week old male White Leghorn chicks. Note the greater amount of "core" in the villi of the conventional chicks when compared to that of germfree chicks. (Gordon and Bruckner-Kardoss, 1961.)

months of age had greater dry weight content than was found in germfree rats (Gordon, 1960a).

The ash content of the wall of the small intestine in White Leghorn chicks was very similar for the two groups (see Table 5.4). Data of Heneghan (1961) indicated there was no difference in the rate of passage of Na^+ or K^+ through the intestinal wall. The fat content of the small intestine of the conventional Leghorn chicks was possibly less than that of germfree birds. There was significantly more nitrogen in the small intestine of conventional Leghorn chicks than in that of germfree Leghorn chicks.

Gustafsson *et al.* (1957b) found much variability in the histamine content of the small intestine of rats and no differences were noted between conventional and germfree categories. Larner and Gillespie (1957) found maltase, invertase, and oligo-1, 6-glucosidase to be present in comparable levels in the intestinal extracts from germfree and conventional rats. The proteolytic activity of intestinal contents appears to be greater in germfree conditions according to the data of Lepkovsky *et al.* (1959) on feces. Lepkovsky and Wagner (1961, personal communication) have recently clarified this concept with data on enzyme levels in different parts of the intestinal tract. In conventional rats, amylase concentrations were higher in the contents of the duodenum, ileum, cecum, colon, and feces than they were in germfree rats. Differences were not found in the pancreas or jejunum contents. More amylase was found in pancreas and cloacal contents of germfree chicks than in conventional chicks, but not in other parts of the intestine. No large differences were found in lipase concentrations, except that the duodenum of germfree rats appeared to have lower levels than conventional rats and pancreatic lipase was higher in germfree chicks than in conventional chicks. Trypsin and total protease activities were similar in the intestine, except for the following: protease in cecal contents and pancreas was present in lower levels in conventional rats than in germfree rats, and conventional chicks had less protease in cecal contents than had germfree chicks. The low trypsin fraction accounted for much of the difference seen in total protease.

The pH of different parts of the intestinal tract for germfree and conventional chicks and rats is given in Table 5.18. Surprisingly, the mouth was the only level where alkaline condition was found. The stomach or gizzard was not very acid under normal fed conditions. No great differences were noted between germfree and conventional animals in pH of the gastrointestinal tract.

TABLE 5.18
pH OF THE INTESTINAL TRACT

White rats		Level	White Leghorn chicks (12 days old)[a]			
Germ-free	Conventional		Germfree (3)		Conventional (2)	
8.5	8.3	Mouth	7.54	(7.0-8.5)	6.54	(6.5-6.6)
—	—	Crop	6.15	(5.9-6.3)	6.35	(6.3-6.4)
—	—	Proventriculus	4.81	(4.6-4.9)	5.63	(5.6-5.7)
2.7	5.8	Gizzard-stomach	4.30	(3.3-5.0)	3.47	(3.4-3.5)
6.3	6.4	Duodenum	6.42	(6.3-6.6)	6.38	(6.3-6.5)
6.3	5.8	Jejunum	—	—	—	—
6.5	7.0	Illeum, upper	—	—	—	—
6.9	7.0	Ileum, lower	6.34	(6.31-6.40)	6.52	(6.51-6.53)
—	—	Cecum	6.38	(6.3-6.5)	6.48	(6.3-6.7)
6.5	6.5	Colon	6.26	(6.1-6.5)	6.37	(6.2-6.5)

[a] Diet 56227 for all except that the individual giving the highest pH in the germfree category was fed 34406. Three germfree and two conventional chicks were used.

Cecum

The gross appearance of the mucosal wall of the ileum and the cecum of conventional birds had a darker color than was found in the germfree birds. The relative weight of the ceca of conventional birds was consistently the same as that of germfree birds in both varieties of chickens in all age groups and all weight groups (Table 5.2). Enlarged ceca were not found in germfree turkey poults.

Nuttall and Thierfelder (1896b) noted that the ceca of germfree guinea pigs were greatly enlarged and distended with a brown liquid containing cheesy particles which was slightly alkaline in pH. Although Glimstedt (1936a) had no serious problem with cecum distension, the total ingesta found was about 50% greater in the germfree guinea pigs than in the conventional animals. The cecum was greatly distended and effectively prevented breeding in the germfree guinea pigs of Phillips *et al.* (1959). Passage through the intestine was not seriously inhibited since normal pellet formation in the large intestine was noted. The wall in the cecal sac in conventional guinea pigs was thick and tough, while in the germfree guinea pigs it was very thin and elastic. Peristalsis of the distended cecum was thought to be ineffectual. The relative weight of the cecal contents was 6.0–14.1% of the body weight in germfree guinea pigs and 5.0–7.1% in conventional animals at 8 weeks (Horton and Hickey, 1961). Since reproduction was obtained by several investigators in germfree guinea pigs when food intake was limited, the problem of the distended cecum was reduced in significance.

Enlarged cecum in the germfree rat was reported by Gustafsson (1946, 1947) who noted that all germfree rats had an enlarged cecum filled with a thin paste-like liquid. At weaning the abdomen was swollen from distension of the cecum. In the first experience of Luckey (unpublished, 1947–1950), enlarged ceca prevented reproduction and the formation of a colony by causing death of the germfree rats before they could mature. The cecum and its contents constituted 20–30% of the body weight and twisted in a counterclockwise direction until intestinal volvulus occurred (Fig. 5.6a and b). Activity decreased and the rats exhibited sporadic lordosis about a week prior to death. Moribund rats lay with little movement for 1–2 days before death. The addition of 3% fiber to the diet alleviated the syndrome. The weight of the cecum and its contents was reduced to 5–10% of the body weight and reproduction allowed the colony to be established (see Chapter 3 for details). The cecum of germfree mice is usually enlarged (4.6–6.4 gm) and filled with dark green-black soup. It is about 10 times the mass of the cecum of conventional mice (0.45–0.52 gm). The volume occupied by the germfree mouse cecum (6.0–7.6 ml) is about 15 times that occupied by the cecum of conventional mice (0.4–0.6 ml) (Fig. 5.6). Gordon (1959b) and Gordon et al. (1960b) reported that the semisolid cecal contents in the germfree, normal-born adult rats and mice were usually 4–8 times that of conventional animals and the weight of the cecal sac in those species was 2–6 times greater in the germfree environment (Table 5.15). Since contamination of the germfree rat resulted in a rapid decrease in cecal contents and a less rapid decrease in the size of the cecal sac, Gordon suggested the main cause of cecal enlargement was reduced muscle tonus. Gustafsson and Malmquist (in Gustafsson, 1959a) found that the weight of the cecal wall of the germfree rat was 0.5% of the body weight while that of the conventional rat was 0.2%. The water content was the same in both categories.

The dry weight of the wall of the ceca of White Wyandotte Ban-

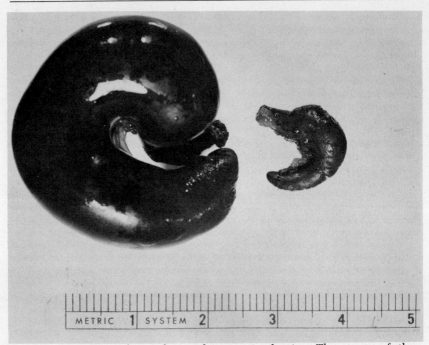

FIG. 5.6a. Ceca of germfree and conventional mice. The cecum of the germfree mouse is 5–10 times more distended than that of the conventional mouse.

tam chicks showed that the values were very similar for germfree and conventional categories at 4 weeks of age and at 46–64 days (Table 5.6). However, in the older age group the cecal wall of conventional birds was 23.3% dry weight, while in the germfree Bantam chicks it was 28.3% dry weight. The quantity of cecal contents was comparable in germfree and conventional Leghorn chicks (Table 5.3). Chemical analysis of the cecal contents (Tables 5.4 and 5.6) was of special interest since it harbors such a large microbial population. The dry weight of the cecal contents of conventional birds was consistently higher than that found in germfree birds. The amount of ash in the cecal contents on the dry weight basis was identical for germfree and conventional Bantam chicks at 8 weeks of age. The quantity of ash present in cecal contents of Leghorn chicks was considerably greater than that of the Bantam chicks, although the amount of mineral in the diet was not significantly greater. The amounts of nitrogen and fat in the cecal contents were not significantly greater in the

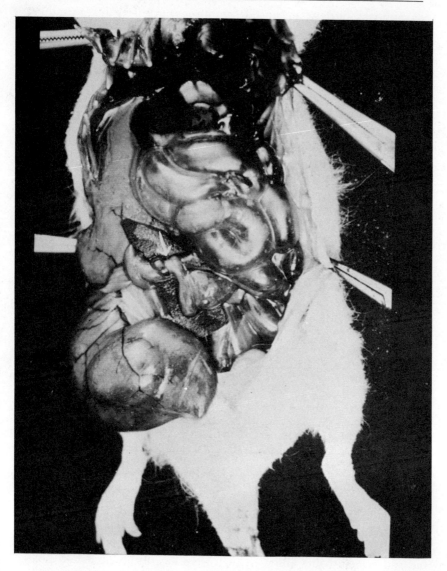

FIG. 5.6b. Intestinal volvulus in a germfree rat. The distended cecum twists counterclockwise until it effectively stops the passage of material through the ileocecal junction. Note also the large amount of gas which accumulated in the small intestine and cecum of malnurtured germfree rats (analysis of the gas indicates aerophagia). Cecum is lower left. Black paper is under ileocecal junction to display volvulus (*arrow*).

conventional birds than in the germfree birds. White Wyandotte Bantam chicks showed no significant difference in thiamine, folic acid, vitamin B_{12}, and riboflavin concentration in the cecal contents. Tremendous differences were noted in the niacin concentration of the cecal contents. The germfree Leghorn chicks had as little as one-twentieth as much niacin as the conventional birds. The younger Bantam chicks of the conventional category had much less pantothenic acid in their cecal contents than was found in the germfree birds. In older White Wyandotte and in Leghorn chicks no differences were seen. Conventional White Wyandotte Bantam chicks typically had more pyridoxine and biotin in their cecal contents than did germfree chicks.

When the concentration of vitamins in the cecal contents of germfree chicks was compared (Table 5.19) with that of the diet on a

TABLE 5.19

APPARENT BIOINCRASSATION IN WHITE LEGHORN CHICKS[a]

	Diet	Cecal contents		Apparent bio-incrassation
		Conventional	Germfree	Germfree
Riboflavin	103	46.6	37.7	3.7
Niacin	92	254	105	1.1
Pantothenate	34	115	264	7.8
Biotin	0.39	8.3	5.9	15.1
Folic	2.8	11.7	10.5	3.8
Vitamin B_{12}	0.033	0.096	0.109	3.3

[a]Data of Luckey (1959c). The data give the average μg vitamin per gram dry material from 8 to 31 chicks.

dry-weight basis, the material in the ceca was found to have greater concentrations of vitamins than the diet; it was suggested that this concentration resulted from a greater proportion of carbohydrate, fat, and protein being absorbed than were less readily absorbed molecules such as vitamins. The net effect was to concentrate the vitamins by taking away other solid material: this phenomenon has been called "bioincrassation" (Luckey, 1958). Since the active excretion of vitamins into the intestinal tract from the tissues had not been taken into account, this evidence gave only the apparent bioincrassation.

Similar phenomena were seen for total ash, calcium, and other minerals. True bioincrassation was seen in the data of Wagner (1959c) in which a nonphysiological material was followed (Table 4.10). Here the dead, readily discernible organism, *M. smegmatis*, was found to be concentrated as carbohydrate, fat, and protein were absorbed from the intestinal lumen.

The cecal contents of conventional rats generally had greater percentage dry weight and ash than that of germfree rats (Table 5.5). On a wet weight basis the biotin and folic acid concentration in cecal contents was similar for germfree and conventional rats. However conventional rats were found to have statistically less riboflavin and more niacin and pantothenic acid in the cecal contents than germfree rats.

Large Intestine

Detailed observations of the large intestine have not appeared. The large intestine of germfree Leghorn chicks may be greater in relative wet weight per 100 gm body weight than that of conventional chicks (Table 5.2). The large intestine and cloaca of conventional and germfree chicks appeared similar by gross observation. Nuttal and Thierfelder (1896b) reported that the large intestine of germfree guinea pigs was slightly acid and free of bacteria, by microscopic and cultural examination. Phillips *et al.* (1959) reported the large intestine to be normal in appearance and function in spite of the enlarged cecum in the germfree guinea pig. The colon of germfree rats and mice contained more material than was seen in conventional animals.

The rectum of germfree mammals rarely contained well formed pellets comparable to those of conventional mammals. Chemical examination of the rectal contents of Leghorn chicks (Table 5.4) indicated no real difference in dry weight between the two categories. The percentage ash of the rectal contents of germfree chicks was almost twice that of the conventional chicks. The anuses of germfree chicks, rats, and mice were normal in appearance and function, while those of germfree guinea pigs had a tendency to prolapse.

Feces

The gross appearance of the feces of conventional chicks and turkey poults resembled that of germfree chicks; the bulk was a dull greenish brown capped with white urates. The germfree birds may be more susceptible to diarrhea and often the excreta of germfree birds was less firm than that of conventional birds fed diet of the same composition. Animals fed synthetic-type diets often had feces which were less well formed than animals fed practical diets. This seemed to be due partially to the increased mineral content of the former and increased fiber for the latter. Balzam (1938) reported the feces of germfree chicks had a honey scent while those of conventional chicks smelled sour; the pH was 6.1 for the former and 6.4 for the latter. The feces of germfree and conventional animals appeared to be qualitatively similar by microscopic observation (Fig. 3.33). Unabsorbed food particles, cellular débris from the intestinal mucosa, and microbial cells were in evidence in feces from both germfree and conventional animals. The major qualitative morphologic difference was that many of the microorganisms were alive in feces of conventional animals, while all were dead in germfree animals. Quantitatively there were usually many more microbial cells seen in the feces of conventional than of germfree animals. However, when 2% of a fermentation residue was fed as a source of possible unidentified vitamins, the dead microorganisms accumulated via bioincrassation to comprise an estimated 50% of the dry weight of the feces in germfree chicks. Nuttall and Thierfelder (1895–1896) reported that in consistency and color (brown or dark green) the feces of germfree guinea pigs were comparable to feces of conventional animals fed unsterile food and water. Cohendy and Wollman (1914) reported no appreciable difference in the total nitrogen or cellulose content of feces of germfree and control guinea pigs. However, few pellets were formed in germfree guinea pigs fed some diets (Phillips et al., 1959). The feces of germfree baby goats were unformed, sticky, and pulpy (Küster, 1913b); Luckey noted the same characteristics in feces of young germfree lambs. The goat feces were sometimes alkaline and sometimes acid. The water content was 75% of the germfree feces and 67% of feces of the control goat. The sugar content was 8.6% in the germfree goat. The stools of germfree monkeys were about the same consistency as that of a human infant (Reyniers and Trexler, 1943b). Feces of germfree rats and mice were less well formed, softer, and more watery than those of conventional animals.

The proteolytic activity of germfree feces from chicks was noted by Schottelius (1899) who used gelatin for embedding samples of material from the germfree experiments. The gelatin remained firm and clear with all samples except the feces, where after 4–8 days the gelatin liquefied into a light green bouillon. This evidence has been verified by Balzam (1938) and Lepkovsky *et al.* (1959). Trypsin and invertase were found in the feces of germfree rats (Borgstrom *et al.*, 1959) while feces from conventional rats had no measurable trypsin or invertase. These enzymes may be partially inactivated by intestinal microorganisms in conventional animals. The amylase content of the feces of germfree animals was slightly greater than that found in conventional rat feces.

When fed a diet with "synthetic corn oil," germfree rats were found to produce feces of which 82% of the neutral sterole was cholesterol (Gustafsson, 1959a). The other steroids were not identified. Taurocholic acid-24 C^{14} was the only metabolite found when germfree rats were fed cholic acid-24 C^{14} by Gustafsson *et al.*, (1957a). The half-life of cholic acid was 11.4 days in germfree rats and 2 days in conventional rats. The germfree rats excreted 0.9 mg of cholic acid per 100 mg body weight (Gustafsson, 1959a). Monoflora rats containing *Aspergillus niger* or *Clostridium perfringens* had the same turnover time for cholic acid that was reported for germfree rats.

Urobilinogens were not found in urine or feces of germfree rats by Gustafsson and Swenander Lanke (1960), while the bilirubin content of feces of conventional rats was lower than the quantity found in feces of germfree rats (4.7 micromoles/kg body/day). Such data, plus the fact that urobilinogens appeared when *Clostridium* sp. was added to germfree rats, would indicate that the intestinal microflora was responsible for the metabolism of bilirubin in the rat. Methyl indole, the compound which typifies fecal odor, is obviously absent from germfree animals. Wagner (1958) found no indole in feces from germfree rats, mice or chicks, while a strong qualitative reaction for indole was found in conventional mice, rats and chicks. Monoflora, *S. faecalis*, rats produced no indole and monoflora, *E. coli*, rats produced indole.

Omentum

The omenta of germfree chicks, rats, and mice were quite comparable to those in conventional animals. The gross appearance of the vessels, nerves, and supporting ligaments were quite comparable in the two groups.

Liver

The macroscopic appearance of the liver of germfree birds and conventional birds was almost identical. The color, consistency, and general appearance, both intact and incised, were the same in all categories of birds where different age groups, body weight groups, and sex were studied. The same statement could be applied to the bilary ducts, the gall bladder, and its contents. The relative wet weight of the liver of conventional birds was consistently higher than that of germfree birds (Table 5.2). A sex difference was seen in the relative weight of the livers of White Wyandotte Bantam birds: the older females had higher values than the males. A similar difference in the liver weights has recently been shown to be statistically significant in White Leghorn chicks by Gordon (1960b) who also noted that the microscopic appearance of the germfree livers presented a much more regular pattern than was found in conventional birds. No difference was noted when the weights of germfree and conventional rat livers were compared (Gordon, 1960b). Phillips *et al.* (1959) found the livers of germfree guinea pigs to be "normal." The values obtained by Glimstedt (1936b) (Table 5.9) showed a decreased weight of the liver in germfree animals when compared to conventional animals. The relative weight of the liver was greater in conventional mice than in germfree mice (Gordon, 1960b).

In the chemical analysis of the livers of germfree and conventional animals, no real differences were noted in the percentage dry weight, nitrogen, ash, or fat for White Wyandotte Bantam chicks at any age category up to 1 year of age (Table 5.6). The conventional birds had somewhat more phosphorus than the germfree birds. Conventional birds had less nonprotein nitrogen in the liver than had germfree birds. In the livers of conventional White Wyandotte Bantam chicks the concentration of thiamine was twice as high as that found in the livers of germfree birds. The riboflavin content of the livers of Bantam chicks at 4–5 weeks of age was similar in both categories. However, 3–4 weeks later the conventional birds had a greater concentration of riboflavin in the liver than was found for the germfree birds. The pantothenic acid content of the liver of conventional birds was usually less than that found for germfree birds. No differences were seen in the pyridoxine, niacin, biotin, or folic acid concentration of the liver of the Bantam chicks in different categories.

In White Leghorn chicks, germfree and conventional birds had comparable relative liver weights (Table 5.2). However, the conventional birds had a greater percentage of dry weight at 4–7 weeks than had the germfree birds (Table 5.7). The percentage of ash on a dry weight basis in the liver of conventional birds was probably less than that found for germfree birds. The conventional Leghorn chicks had a greater amount of fat in the liver at 4–7 weeks of age than was found in the germfree birds. No difference was seen between the two groups of 10 week old birds. Kritchevsky et al. (1959) found that the non-saponifiable fraction of the liver lipids and the cholesterol were present in highest quantity when the birds were fed starch as the carbohydrate. These values were usually lower in conventional chicks than in germfree chicks (Table 5.20). The phosphorus content of the liver of germfree and conventional birds was similar in the 4–7 week age categories. The nitrogen content of the liver was similar in the 10 week old birds. The thiamine content of the liver indicated the possibility of less thiamine in the conventional birds at 4–7 weeks than was found in germfree birds. No difference was found in the two categories with respect to riboflavin, niacin, pyridoxine, and biotin. The germfree chicks had 50% more pantothenic acid in the liver than was found for conventional birds. This difference confirmed that found with Bantam chicks. Germfree Leghorns were also found to have more folic acid and vitamin B_{12} in the liver than had conventional birds. The vitamin C in the liver of conventional birds was approximately four times that found in germfree birds. When the concentration of B vitamins in the liver was considered with respect to maturation of germfree chicks, the data showed a decrease with age for pantothenic acid and riboflavin, while folic acid remained nearly constant.

Carnitine was found to be present in the liver of germfree birds (22.4 μg/gm dry tissue) by Fraenkel (1954) in quantities comparable to those found in conventional chicks. Its presence there may have little significance since some of the dietary ingredients, i.e., casein, contained carnitine. A. W. Phillips (1960) found the monoamine oxidase content of livers of 4 week old conventional chicks to be only one-half of that found in germfree chicks.

Analysis of the liver indicated no difference in the amount of dry weight of this organ in germfree and conventional rats. (Table 5.5). The ash content of the liver of germfree and conventional rats was similar at 29 days and at 67 days. However, at 162 days the germfree rats were found to have significantly less liver ash than was found in conventional rats. The fat content of the liver of germfree and conventional rats was very similar except in the older categories. At 256 days the conventional rats were found to have less liver fat than was found for germfree rats. The nitrogen content of the liver of germfree

TABLE 5.20

LIVER LIPIDS IN 28-DAY-OLD CHICKS FED 3% CHOLESTEROL AND 5% CORN OIL[a]

| Diet | | Nonsaponifiable (mg/gm) | | | | | | Cholesterol (mg/gm) | | | | | |
| | | Germfree | | | Conventional | | | Germfree | | | Conventional | | |
Protein, 25%	Carbohydrate, 54%	No.[b]	Mean	Range	No.	Mean	Range	No.	Mean	Range	No.	Mean	Range
Casein	Glucose	11	498	380-754	10	343	191-478	11	111	35-201	10	86	32-150
Casein	Sucrose	10	426	295-679	10	426	302-782	10	104	79-183	10	121	72-260
Casein	Starch	10	1300	859-1906	10	846	520-940	10	467	279-598	10	202	170-248
Promine (soya protein)	Starch	10	599	245-1000	10	480	300-777	10	233	65-452	10	152	98-255

[a]Data of Kritchevsky et al. (1959).
[b]Number of observations.

rats tended to be somewhat higher than that of conventional rats. The difference approached significance in the younger rats; as the rats matured, the difference disappeared. The concentration of B vitamins in the liver of rats 162 days old is presented in Table 5.5. It is seen that the concentration of each was somewhat lower in conventional rats than in the germfree rats. The difference was significant only in the folic acid comparison. Meister (1960) found D-amino acid oxidase in germfree and classic mouse livers. This evidence suggests the presence of the enzyme is not a result of adaptive enzyme formation in response to D-amino acids produced within the intestine.

Küster (1914) found no difference in liver dry weight when germfree and conventional goat twins were compared. Germfree pups fed diet L-102 were found to have 25.9% (20.8–26.4%) dry weight and 6.32% (6.32–6.33%) fat in the livers.

Differences in the composition of the livers with respect to maturation and aging may be compared on a 100 gm body weight basis. The total liver ash dropped markedly with age in the germfree White Wyandotte Bantam chickens; and although the liver ash dropped in the conventional chicks, the change was less dramatic. The concentration of riboflavin and folic acid per 100 gm body weight dropped markedly in both germfree and conventional birds. In germfree chicks the quantity of pantothenic acid in the liver decreased with age when expressed on a 100 gm body weight basis, while it increased with age in conventional birds. A regular decrease was noted for the pyridoxine content of the liver as germfree White Wyandotte Bantam chicks matured: this difference was not comparable to the data from conventional birds. Since the patterns seen in the change of tissue composition during maturation were more regular in germfree conditions, it would be interesting to continue these studies into senescence for germfree animals.

Bile

The gross appearance of the gall bladder and dark green bile was similar in germfree and conventional chicks. When the birds were malnurtured or starving, bile engorged the gall bladder. In well nurtured birds the quantity of bile was about the same in germfree and conventional birds (see Table 5.2). The straw colored bile of guinea pigs and mice looked the same in both germfree and conventional animals. The gall bladder of germfree guinea pigs showed good tonus (Phillips *et al.*, 1959).

Chemical analysis of the bile of Leghorn chicks indicated the dry weight of bile of conventional birds was higher than that of germfree chicks. No difference was seen in the per cent of ash or nitrogen on a dry basis, nor were differences found in the concentration of niacin, pantothenic acid, or folic acid of the bile between the germfree and conventional chicks. However, the conventional chicks had much less riboflavin and biotin in their bile than had germfree birds.

Excretory System

Kidney

The gross morphology of the kidneys of conventional chicks was very similar to that of germfree chicks. The total weight, about 0.09% of the body weight, was comparable in both groups. The weight of the kidney relative to total body mass might have been greater in conventional than in germfree guinea pigs at 1 and 2 months of age according to the data of Glimstedt (1936b) (Table 5.9). However, there was overlapping between the groups. The urinary system of the germfree guinea pigs was found to be normal by Phillips et al. (1959). A similar statement could be made regarding the excretory system of germfree rats and mice.

The percentage dry weight in the kidney was identical in germfree and conventional birds (Tables 5.6 and 5.4). There was a persistent tendency ($p = 0.08$) for the conventional White Leghorn birds to have a lower kidney ash in comparison with that of germfree birds. There were no differences in the fat or nitrogen content of the kidney between germfree and conventional birds.

No differences in dry weight of kidney of germfree and conventional rats were seen at any age category (Table 5.5). The ash content of kidney of germfree rats was lower than that of conventional rats for most age groups. The fat and nitrogen content of kidney of young germfree and conventional rats were very similar. However, at 265 days the conventional rat kidney was higher in fat than was found for germfree rats and the nitrogen of the kidney of the germfree rat was somewhat higher than that of the conventional rat. The dry weight and fat content of kidney in germfree pups was 18.6 (17.5–19.7)% and 4.5 (4.54–4.59)% respectively. Küster (1914) found the kidney of germfree and conventional goats to have the same dry weight. D-Amino acid oxidase was found in similar concentrations in germfree and conventional mouse kidneys (Meister, 1960).

Urine

Urine of germfree and conventional mammals appeared to be similar by visual observation. The straw colored liquid had the same color, fluidity, and clarity in both categories. The volume varied with the fluid intake and composition, and the diet composition. When sugar water was fed, as in the dental caries experiments, much fluid was consumed and excreted. When distilled water was given, less was consumed than when tap water was fed; such was reflected in the urinary output. Accepting such variation, it was generally found that conventional rats used less water and passed less urine than germfree rats (see data of the metabolism study in Chapter 4) fed diets of the same composition.

The urine of germfree guinea pigs contained aromatic oxy acids and no phenol, cresol, indole, skatole, or pyrocatechin (Nuttall and Thierfelder, 1896b). Analysis of urine of germfree goats (Küster, 1913b) (see Table 5.21) showed that most of the nitrogen was in the form of urea and about one-fifth of that amount occurred as ammonia. His comparisons may not be valid since the number of values for "normal" is small, the fluctuation was great, and the urine was not preserved aseptically during the collection periods. The ammonia in the urine of germfree goats appeared to decrease with age. Küster found ethyl sulfates in the urine of germfree goats. Protein, leucocytes, and coffin-lid shaped crystals appeared in the urine when the kid was suffering from formalin toxicity.

Gustafsson *et al.* (1957b) found urinary histamine to be excreted in equal quantities in germfree and conventional rats. Male rats excreted histamine primarily in conjugated form. Germfree female rats excreted both free and conjugated histamine, while conventional female rats excreted primarily free histamine. No urinary indican was found in germfree mice, rats, and chicks, or conventional chicks by Wagner (1958), while conventional rats and mice gave a strong positive urinary indole test. Part of the difference in odor of germfree animal cages and conventional animal colonies was thought to be due to the lack of ammonia excretion by germfree animals. This was confirmed by Levenson *et al.* (1959) who found only C^{14} urea was excreted by germfree rats while conventional rats excreted 2% of the C^{14} urea carbon as $C^{14}O_2$ within 6 hours. Such results supported the hypothesis that enzymatic hydrolysis of urea in mammals was effected by the urease of associated microorganisms.

TABLE 5.21
COMPOSITION OF GOAT URINE[a]

Animal condition	Total nitrogen	Urea + NH₃ N (%)	NH₃/N (%)	Urea N (%)	NH₃ N[b] total N	Urea + NH₃ N[b] total N	Urea N[b] total N
Germfree	0.28	0.23	0.048	0.18	17	82	64
	0.254	0.21	0.039	0.17	15.4	82	67
	0.14	0.07	0.028	0.042	20	50	30
	0.140	0.089	0.014	0.075	10	63	53
	0.202	0.155	0.005	0.149	2.5	76	73
	0.500	0.393	0.078	0.315	14	64	50
	0.311	0.224	0.015	0.209	5	71	66
	0.272	0.151	0.0168	0.138	6	56	50
Germfree; Hay bacilli plus E. coli contaminated	0.208	0.149	0.034	0.115	17	72	55
	0.208	0.143	0.044	0.099	207	69	48
	0.322	0.308	0.042	0.266	13	85	72
Normal	0.258	0.197	0.014	0.183	5.4	76	71
	0.205	0.146	0.123	0.023	60	71[c]	11[c]
Contaminated urine	0.143	0.115	0.104	0.011	72.5	81[c]	8[c]

[a] Kuster (1915).
[b] Ratio x 100
[c] Urine contaminated by bacterial action.

Nervous System

Conventional and germfree birds were much alike as judged from examination of brain, spinal cord, and peripheral nerves at autopsy. The relative net weight of the brain (Table 5.2) was similar in the two groups, although it did decrease with age. Germfree guinea pigs (Phillips *et al.*, 1959), rats, and mice had "normal" nervous system by gross observation.

The percentage dry weight, nitrogen and fat of brain of conventional and germfree birds was almost identical for all age categories (Tables 5.4 and 5.6). The percentage of ash on a dry weight basis was found to be somewhat higher in the germfree Leghorn chicks than in the conventional Leghorn chicks. Brains of conventional and germfree Leghorn birds had similar concentrations of riboflavin, niacin, biotin, folic acid, vitamin B_{12}, and vitamin C. The main difference noted was that the conventional birds had a greater concentration of pantothenic acid than was seen in the germfree birds.

The percentage dry weight of the brain was somewhat greater in conventional rats than in germfree rats at 29 days but not in older rats. No differences were noted between the amount of ash in the brain of conventional and germfree rats, excepting at 65 days the conventional rats had somewhat less brain ash than had the germfree rats. The conventional rats had less fat in the brain than was found for germfree rats at 4 weeks but this difference was not seen in older rats.

Sensory Organs: Nose, Ear, Eye, Tongue

The noses, ears, eyes, and tongues of germfree and conventional chicks and mammals were identical by macroscopic observation. The eyes were bright, lustrous, and had good color in all cases. The weight of the eyes of germfree and conventional Leghorn chicks were very similar (Table 5.2). Relative to the body weight, the size decreased with age. The eyes of Cesarean born, hand-fed, germfree rats opened at the same time (2 weeks) as those of normal born rats in either germfree or conventional environments. The light red retinal plexus typical of the albino rat was seen with equal clarity in the germfree albino rat. The eyes of conventional mice often show signs of irritation, sometimes with half-closed lids (or lids closed with exudate). These conditions were not seen in germfree mice which appeared to be more "wide-eyed."

The beaks of germfree chicks were well developed, and the color

of the beak varied with the constituents of the diet. The mucous lining
of the mouth of chicks appeared to be quite normal in germfree birds.
The glistening red surface was very similar to that of birds containing
microorganisms. The tongue of the germfree birds appeared from
macroscopic observation to be healthy with well defined papillae.

The external auditory organs of all the birds examined were identical from a gross viewpoint. Kelemen (1960) found the ears of germfree rats to be free of any signs of infection. The spaces of the internal
ears were very free; Reissner's membrane was stretched normally, and
the sensory organs were in satisfactory condition.

Lymphatic System

Those organs and tissue which are removed from daily intimate
contact with microorganisms are comparable in germfree and conventional animals; those organs and tissues functioning against the
interminable activities of microorganisms show a greater development
of the elements of defense. Glimstedt (1932) noted that the lymphatic
system of germfree guinea pigs was grossly underdeveloped. His
data (Table 5.9) showed that lymph nodes serving cervical, bronchial,
and mesenteric areas were 3–5 times greater in conventional than in
germfree guinea pigs, while the lymphatic development in the scapu-
lar, inguinal, and pancreatic areas were only 2-fold greater in conventional than in germfree animals. He found the cellular composition
of the lymphatic tissue in both categories to be similar, except for the
great reduction in lymphocyte number and the absence of secondary
nodules in germfree guinea pigs. Inside the lymph node the parenchyma was rarefied and the number of lymphocytes was greatly
decreased. Glimstedt's findings were echoed by Tajima (1955),
Miyakawa (1957c), and Phillips et al. (1959) who found especially
poor development of mesenteric lymph nodes and Peyer's patches.
Little reaction of cortisone or ACTH was seen in the depression of
small lymphocytes or their nuclear division in germfree guinea pigs
(Miyakawa et al., 1957a). Tajima (1955) noted the ratio of large to
small lymph nodes to be 8.9, 3.0, and 2.2 for naturally reared, artificially reared, and germfree guinea pigs, respectively. Miyakawa et al.
1957a) gave a detailed description of the number and development of
Peyer's patches and lymph nodes in other areas. No clear-centered
secondary nodules were seen histologically, but plasma cells were
seen on the medullary cord. Clear centered, secondary nodules appeared when the guinea pigs were inoculated with a single species of

microorganisms. A single injection of egg albumin caused the appearance of numerous large cells containing a large nucleolus, but no clear-centered secondary nodules were seen.

With the ileocecal tonsil of the birds being used as an index of the lymph node development generally, a great difference was found (Reyniers *et al.*, 1960a; Gordon, 1960b) between germfree and conventional chickens. Conventional birds had a tonsil of much greater size and a much fuller and more turgid organ than was found in germfree birds. The ileocecal tonsils of the germfree birds were flabby, inconspicuous, and pale in this comparison. The difference between the two was seen at 1 month, and this difference persisted until approximately 5 months. From then on the difference became less conspicuous; the lymph node development of the germfree birds approached that of the conventional birds, while the well developed reddish, firm tonsils of the conventional birds gradually became dulled with advancing age. The relative weight of the trident at the ileocecal valve which contains both ileocecal tonsils was consistently and substantially smaller in germfree birds than in conventional birds. The concentration of lymphocytes in the ileocecal tonsils of the germfree birds was from one-fifth to one-twentieth of that found in the birds harboring live bacteria. It was quite apparent that the presence of living microorganisms contributed greatly to the development of the ileocecal tonsil in birds as well as in mammals.

Thorbecke (1959) found no plasma cells or secondary nodules in the ileocecal-colic junction of germfree chicks at 2, 4, 8, and 14 weeks (Table 5.32). They were found in conventional chicks of all ages and in germfree chicks 6 weeks of age. She found plasma cells and secondary nodules to be less numerous in the mesenteric lymph nodes and intestinal mucosa of germfree rats than in conventional rats. Gordon (1960b) found twice as many Peyer's patches in conventional rats as in germfree rats: both the number and weight of Peyer's patches were decreased in germfree rats. Gustafsson (1948) had previously noted the general underdevelopment of the lymphatic system in young germfree rats.

In conventional rats at 3 months of age the weight of the ileocecal lymph nodes was about 2.5 times that of germfree rats. A similar pattern was found by Gordon (1960b) for Swiss mice at 48–66 days of age. Similar data for cecal lymph nodes is seen in Table 5.16; however, the number of lymphocytes per mm^3 was the same for germfree and conventional rats. A comparative study of these relationships is pre-

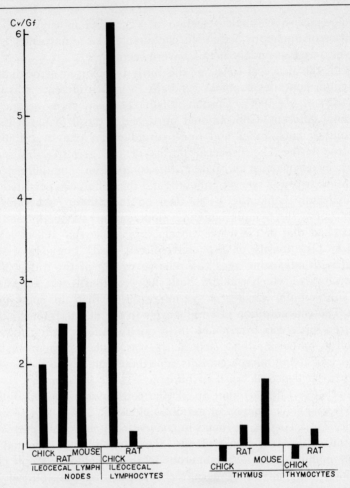

Fig. 5.7. Comparison of the relative weights of lymph nodes and thymus. The vertical bars indicate the ratio obtained by comparing the conventional to the germfree values. (Gordon, 1960b.)

sented in Fig. 5.7. The chick had about 6 times more ileocecal lymphocytes in the conventional state than in the germfree state while surprisingly, the rat showed no significant difference.

In a detailed study of the development of the nasal lymphatic system, Miyakawa (1959b) found that prenatally formed lymphatic tissue developed on the floor of the nasal cavity. The postnatal development of lymphatic tissue in germfree guinea pigs developed little beyond this stage. Lymphatic tissue was found in small amounts, few nodules with solid centers were seen, and no clear-centered, secondary nodules (Fleming nodules) were found in germfree guinea pigs at 40 days. In conventional guinea pigs at 40 days he found well developed lymphatic tissue with solid secondary nodules and the ciliated epithelium in the mucous lining had become stratified. Miyakawa also noted the lymphatic tissue in the sinus maxillaris of 40 day old germfree guinea pigs showed little development when compared to that of conventional and monoinoculated guinea pigs. Again, no secondary nodules or lymphatic infiltrations were seen, and the ciliated epithelium of the mucous membrane had not become stratified in germfree guinea pigs, whereas conventional guinea pigs had a well developed lymphatic system in the sinuses. Gordon (1960b) reported the submaxillary lymph nodes of 3 month old Wistar rats had about 4 times greater relative weight in the conventional state than in the germfree environment.

The bursa Fabricius of the chick was expected to be similar to the ileocecal tonsil which it has been thought to resemble in character, function, and location. It is also similar to the thymus in that it undergoes complete involution as the birds approach sexual maturity. Therefore, it was an organ of special interest from several viewpoints. Macroscopically, Gordon (in Reyniers et al., 1960a) found the bursa of White Leghorn chicks of all categories presented the same qualitative and quantitative picture. In White Wyandotte Bantam chicks the bursa of conventional chicks was larger per 100 gm body weight than that of germfree chicks although the variability of the organ was great in all categories of birds studies. The dry weight of the bursa of the Bantams was found to be the same in both germfree and conventional birds. This view agreed with that presented by Thorbecke (1959) who concluded that the bursa of Fabricius must differ in development as well as in function from other lymphoid nodules. Thorbecke et al. (1957) found no plasma cells in the bursal follicles.

Spleen

Macroscopic observation of the spleen indicated that the general structure, color, and consistency of both the peripheral and the cut surfaces were similar in condition and development in germfree and conventional chicks. The relative size of the spleen was found to be lowest in some of the germfree birds (Table 5.2). This difference was particularly noticeable in the germfree White Wyandotte Bantam chicks under 2 months of age. In the White Leghorn chicks, the spleen of the germfree birds tended toward a lower weight than was found in conventional birds (Table 5.13), but the difference was not statistically significant. The lymphocyte concentration in the spleen of conventional birds and that of germfree birds was found to be approximately equal. This conception is open to question since Thorbecke *et al.* (1957) stated that spleens of germfree animals "show

TABLE 5.22

ESTIMATION OF THE FREQUENCY OF OCCURRENCE OF
PLASMA CELLS IN WHITE LEGHORN CHICKS[a]

	Age (weeks)	No. of chicks	Spleen	Thymus	Ileocecal junction
Germfree	4	6	2(1 — 3)	1(0 — 1)	0(0 — 0)
	8	5	3(2 — 4)	2(1 — 2)[b]	1(0 — 2)
Control	4	5	3(3 — 4)	2(0 — 2)	3(2 — 4)
	8	5	3(3 — 4)	3(2 — 4)	4(3 — 4)

[a]From Thornbecke (1959).
[b]Only 3 observations.

little development of the lymphoid tissue." Plasma cells were found in the spleen of germfree White Leghorn chicks in number equal to those found in conventional chicks. These cells were found less often in the thymus and ileocecal junction of the germfree chick than in the conventional chick (Thorbecke, 1959) as shown in Table 5.22.

The spleens of germfree guinea pigs were small but showed normal distribution between the red and white pulp (Phillips *et al.*, 1959). Glimstedt (1936a) found the spleen was smaller in size (Table 5.9) and contained less white pulp in germfree animals. The spleen of germfree male rats at 3 months of age was found to be about one-half as large as that of conventional control rats by Gordon and Wostmann (1960a) (Table 5.15). Thorbecke (1959) found fewer plasma cells and secondary nodules in the spleens of germfree rats than in conventional rats. Figure 5.8 shows a large reaction center with secondary nodule in the spleen of a germfree rat. The spleens of conventional mice were 2–3 times larger and had a deeper red color when compared to spleens of germfree mice.

The dry weight of the spleen of germfree and conventional Bantam chicks was identical until 7–8 months when the conventional birds showed a somewhat smaller percentage dry weight than was found in

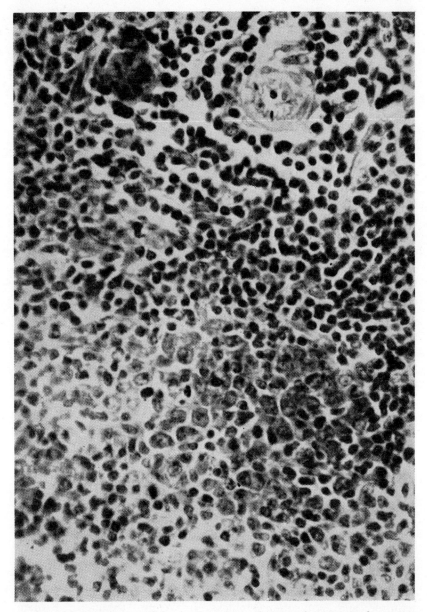

FIG. 5.8. Secondary nodules in the spleen of a germfree rat. Such reaction centers are found in conventional guinea pigs but not in germfree guinea pigs. They are occasionally seen in germfree chicks. (Thorbecke and Benacerraf, 1959.)

the germfree birds. This difference was not seen in birds at 1 year of age. Analysis of the spleen of germfree and conventional rats indicated no difference in the dry weight between the two groups (Table 5.5). The percentage of ash in the spleen of conventional rats was variable; at 29 days it was significantly greater than that of germfree rat spleens. The reason for fluctuation in the ash in the spleens of conventional rats was not apparent.

Thymus

The thymus data indicate that changes in the thymus were similar to those described for the bursa of Fabricius. No macroscopic difference was seen between the thymus of the conventional birds and that of the germfree birds in either qualitative or quantitative examination. The weights presented (Tables 5.3 and 5.4) showed very little variation and no consistent difference between animals with or without microorganisms. Microscopically, the thymus appeared very similar and thymocytes were equally abundant in both groups of birds. Thorbecke (1959) found plasma cells less numerous in the thymus of germfree birds than in conventional birds. No secondary nodules were found in either groups at 2–8 weeks of age.

Glimstedt (1936a) noted a decreased size in the thymus of germfree guinea pigs when they were compared to conventional guinea pigs (Table 5.9). The thymus of germfree guinea pigs was found to be small and "fatty" by Phillips et al. (1959). In 3 month old Wistar rats the relative weight of the thymus was smaller in germfree rats while the number of thymocytes per mm^3 tended to be greater ($p = 0.06$) in conventional than in germfree animals (Gordon and Wostmann, 1960). The relative weight of the thymus of Swiss mice at 48–66 days was not significantly greater in conventional mice (Gordon, 1960b). Thorbecke (1959) stated that neither large plasma cells aggregates nor secondary nodules were present in the thymus of germfree mammals.

Endocrine Glands

Thyroid Gland

The general appearance of the thyroid gland was very similar in germfree and conventional chicks. In White Wyandotte Bantam chicks, there was no difference in wet weight, total weight, or relative weight of the thyroid gland of germfree and conventional chicks, irrespective of sex, body weight, or age groups. In the few White Leghorn chicks studied the relative size of the thyroid of the germfree birds was less than one-half the value reported for conventional birds (Table 5.2). It would be interesting to obtain information on thyroid size in germfree mammals.

Adrenal Gland

The adrenal glands of conventional chicks were identical to those of germfree birds by gross observation. The total mass showed no difference using either wet or dry weight data in White Leghorn or White Wyandotte Bantam chicks. Adrenal glands in germfree guinea pigs (Phillips *et al.*, 1959) and mice resembled those of conventional animals. Glimstedt (1936a) found no difference in the relative weights of adrenals from germfree and conventional guinea pigs (Table 5.9) at 30 days of age. The data from 60 day old guinea pigs were less easily interpreted. Gordon (1960b) reported the wet weight of adrenal glands per 100 gm body weight was greater in germfree rats than in conventional rats (Table 5.15).

Adrenal cholesterol was found to be higher in conventional Bantam chicks than in germfree birds at 2 weeks of age. This difference disappeared and was not seen in chicks from 1 month to 1 year of age. The ascorbic acid content of adrenal glands was the same in germfree and conventional Leghorn chicks.

Gonads

The testicles of White Leghorn and White Wyandotte Bantam conventional birds were very similar in over-all appearance, relative weight, wet weight, and percent dry weight to those of germfree birds. Although some possible differences were indicated, the variability found in the birds precluded their being statistically valid.

The male reproductive glands were normal in the germfree guinea pig, and Phillips *et al.* (1959) observed abundant viable spermatocytes and sperm in the epidydimus and ductus deferens. The penis, testes, prostate, and epidydimus appeared to be comparable in germfree and conventional mice.

The ovary in young Leghorns showed no gross difference between conventional and germfree birds. The mass of the ovary was almost identical in the two groups, on both an absolute and relative-to-body-weight basis (Tables 5.2 and 5.13). The variability in the groups was rather great for these organs. The same statements could be made for the Bantam chicks observed (see Table 5.14). Detailed studies have not been reported on mature functioning ovary or oviduct in the germfree hen. Germfree White Wyandotte Bantam hens layed eggs at the same age and rate as did conventional hens fed the same diet. Reyniers and Sacksteder (1960a) report egg production in germfree quail. The ovaries of the germfree guinea pigs of Phillips *et al.* (1959) appeared anemic: numerous ova were seen, no corpus luteum was seen, and no sign of recent ovulation were seen in 3 females over 1 year of age. This picture was considerably altered by reports of reproduction in germfree guinea pigs (Teah, 1959). Reproduction in germfree mice, rats, and rabbits is good evidence for a functioning ovary in these species.

Since the vagina is susceptible to secondary infection by its normal but potentially pathogenic flora, Beaver (1960) studied the exudative phase of the estrous cycle by injection of progesterone into germfree mice. These mice were found to have the typical inflammatory response with extensive neutrophil infiltration of the vaginal mucosa and exudation of cells into the lumen. Micro abscesses and isolated examples of cellular degeneration were seen histologically. The leucocytic attraction to this area was a striking exception to the lack of activity by the "uneducated" leucocytes during infection and wound healing in germfree animals.

Pituitary

The size of the pituitary gland relative to body weight in germfree and conventional White Leghorn chicks was nearly identical (Table 5.2). The pituitary of germfree guinea pigs was comparable to that of conventional guinea pigs (Phillips *et al.*, 1959).

Defense Mechanisms

In presenting the body defense mechanisms in as broad a pattern as proposed, difficulties arise in trying to distinguish an over-all effect of a single organism upon the host. Certain aspects of the interaction between the microorganisms and the host may be to the benefit of the host and certain others might be detrimental. With innocuous microorganisms, it may be improper to call the host response a defense mechanism since the over-all effect of the microorganism may be beneficial to the host. For the sake of clarity, each microorganism inoculated into or presented to a germfree animal will be considered as if it did stimulate one or more defense systems.

Physiological defense mechanisms include the active excretion of microorganisms via nasal-oral-fecal-urinary discharge, the production of fevers, the increased blood flow to active areas of invasion, and the various aspects of phagocytosis. Much of the physiological action might be brought to a biochemical basis and most of the information given under serology is based upon biochemistry. The biochemical defense mechanisms are primarily of protein nature—lipoproteins decrease the permeability of skin; serum antibodies are effective against foreign antigens; cathepsins and enzymes such as lysozyme are effective in destroying microorganisms. Nonprotein antimicrobial compounds include the acid of the stomach and a variety of other compounds produced by the tissues. Such compounds are major components of natural resistance—that element which prevents microorganisms from producing disease in some individuals or species when they are virulent pathogens for others.

Anatomical

The obvious and most probably the best studied parts of the body defense system are the anatomical structures. The integrity of the skin and the mucosal surface of the mouth, respiratory, gastrointestinal, and urinary genital systems provide the first line of defense against invasion of microorganisms to the tissues. The specialized structures of some of the cells and the subsurface units are contributory to the over-all effectiveness of this first line of defense; i.e., the cilia of the epithelial cells which move in such fashion as to dislodge any particles toward the outside of the body cavities. Secondly, we must consider the phagocytes which exist in most tissues, blood, and in the epidermal layers. The variety of the cells capable of phagocytosis, the differences in their origin, and the effectiveness of their action will be discussed under phagocytes as such. Part of this picture is the development of the lymphatic system and the lymph nodes and the effectiveness of the nodes in storing and providing new phagocytes of different cytological or morphological species.

The first and possibly still the greatest amount of work done in the area of anatomical development with respect to defense mechanisms was that of Gosta Glimstedt (1936a) in the investigation of the development of the lymphatic system of the guinea pigs. He was particularly interested in the Hellman reaction centers, the secondary development of the inner lymph nodes. His work and subsequent morphological investigation by Thorbecke, Miyakawa, and Gordon were presented under the headings of spleen, thymus, lymph nodes, and blood.

The reduction in size of the ileocecal tonsil in the White Wyandotte Bantam chicken (Gordon, 1955) was shown by quantitative histological techniques to be paralleled by the reduction in the number of lymphocytes present in it; only one-tenth as many ileocecal lymphocytes were present in the germfree bird as were found in the conventional birds. Gordon found no differences in the lymphocyte count of the spleen while the blood had only one-half as many lymphocytes in the germfree animals as in the conventional animal. By analyzing the lymphocyte concentration in arterial and venous vessels connected to different organs, Gordon found that in the conventional rat a large number of lymphocytes were removed from the blood by the upper intestine while a lesser quantity were taken by segments of the lower intestine (due, in part, to the greater lymphopoietic capacity of the lower intestine). In germfree rats, the segments from the upper intestine were found to relieve the blood of very few lymphocytes, and in segments of the lower gut more lymphocytes were found in the venous than in the arterial blood. These results could be interpreted to mean that with no bacteria in the intestine, few lymphocytes were removed from the blood for defense mechanisms. In the lower gut of germfree rats lymphopoiesis progressed at a low rate. Similar analysis of the splenic blood showed this organ to be a major contributor to blood lymphocytes. The spleen of the germfree rat showed reduced lymphopoiesis when compared to that of conventional rats. When germfree animals were contaminated lymphopoiesis increased 7-fold within a 3 week period.

Serology

Serum bactericidal power. The serum of germfree guinea pigs was found to have little bactericidal power against *Salmonella typhi* while that of conventional guinea pigs killed 80% of the organism within 6 minutes according to the work of Togano (1958), Tanami (1959), and Ootaka (1959). Similar results with *S. typhi, Shigella dysenteriae,* and *E. coli* were obtained by Sacquet *et al.* (1961). Other bacteria tested by respiration studies showed no difference. The effects of specific microorganisms on the bactericidal action of serum is presented in Chapter 6.

Antibodies. In tests for agglutinins for foreign species erythrocytes, Wagner (in Reyniers *et al.*, 1960a) found that rabbit erythrocytes were not agglutinated by the serum of germfree and conventional chicks at 1 day, nor at 10–14 days. The reaction at 30–40 days was almost as strong as that of older birds, and no difference was found between germfree and conventional birds. When the agglutinins in germfree and conventional chicken serum were challenged with rat erythrocytes, the reactions were very similar to those observed with rabbit red blood cells, although titers were somewhat lower (see Table 5.23). Germfree chicks showed no reaction with erythrocytes from sheep, horse, Leghorn chicken, and human (type O, A, and B) erythrocytes. This same pattern was seen in conventional chicks with the exception that occasionally an older chick would react with horse erythrocytes at 1 to 2 dilution. Similar response was seen by Wagner (Reyniers *et al.*, 1949d) in White Wyandotte Bantam chicks (Table 5.24). Precipitants for dietary protein such as gelatin, hog protein, casein, or yeast extract were consistently negative in both germfree and conventional birds in all age categories. Complement was found in germfree Bantam chicks, the Mazzini reaction was positive and the Kahn reaction was probably negative. Wagner discussed the discrepancy between his data and that of others using conventional chicks and suggested that it was due to differences in diet, source or breed of chicks, environment, technique, or interpretation. Since the reactions in germfree and conventional chicks were similar it was probable that the production of heterohemagglutinins was not dependent upon the presence or activity of viable microbial forms. Wagner (1959b) suggested that the anti-rat and anti-rabbit hemagglutinins in germfree chickens were probably produced in response to some as yet unrecognized antigenic components of the diet which illicit the response noted. This would be in keeping with the finding of Springer *et al.* (1959a,b) that germfree chicks had hemagglutinins for type B erythrocytes. They also concluded that the so-called natural heteroagglutinins and antibacterial agglutinins which were observed in conventional chicks probably arose by immunogenic reaction rather than spontaneous reaction. The spontaneous origin of the agglutinins seemed to be a remote possibility.

Germfree rats had no heterohemagglutinins in the serum against the erythrocytes of bovine, human, rabbit, sheep, chicken, or horse. No response was obtained in conventional rats under similar conditions in the experience of Wagner (1959b). However conventional rats older than 300 days did show a low titer. It is important to remember that the germfree animals used to date were not entirely antigen free.

TABLE 5.23
HEMAGGLUTININS IN DILUTED SERUM OF GERMFREE AND CONVENTIONAL WHITE LEGHORN CHICKS[a]

Agglutinin for	Germ status	Age 31-39 days					Age 50-67 days					
		No. runs[b]	1/2	1/4	1/8	1/16	No. runs[b]	1/2	1/4	1/8	1/16	1/32
Rabbit erythro-cyte	Gf	6	0	4	2	0	10	0	2	5	3	0
	Cv	2	0	2	0	0	7	0	0	4	3	0
Rat erythrocyte	Gf	6	4	1	0	0	10	3	5	2	0	0
	Cv	2	2	0	0	0	7	1	5	1	0	0
Paracolobactrum aerogenoides	Gf	6	0	0	0	0	10	0	0	0	0	0
	Cv	2	0	2	0	0	7	0	0	2	4	1
Escherichia coli	Gf	5	0	0	0	0	10	0	0	0	0	0
	Cv	2	1	1	0	0	7	1	5	1	0	0
Lactobacillus sp. (fecal)	Gf	6	0	0	0	0	10	0	0	0	0	0
	Cv	1	0	0	0	0	7	0	3	3	0	0
Lactobacillus sp. (diet)	Gf	5	0	0	0	0	10	0	0	0	0	0
	Cv	2	0	0	0	0	7	1	1	0	0	0
Lactobacillus sp. (human)	Gf	4	0	0	0	0	10	0	0	0	0	0
	Cv	2	0	0	0	0	7	1	0	0	0	0
Micrococcus pyogenes	Gf	4	0	0	0	0	10	0	0	0	0	0
	Cv	2	0	1	1	0	7	5	1	0	0	0
Micrococcus epidermidis	Gf	6	0	0	0	0	10	0	0	0	0	0
	Cv	2	0	1	1	0	7	0	2	3	2	0

Agglutinin for	Germ status	Age 150-168 days								
		No. runs[b]	1/2	1/4	1/8	1/16	1/32	1/64	1/128	1/256
Rabbit erythro-cyte	Gf	5	0	1	3	0	1	0	0	0
	Cv	2	0	0	0	0	0	2	0	0
Rat erythrocyte	Gf	5	2	1	0	1	0	0	0	0
	Cv	2	0	0	1	1	0	0	0	0
Paracolobactrum aerogenoides	Gf	5	0	0	0	0	0	0	0	0
	Cv	2	0	0	0	0	0	0	2	0
Escherichia coli	Gf	5	0	0	0	0	0	0	0	0
	Cv	2	0	0	1	1	0	0	0	0
Lactobacillus sp. (fecal)	Gf	5	0	0	0	0	0	0	0	0
	Cv	2	0	0	0	2	0	0	0	0
Lactobacillus sp. (diet)	Gf	5	0	0	0	0	0	0	0	0
	Cv	2	2	0	0	0	0	0	0	0
Lactobacillus sp. (human)	Gf	5	0	0	0	0	0	0	0	0
	Cv	2	1	1	0	0	0	0	0	0
Micrococcus pyogenes	Gf	5	0	0	0	0	0	0	0	0
	Cv	2	1	1	0	0	0	0	0	0
Micrococcus epidermidis	Gf	5	0	0	0	0	0	0	0	0
	Cv	2	0	0	0	0	1	1	0	0

Agglutinin for	Germ status	Age 200+ days						
		No. runs[b]	1/2	1/4	1/8	1/16	1/32	1/43	1/128
Rabbit erythro-cyte	Gf	3	0	1	0	0	1	1	0
	Cv	2	0	0	0	0	2	0	0
Rat erythrocyte	Gf	3	0	1	1	1	0	0	0
	Cv	2	0	0	1	0	0	0	0

TABLE 5.23 (Continued)

Agglutinin for	Germ status	No. runs[b]	Age 200+ days (continued) Titer						
			1/2	1/4	1/8	1/16	1/32	1/43	1/128
Paracolobactrum aerogenoides	Gf	3	0	0	0	0	0	0	0
	Cv	2	0	0	0	2	0	0	0
Escherichia coli	Gf	3	0	0	0	0	0	0	0
	Cv	2	0	0	0	1	1	0	0
Lactobacillus sp. (fecal)	Gf	2	1	0	1	0	0	0	0
	Cv	1	0	0	0	1	0	0	0
Lactobacillus sp. (diet)	Gf	3	0	1	2	0	0	0	0
	Cv	2	0	0	2	0	0	0	0
Lactobacillus sp. (human)	Gf	3	0	0	0	0	0	0	0
	Cv	2	2	0	0	0	0	0	0
Micrococcus pyogenes	Gf	3	2	1	0	0	0	0	0
	Cv	2	0	0	1	1	0	0	0
Micrococcus epidermidis	Gf	2	0	0	2	0	0	0	0
	Cv	2	0	0	0	0	1	1	0

[a]Data of Wagner from Reyniers *et al.* , (1960a).
[b]One or more chicks for each run.

The diets used contained many antigens and these included bacterial antigens from dead microorganisms in the diet. It is possible that some of these antigens caused production of heterohemagglutinins in germ-free chicks.

Wagner's (1959b) study of lactobacilli agglutinins indicated that a chicken fecal strain of lactobacillus did not agglutinate serum from germfree chicks until the 24th week when low activity was found. The conventional chicken serum agglutinated this strain of *Lactobacillus* at the age of 9 weeks. When a lactobacillus obtained from a human dental caries patient was tested against germfree serum, no reaction was found even in the oldest age birds, while there was activity in conventional birds at 7 to 8 weeks. When a lactobacillus and two species of micrococci were isolated from the diet and used as agglutinins, no reaction was found in the germfree group except in the birds over 30 weeks of age, while some reaction was noted in conventional birds beginning at 5 weeks and in all older categories. When dead bacteria were incorporated into the diet of germfree animals, Wagner found antibacterial agglutinin production was quite active. Therefore, the low levels of antibodies against microbial antigens in germfree chickens was not due to an innate inability to activate the lymphatic system or form different kinds of γ-globulin. When germfree birds were fed 1% autoclaved *Paracolobactrum aerogenoides* for 21 days, agglutinin titer was developed against this particular organism, but

TABLE 5.24
WAGNER DATA ON SEROLOGY IN ADULT GERMFREE AND
CONVENTIONAL WHITE WYANDOTTE BANTAM CHICKENS

Serological reaction		Chicken group	
		Germ-free	Conventional
Natural hemag-	Rabbit	1:4	1:16
glutinins for	Rat	1:4	—
foreign	Horse	1:2	1:2[a]
erythrocytes	Sheep	—	—
	Human	—	—
Natural anti-	*Paracolobactrum aerogenoides*	—	1:32
bacterial	*Escherichia coli*	—	1:32
agglutinins	*Staphylococcus albus*	1:2	1:8
	Lactobacillus L-301	1:4	1:4
	Lactobacillus L-652	—	1:2
Precipitins for casein		—	—
Complement[b]		1:16	1:8
Kahn reaction		Doubtful	Negative
Mezzini reaction		Positive	Positive

[a] Partial reaction in lowest dilution tested.
[b] Titrated against 2.5% sheep erythrocytes in the presence of three anti-sheep hemolysin. Reyniers, *et al.*, (1960a).

the response to the micrococcus remained negative (Table 5.25). The response of conventional animals to these two organisms was very similar irrespective of the presence or absence of added *P. aerogenoides* in the diet. Presumably both organisms were present in the intestinal tract of conventional chicks. It was therefore suggested that germfree chicks respond slowly to dead microorganisms in the diet and that many of the antibacterial agglutinins present in the serum of conventional chicks occur in response to the presence of living microorganisms in the digestive tract during the life of an animal.

Wagner also studied the production of antibody in germfree chickens which had been injected intravenously with killed *Salmonella pullorum* or sterile beef serum. The results, summarized in Table 5.26, showed that the production of antibody in response to injected antigen was as fast and as great in germfree birds as it was in conventional birds. The germfree state apparently did not interfere with antibody production under these conditions. Miyakawa (1955c) found good

TABLE 5.25

BACTERIAL AGGLUTININ RESPONSE IN WHITE LEGHORN CHICKS

Agglutinin	Germ status	Age (days)	Days with 1% antigen in diet	No. of chicks	Titer[a]	
					Anti Paracolon	Anti Micrococcus
Paracolobactrum aerogenoides Germfree	Germfree	52	0	1	0	0
	Germfree	52	21	3	1:8	0
	Coventional	51	0	3	1:16	1:32
	Conventional	51	21	3	1:16	1:32

[a] The lowest titer found is expressed. Data of Wagner.

antibody production in germfree guinea pigs which had been injected with typhoid vaccine into a foot pad. However, the titer was not as great as that found in classic guinea pigs.

Both germfree and conventional rats fed syntype diets showed no activity against bacterial antigens up to 30 days of age (Wagner, 1959b). From 30 to 250 days of age the germfree rats showed no activity against the antigens in *Escherichia coli, Streptococcus faecalis,*

TABLE 5.26

ANTIBODY RESPONSE OF GERMFREE AND CONVENTIONAL WHITE LEGHORN CHICKS TO INJECTED ANTIGEN[a] AT 58 DAYS

Antigen Injected	Germ Status	Animals	Anti-S. pullorum	Anti-beef serum
Salmonella pullorum	Germfree	3	1/128	0
	Conventional	4	1/64	0
Saline	Germfree	3	0	0
	Conventional	4	Trace	0
Beef serum	Germfree	3	0	1/4096
	Conventional	4	0	1/2048

[a]At 48, 50, and 52 days, 0.5 ml of microbial serum or 0.1, 0.2, and 0.4% beef serum administered parenterally. Data of Wagner.

Lactobacillus (heterofermentative), or *Lactobacillus* (homofermentative) (Table 5.27), while conventional rats shown a titer against all of these with the exception of the homofermentative *Lactobacillus*. Of some importance would seem to be the fact that some bacteria could be inoculated into germfree rats and illicit no antigenic response. This was true of a pleomorphic rod and a proteolytic rod found as contaminants.

When germfree rats were inoculated at weaning with homofermentative lactobacilli, the titer was just as high as, or higher than, that of conventional rats (Wagner, 1959b). Further work with the homofermentative *Lactobacillus* organism was most interesting. Twelve first generation germfree rats inoculated with the *Lactobacillus* at birth showed an average titer of 1:16 at 6 months of age, while no response was found in second and third generation offspring which were exposed to this single organism at birth. Fourth generation germfree rats were inoculated with the organism after 48 days of germfree existence. Those rats also showed a titer of 1:16 against the *Lactobacillus*. Wagner speculated that these findings may be explained by embryonic tolerance to the organisms.

Landy *et al.* (1962) found that germfree and classic mice reacted similarly in the following; LD_{50} of endotoxin (*Shigella flexneri*), increased resistance to infection by *Salmonella enteritidis* following treatment with endotoxin from that organism, susceptibility to infection with *Salmonella typhosa*, elevation in antibody levels following inoculation with gram negative bacteria, and increased glycolysis and acid formation from treatment with *Salmonella enteritidis* endotoxin.

TABLE 5.27

ANTIBACTERIAL AGGLUTININ TITERS IN SERUM OF GERMFREE
AND CONVENTIONAL RATS [a,b]

Antigen	Germ status	Age in Days		
		30	30-99	100-250
Micrococcus epidermidis	Germfree	0	0	0
	Conventional	0	1/4-1/64	1/8-1/256
Micrococcus epidermidis (after 1955)	Germfree	0	1/32-1/64	1/32-1/64
Escherichia coli	Germfree	0	0	0
	Conventional	0	1/4	1/2-1/16
Streptococcus faecalis	Germfree			0
	Conventional		1/2-1/4	1/2-1/256
Lactobacillus (hetero.)	Germfree		—	0
	Conventional		0	1/8-1/16
Lactobacillus (homo.)	Germfree		—	0
	Conventional		0	0

[a] Data of Wagner (1959).
[b] Germfree rats, 3 to 23 rats in each group; 3 to 38 rats in conventional studies. Fed pelleted diets.

Complement. Wagner's study (1959b) included titration of serum for hemolytic complement with germfree Bantam and Leghorn chickens. Conventional and germfree chicks had very similar complement components in their serum from 1 month of age to 1 year of age. Age apparently made very little difference in the concentration of hemolytic units of complement. These results agree with those of Tanami (1959) and Newton *et al.* (1960a) who found similar titers of complement in germfree, monoflora, diflora, and conventional guinea pigs.

However, Saquet *et al.* (1961) found lower serum complement in germfree than in classic rats.

Properdin. Pillemer (1956) found properdin to be present in the serum of germfree rats. This experiment was elaborated by Wagner (1959b), whose data (Table 5.28a) indicated the quantity of properdin in germfree rats was almost as great as that found in conventional

TABLE 5.28

A. PROPERDIN, COMPLEMENT, AND COMPLEMENT-COMPONENT TITERS IN NORMAL SERA OF GERMFREE AND CONVENTIONAL RATS[a]

Serum no.	Properdin (units/ml)	Complement (units/ml)	Complement components (units/ml)			
			C'1	C'2	C'3	C'4
GF-134	48	50	700	90	700	45
GF-135	48	50	1000	90	1000	45
GF-139	48	50	700	90	700	45
C-1001	48	65	1400	90	1400	60
C-1002	56	80	1400	120	1000	60
C-1006	56	80	1400	120	1000	60

B. PROPERDIN TITERS IN SERA FROM GERMFREE AND CONVENTIONAL ANIMALS[b]

Category	No. animals	Units properdin per ml	
		Mean	Range
Germfree	9	3.3	4-4
Ex germfree 14 days	9	7.1	2-16
Ex germfree 42 days	9	9.8	4-16
Conventional -1	9	17.6	2-32
Conventional -2	9	14.0	4-32

[a]Data of Wagner (1959).
[b]Data of Gustaffson and Laurell (1960).

rats. When Gustafsson and Laurell (1960b) repeated this work (Table 5.28b) they found properdin titers in germfree rats were significantly lower than those of conventional rats. Exposure of the germfree rats to a stock colony flora for 2 weeks increased properdin titer 2-fold. After 42 days the titers in the previously germfree rats were almost as great as those found in conventional rats fed the same diet. From the similarity of this data to that of plasma globulins, these authors suggested that properdin be categorized with the β- and γ-globulins. All groups agree that properdin was present in germfree rats. The quantitative differences between the results cannot be easily rationalized.

Ward (1959) reported about two-thirds of the sera of 27 germfree mice were shown to possess complement fixing antibodies against the polyoma virus of Stuart and Eddy. This antigen or one related to it must have been in the germfree mice. Other work indicates the absence of viral antigens (see Chapter 6).

When typhoid vaccine was injected into the pad of guinea pigs, agglutination titer was positive in germfree guinea pigs at 1:320, while serum from conventional guinea pigs was active at 1:640. This and the native reaction seen to thrice-injected egg albumin were the bases for Miyakawa et al. (1958b) to conclude the "productivity of antibody is apparently declined in the germfree guinea pigs but not yet entirely stopped." Since detailed data were not given, it would be difficult to agree with their statement. Certainly, other work indicates no serious difficulty with antibody production in germfree animals if the antigen were presented after maturation of the synthesizing apparatus.

Immunologic Reactions

The relative inactivity of the immunological apparatus of germfree animals has allowed acceptance of homologous and heterologous tissue in transplants made into germfree animals. Miyakawa et al. (1958b) transplanted sections of guinea pig ear subcutaneously into another guinea pig. In the germfree state the transplant became established with active proliferation at 15 days. In conventional animals necrosis was seen at 48 hours and was almost complete in 6 days. Miyakawa (1957b, 1959a) injected rat Yoshida sarcoma into the abdominal cavity of guinea pigs. The cells grew rapidly and caused little exudation in the germfree animals, but in the conventional guinea pig very few sarcoma cells could be found among the tremendous amount of ascites with neutrophils and large mononuclear cells at the side of injection. Sterile human breast cancer was transplanted subcutaneously into guinea pigs. In conventional animals the transplant caused marked exudation and after 8 days the necrotic cancer cells were encapsulated. In germfree guinea pigs the architectural features of the cancer were intact at 25 days and no marked tissue reaction had occurred. Human skin melanoma was well preserved 19 days after being transplanted into germfree guinea pigs while in conventional guinea pigs it was necrotic and had abscesses by the seventh day.

In another experiment Miyakawa (1959a) injected 2 ml of 1% sterile agar into the abdominal cavity of guinea pigs. Most of the conventional animals died while no specific reaction was seen in the germfree animals.

Phagocytosis

Reticular cells in the lymph nodes are fewer in number and their phagocytic activity was shown to be very feeble by Miyakawa (1957b). The phagocytic activity of circulating leucocytes from germfree rats was found to be less for some bacteria than that found in lymphocytes from conventional rats (J. P. Doll, quoted by Trexler, 1959b). C. Hyman and H. A. Gordon (quoted by Thorbecke and Benacerraf, 1959) found that the Kupffer cells in the livers of germfree animals took up materials such as Evans blue and thorium dioxide in suspension. Sterile black ink was taken up at a much slower rate in reticulum cells of the abdominal inguinal and popliteal lymph nodes in germfree guinea pigs than it was in conventional guinea pigs (Miyakawa et al., 1957c). These investigators found no difference in phagocytic activity of parenchyma reticulum cells in animals from the two environmental categories.

The clear experiments of Tanami (1959) indicated that leucocytes ingested fewer *Staphylococcus aureus* and the proportion of phagocytosing leucocytes was lower in germfree than in conventional guinea pigs. The phagocytic index and the phagocytic percentage of diflora guinea pigs was between that of the germfree and the conventional guinea pigs.

Blood Clearance

Germfree mice cleared intravenously injected carbon from the blood at approximately the same rate as did conventional mice (Thorbecke and Benacerraf, 1959). When dead P^{32}-labeled *Staphylococcus aureus* were injected intravenously into germfree and conventional mice, the clearance from the blood was complete in both within 11–12 minutes. When heat-killed P^{32}-labeled *Escherichia coli* was injected, the 40 day old germfree mice cleared the blood at a slower rate than did conventional mice. The time for 50% clearance in germfree mice was 47 minutes whereas in conventional mice, immunized with *E. coli* 8 days prior to the clearance test, all organisms were cleared in 11 minutes. These authors suggested that the rate of clearance depended upon the amount of antibody present in the animal. Unfortunately the fast clearance of S. *aureus* was not correlated to data regarding the antibody titer of these mice for this particular organism. The average percentage of P^{32}-labeled bacteria in various organs and blood of mice sacrificed at the end of the blood clearance experiments by Thorbecke and Benacerraf (1959) is given in Table 5.29. The greatest quantity was found in the liver. When mice were immunized with *Escherichia*

TABLE 5.29
PERCENTAGE DISTRIBUTION OF RADIOACTIVITY IN
MOUSE ORGANS AND BLOOD AFTER BLOOD
CLEARANCE OF P^{32} - LABELED MICROORGANISMS[a]

Organ	*Eschericha coli*		*Staphylococcus aureus*	
	4 Germfree (average, %)	4 Conventional (average, %)	2 Germfree (average, %)	3 Conventional (average, %)
Liver	21.4	25.0	63.5	74.0
Spleen	14.8	15.4	7.5	5.5
Lungs	7.0	4.9	4.5	1.0
Kidneys	2.5	1.6	0.7	0.3
Blood	30.2	23.8	6.2	4.5
Total re-covered	75.9	70.7	82.4	85.3

[a]Data from Thorbecke and Benacerraf (1959).

coli, the livers of both germfree and conventional mice took up about 75%: this is comparable to the amounts found in the livers in the *Staphylococcus aureus* experiments. This data would suggest either of two possibilities: (1) the mice used were preimmunized (by dead bacteria in the diets) for S. *aureus* or (2) different mechanisms were active in the deposition of killed microorganisms into the tissues.

Abnormalities in Form and Function

The low state of development of mechanisms of defense and the absence of infections in germfree animals makes them exceptionally useful for the study of disease. Germfree animals may be inoculated with one, two, or more known organisms to study infection. Such studies will be reported in the final chapter. Germfree animals best show the course of noninfectious diseases; acute diseases often could progress further and chronic disease could be studied without the complication of infection. Physiological disease might be most clearly defined and studied with germfree animals. Abnormalities associated with specific nutritional disease have, for the most part, been placed in the chapter on nutrition. The material presented includes syndromes of the vitamin deficiency states, the abnormalities seen in hand-fed suckling rats, and studies on such nutritional problems as induced hemorrhagic liver necrosis. Details of general malnutrition caused by a lack of proper feeding are not reported. These can be found wherever failures to rear healthy germfree animals are reported.

Anoxia

Asphyxia was a problem which obviously has no direct connection with the germfree status of an animal; it was seen on occasion, due to one or two causes. The first was simply human error in not providing adequate ventilation, or failure of air pumps. Animals in this condition could be readily recognized by the gasping, the general weakness, and usually the high humidity in the isolator. Whether death was due to anoxia or to carbon dioxide poisoning is open to question. The second place where asphyxia was sometimes seen was following the Cesarean operation. If the newborn animal did not get all the mucus away from its nose and mouth within a few minutes after extirpation of the uterus, it would become weak from anoxia and die. The techniques of operation of small mammals has been developed to the extent that few deaths occur from the Cesarean operation. When the mother was heavily anesthetized, the problem of getting the young to breathe became greater. This was the main reason why light anesthesia or no anesthesia was used for most Cesarean operations. With larger animals, asphyxiation during the Cesarean operation was a more serious problem. In lambs, enough mucus was sometimes swallowed by the young during the operation that it was very difficult to clear the pharynx for easy passage of the air. Aseptic pneumonia in a germfree kid was seen by Küster (1913b) following accidental formalin vapor administration. Severe corrosion of the respiratory tract preceded the pneumonia. No fever was detected.

Malnutrition

Many of the germfree animals reared prior to 1940 were malnurtured due to a lack of knowledge of nutrition and the effects of steam sterilization upon the destruction of vitamins and amino acids. Germfree animals had a tendency to compensate for a dietary deficiency by overeating, while conventional animals exhibited anorexia in similar circumstances. A description of malnurtured guinea pigs was given by Reyniers (1946a). The animals' appearance was essentially that of starvation. Such animals were more susceptible to purgative drugs than conventional animals.

The orexis of germfree birds fed a protein-deficient practical diet surpassed that of conventional chicks many times. This was probably the condition of the chicks of Schottelius (1902):

> Another equally interesting phenomenon is seen in the fact that the sterile raised chick is permanently hungry and continuously eats and digests and drops excrement. This takes place in sterile chicks to a greater extent than in normally nourished animals. Even in the latter, the gut canal (as one can convince himself from any hen yard) shows an enviable conductivity. But these sterilely-raised animals surpass in their ravenousness and in the evacuation of the gut contents the normal animals by many times.

Cohendy (1912a) agreed that defecation was more frequent and abundant in the germfree birds than in conventional chicks fed the same sterilized diet. In the author's experience, no difference was noted between healthy conventional and germfree chickens when the diet is adequate.

Newly hatched chicks sometimes starve to death because they do not find the food or never learn to eat. Older chicks may starve from an accumulation of certain diets within the beak. A combination of the casein and carbohydrate occasionally made a sticky material upon contact with the saliva which became stuck on the beak. This started a vicious cycle in which more material accumulated as the chicken tried to eat. Eventually, the chicks reached the point where they could not eat effectively and died if this material was not removed from the beak.

One of the interesting abnormalities in germfree rats, discussed under nutrition, was the spontaneous fracture which occurred shortly after they had begun to eat solid diet and were walking with greatly distended abdomens. The composition of their bones was particularly low in calcium when compared to the bones of rats from conventional colonies.

Oral Abnormalities

Depending upon the definition, oral calculus has been observed by Fitzgerald and McDaniel (1960) and Baer and Newton (1960) in germfree rats and mice respectively. The scale-like material seen on the teeth of germfree rats was much more easily pulled from the

tooth than the usual calculi. The calculi in mice were hard and
contained calcium. X-ray diffraction patterns typical of apatite were
obtained from this material. It seems probable that at least part of
the process of calculus formation was seen in germfree animals;
perhaps another part, the formation of the physical bond between the
tooth and the scale, has a microbial vector. Peridontal disease was
seen in all germfree mice older than 6 months examined by Baer and
Newton (1959). The onset of changes began at 3–4 months with the
downward growth of the epithelial attachment and loss of alveolar
bone. Inflammation was not prominent in germfree mice. Teeth of
germfree animals may fragment from pressure or other causes and
the usual wear and abrasion was seen. Fitzgerald *et al.* (1960b) found
that impacted hairs in germfree rats caused oral exudative, ulcerative
lesions similar to those found in conventional rats. Dental caries do
not occur in germfree rats (Orland *et al.*, 1954): results with monoinoculated rats are presented in the final chapter.

Cecum Distension

The most distressing abnormality seen in germfree mammals was
the distended cecum. Presumably, this was not a necessary characteristic of the germfree animal since germfree chickens, turkeys, and
some germfree rats had ceca quite within the size range found for
the conventional animals. The major problem with the distended
cecum began when the young first learned to eat solid food. With-
holding some food was found to be partially effective in hand-fed
animals.

No one has thoroughly studied the cause of the enlarged cecum.
Wostmann and Bruckner-Kardoss (1959) found that the cecum was 4
times enlarged at 16 days in germfree rats. This work confirmed that
of Reyniers *et al.* (1946) in which a wide variety of milk formulas
were fed to germfree rats until weaning, and most of them showed
enlarged ceca. In Chapter 4 the enlargement of the ceca in germfree
rats was noted as a causative factor in the premature death of these
animals. Details about the cecum and its contents have been presented in this chapter under the heading *Gastrointestinal Tract*. The
cecum became so large that it was not easily mobile and turned in
one direction. The twisting stopped the flow of intestinal material
(Fig. 5.6). The animal became sluggish and exhibited seizures of
pain as exhibited by lordosis. The cause of death was not known.
Obviously, if death was attributed to toxins, these would be nonbac-

terial in nature. Second and subsequent generation germfree rats had enlarged ceca which showed that the hand-feeding problems were not the basic cause of cecum distension. Histologically, the dilated cecal wall of the germfree guinea pig (Glimstedt, 1933; Gustafsson, 1948) showed a widening of Lieberkuhns crypts, with reduced number of free cells in the epithelium and in the subepithelial connective tissue.

Anal Blockage

Anal blockage in chicks was seen on two occasions in several years experience with germfree chicks. On both occasions anal blockage was observed in conventional chicks as well as in the germfree chicks.

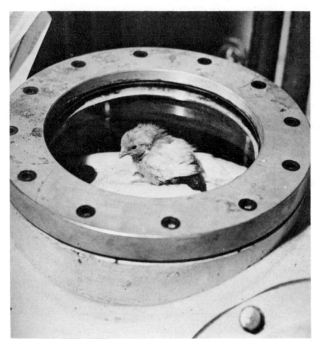

Fig. 5.9. Anal blockage in a germfree chick. The occurrence of anal pasting in germfree chicks eliminates microbes as the main etiological factor. (Luckey, 1959.)

The occurrence of anal blockage (Fig. 5.9) in germfree chicks showed rather conclusively that this disease did not depend upon bacterial manifestation. Therefore, it must be related to the condition of the chicks at hatch, viral infection, or diet. Since it did not occur regularly the dietary vector is probably minor.

Tumors

Spontaneous tumors have not been seen in germfree animals, with one or two possible exceptions wherein a virus infestation was suspected. One example, known as the "jitters" in germfree chicks, was reported by Gordon *et al.* (1959). Here, the unsteadiness exhibited by the birds was related in most cases to a cellular proliferation in the brain of microscopic proportions. This was not found in all of the birds despite the fact that whenever the disease appeared in the germfree cage all of the birds were affected. Tumors have been induced in germfree birds by the injection of methylcholanthrene in benzene. These fibrosarcomas were not transmissible from conventional chicks but they were transmissible when induced in germfree chicks (Reyniers and Sacksteder, 1959b). This group isolated particles from such tumors in germfree mice. The infectivity of these particles has not been shown unequivocally. Ward (1959) reported 17 specimens of a wide variety of spontaneous tumor from germfree mice and rats. No details were reported. He found (1961) the rate of spontaneous tumors to be similar in germfree and conventional and germfree rats and mice. Dougherty and Solberg (1961) can induce tumors in axenic *E. fragmentosus* by trapping them temporarily in water.

The possibility of virus disease was evidenced in the collapsed lungs of young rats and mice (Pleasants, 1959; Reyniers and Sacksteder, 1958c). This was another case where death was presumably due to asphyxiation since there was not enough lung inflated to properly aerate the venous blood. While no definite etiology was shown in the lung collapse, virus infection remained one of the possibilities. Beaver (1960) found a lipoid pneumonia with xanthoma cells in the lungs of germfree rats. This was not seen in conventional rats reared inside the steel cage; he concluded only that the phenomenon was not caused by environmental factors such as oil droplets in the air line.

Radiation Damage

Germfree chicks survived X-irradiation better than did conventional chicks when the dosage was below 800r, at the rate of 32r per hour (McLaughlin *et al.*, 1958). When doses larger than 800r were used, no significant difference was seen in the percent survival of the groups, but the survival times of the conventional chicks was shorter than those of germfree chicks. Reyniers *et al.* (1956) found the average survival time of conventional rats given 400r X-radiation was only one-half that of germfree rats treated in like manner. Symptoms of radiation sickness were comparable in the two groups, excepting the bacteremia of conventional rats. Similar results with germfree mice compared to classic mice were reported by Wilson and Piacsek (1961).

Shock

Since pretreatment with antibiotics circumvents the irreversible features of shock, Zweifach (1959) resorted to the use of germfree rats in order to determine the importance of the bacterial vector in this syndrome. Hemorrhagic hypotension was induced by carotid bleeding under pentobarbital anesthesia. No significant differences were seen by Zweifach *et al.* (1958) in the response of germfree and conventional or monoinoculated or recently polycontaminated rats. Results were similar with germfree rats fed syntype diets or practical diets. Germfree rats having enlarged ceca showed extensive cecal hemorrhage but otherwise reacted in the same manner as germfree rats having a normal size cecum. The autopsy of germfree rats subjected to hemorrhagic shock showed the liver to be small, contracted, and pale. The liver of conventional rats in shock was distended, dark, and congested. Gastrointestinal hemorrhage and mucosal damage were similar in germfree and conventional animals. Bacteremia was present in conventional rats and, of course, absent in germfree rats. Zweifach concluded that the bacterial contribution in irreversible shock was of secondary importance. Horowitz *et al.* (1960) and McNulty (in György, 1959) also reported no difference in mortality between germfree and conventional animals subjected to hemorrhagic shock within the confines of a germfree tank. Such results leave open to question the interpretation of the antibiotic alleviation of detrimental action in shock which considers only the antibacterial action of antibiotics. The experiments of Friedman *et al.* (1957) using antibiotics in shock need to be repeated using germfree rats.

Heat shock, studied by Ward and Lindholm (1960), was more harmful to germfree mice than conventional mice. When placed in water at 70°C, germfree mice were killed more quickly than conventional mice. Rosenthal *et al.* (1961) continued this study and found lower antitoxin titers in germfree rats than were found in conventional rats. This study indicated that the toxin of burns was not of bacterial origin. Such results suggested that bacteria and infection did not play a primary role in experimental shock. Germfree chicks showed a greater mortality at 24 and 48 hours following tourniquet shock than did classic chicks (Levenson *et al.*, 1959).

Miscellaneous Abnormalities

Heavy accumulation of fat around the heart, ovaries, and uterus and in the abdominal cavity was found by Reyniers *et al.* (1946) in rats contaminated for 3 weeks after 3–8 months in the germfree state. Levenson *et al.* (1960a) found that germfree rats developed liver cirrhosis faster than did conventional rats fed the "cirrhogenic" diet. Luckey *et al.* (1954a) reported that germfree rats showed massive hemorrhagic liver necrosis when fed the Himsworth diet with limited food intake.

Reparative Processes

Wound healing in germfree animals has been studied by few investigators, and only one systematic report, that of Miyakawa, has been published to date. Küster (1913b) noted that wound healing was slow in germfree goats. After 10 days a small cut had no tissue united to it and the wound could be reopened with a slight pull. Similar cuts in the control goat had healed quickly. Preliminary work by H. A. Gordon (personal communication) at the University of Notre Dame indicated that skin wounds of germfree animals heal in somewhat less time than in conventional animals. There was apparently less cellular activity in removing debris and very little, if any, phagocytosis during the cleansing process. Similar work has been done by Dr. Malmo and Dr. S. Levenson (personal communication) at the Walter Reed Army Institute of Research.

Observation of a wound cut into the subcutaneous tissue of the germfree guinea pigs showed that the exudative process was weaker in the germfree condition than in conventional animals (Miyakawa *et al.*, 1958a). In the germfree guinea pig experimental wounds were closed within 48 hours with an epidermal bridge, and within 6 days regenerative mesenchymal tissue filled the space between the epidermis and the mesenchymal tissue. Few capillaries formed in this new tissue. In contrast, in conventional animals granulation tissue was formed in the open wound before regenerating epidermis covered it and the regenerated mesenchymal tissue had many new capillaries. The reduced blood vessel formation in new tissue of germfree guinea pigs was confirmed (Miyakawa, 1959a) by introduction of sterile sponges into subcutaneous tissue. Proliferation of mesenchymal cells was noted within 24 hours. In 6 days the sponges were penetrated and encapsulated by mesenchymal tissue with the penetration of no blood vessels. Conventional guinea pigs encapsulated the sponge with granulation tissue having newly formed blood vessels.

Itaya (1958) reported histological changes in response to irritants by tissues of germfree guinea pigs. The initial inflammation showed less exudative changes occurring in germfree guinea pigs than in conventional guinea pigs. When leucotoxin-like substances of germfree guinea pigs, extracted by saline from skin and muscle following mechanical trauma, were injected into rabbits, the rabbits reacted with acute inflammation, increased permeability, and polymorph migration: this response was the same as that obtained when rabbits were injected with extracts from conventional guinea pigs.

Senescence

Knowledge of aging in germfree animals is important because longevity studies with conventional animals involve infectious diseases and changes other than physiological aging. Germfree animal studies to date on ontogenetic development—morphological, biochemical, and immunological—have not been carried into the aged category. Space in germfree cages has been too valuable to allow animals to accumulate for longevity studies. Germfree male mice of the C3H strain lived longer than do germfree females which were more susceptible to kidney metastatic calcification according to one study by Reyniers (1959b). The condition was not seen in the germfree males or conventional female mice fed the same diet. More germfree female mice died from volvulus and other causes up to 600 days than did conventional female mice. It should be recalled that germfree flies had a greater longevity than classic flies.

Death and Post-Mortem Changes

Premature death of germfree animals may be caused by physiological diseases or external agents. Death from natural aging processes has not been studied systematically. Schottelius (1902) noted that malnurtured germfree chicks may lie unmoving in the cage 1 or 2 days in such weakened condition that it is difficult to determine the time of death. His death watch consisted of close observation with field glasses for breathing and heart action. Germfree chicks dying at

29 days lost 29% of their body weight. The physiologic deaths in germfree mammals observed at autopsy by W. Scruggs (see Ward and Trexler, 1958) is summarized in Table 5.30. Respiratory deaths were the most numerous, which indicates that the lungs were one of the weakest systems of the body.

TABLE 5.30
PHYSIOLOGIC (NONINFECTIVE) CAUSES OF DEATHS[a] IN
GERMFREE MAMMALS

Diagnosis	Rats (% deaths)[b]	Swiss mice (% deaths)[c]
Asphyxia	42.5	59.1
Cecum volvulus	27.4	—
Lung hepatization	6.0	18.2
Pulmonary edema	9.0	6.7
Pneumonia	6.0	9.1
Liver disease	3.0	2.6
Arteriosclerosis	3.0	2.2
Ruptured viscus	3.0	—
Pancreatic necrosis	—	2.2

[a]No deaths due to failure of apparatus are included.
[b]Data of Ward and Trexler (1958) for 33 rats
[c]Data of Ward and Trexler (1958) for 44 mice.

Post-mortem changes in dead germfree animals revealed three main patterns. First, putrefactive changes are minimum. There is no disagreeable odor to dead germfree animals. Second, autolysis occurs, particularly in the intestinal area. The digestive enzymes and cathepsins quickly distorted any semblance of the beautiful patterns seen in life. If the intestinal contents are present in great quantity, the entire body cavity may become liquefied within 2–3 days and the outer surface shows the discoloring effects of post-mortem changes. Third, drying and mummification occurs in emaciated animals which have a decreased amount of abdominal mass. Schottelius noted (1902) that if the air were dry and there was not too much material in the intestine, mummification occurred rapidly and effectively. Although rigor mortis has been seen in germfree rats and chicks by the author, Reyniers (1946a) reported no rigor mortis in germfree guinea pigs.

When germfree C3H mice (Reyniers, 1958) and rats (Luckey, 1959c, p. 380) were taken directly from a germfree environment to a conventional animal colony, most of them died within 1 week. There was a general microbial flooding of the intestinal tract, blood, and tissues which showed no set pattern for the determination of the cause of death. When germfree rats were placed in an office for 5–7 days before being taken to the conventional animal room, they survived. Germfree chicks and turkey poults did not die when taken directly to conventional rearing pens.

Summary

The characteristics of germfree animals are summarized from the viewpoint of morphology, biochemistry, immunology, and pathology. No summary of classic physiology of germfree animals is possible, since systematic studies have not been made in this area. Information in Chapter 2 indicates that the growth and reproduction of germfree animals is comparable to that of conventional animals wherever the enlarged ceca do not interfere. Information is presented in Chapter 4 on the nutritional requirements and the growth characteristics of animals fed different diets.

Morphology

Differences in morphology indicate that organs in continuous intimate contact with microorganisms are enlarged or more active in conventional than in germfree animals. Examples of this are the increased weight, cellular tissue, and length of the small intestine, and the size of lymph nodes of the intestinal wall. In contrast, lymphatic organs such as thymus and bursa Fabricius, which are removed from the first line of defense against the myriad microinvasions, show no consistent increased size or lymphatic activity. Organs which have less direct function in defense against invasion and which are also removed from the continuous intimate contact with microorganisms, such as bone, heart, brain, or endocrine glands show great similarity between germfree and conventional animals. These internal organs and tissues are usually germfree in the body of a conventional animal. Microorganisms rarely penetrate the body defenses to reach these tissues. The realistic study of internal organs in a microbial environment would use animals with a chronic infection where microorganisms were in intimate, prolonged contact with the organ being studied.

The general characteristics of germfree animals resembled those of conventional animals. Gross appearance gave no consistent clue to indicate whether the animal was a germfree animal or a polycontaminated animal. The growth rate and size was comparable in the two groups, although germfree birds apparently grew at a slightly faster rate than did conventional birds. The feathers of germfree birds were well developed and the fur coat of germfree mammals is often luxurious. The skeletal system of germfree animals was quite comparable to that of conventional animals. However, there was an indication that conventional animals had less osseous material than had germfree animals. The musculature of germfree chicks was found in the same quantity as that in conventional controls. Similar studies have not been made for germfree mammals. There was good evidence that the musculature of the intestinal mucosa, particularly the cecum of mammals, had inadequate tonus. The circulatory system of conventional and germfree animals was identical as far as heart and vascular system are concerned. The hemoglobin values and red blood cell counts of conventional and germfree animals were comparable. The major difference in the blood morphology of the two groups of animals was the increased number of lymphocytes found in conventional animals. The percentage of neutrophils in conventional guinea pigs was found to be lower than that of germfree guinea pigs. The circulating heterophils were the same in conventional and germfree birds, while the neutrophil count in conventional animals was twice that of germfree animals. Basophilic cells sometimes appeared to be more rare in germfree mammals but there was no consistent difference in numbers of circulating eosinophils and basophils between germfree and conventional chicks. The absolute number of monocytes was greater in conventional than in germfree birds; this pattern was also found in guinea pigs, but no difference was seen in the two categories of rats. Macroscopic similarity was seen in the respiratory systems of the two groups of animals; however, the epithelial cells of the conventional guinea pigs developed cilia and became stratified, while germfree guinea pigs showed little development of the respiratory epithelial lining or lymphatic tissue beyond that of newborn animals. Gross observation of the pancreas indicated no difference between germfree and conventional animals. The small intestine was found to be greater in length and somewhat thicker and heavier in

conventional than in germfree animals fed the same diet. Part of this
decrease in the germfree animals was due to less lamina propria. The
over-all picture seen was that the intestinal mucosa of germfree
animals remains specialized for absorption, while that of conventional
animals serves a dual purpose of absorption and defense against
invading microorganisms. The germfree animals had less total absorptive area but this was apparently more efficient since it also had
less connective tissue in the mucosa. The cecum of germfree and
conventional birds appeared to be very similar by gross observation.
The enlarged cecum of germfree mammals was the major macroscopic
difference between germfree and conventional mammals. In the early
work the size of the cecum would be as great as 25–35% of the total
body weight. Presently the cecum size is usually below 5% of the body
weight of germfree rats. The enlarged cecum was a deterrent to
reproduction and was the principal cause of death in the early
attempts to rear colonies of germfree animals. The wall of the cecum
was greatly distended with a large quantity of brown liquid with
small cheesy particles. No macroscopic difference was seen between
the large intestine of germfree and conventional animals. Microscopically there was a great difference in the contents of the intestinal
tract of the two groups of animals. Approximately 50% of the contents
of conventional animals was microbes or microbial debris, while less
than 1% ingesta from syntype diets in germfree intestinal tract was
dead microbes. The contents of the rectum and the appearance of
the feces were generally different between the two categories. The
stools were usually more soft and less well formed in germfree animals
than in conventional animals. The tendency for diarrhea was greater
in germfree animals than in conventional animals. The omentum of
germfree animals was comparable to that seen in conventional animals.
However, the general view of the internal abdomen was usually
different owing to the fact that much more ingesta was present in the
intestine of germfree mammals than in conventional animals. The
macroscopic appearance of the livers of germfree and conventional
animals was almost identical; the liver size in germfree birds was
somewhat lower than that of conventional birds. This difference was
not seen in rats. The amount and color of the bile was identical in
animals from germfree and conventional environments. No differences
were seen in the excretory system, the kidney, uterus, and bladder
between the two groups of animals. The quantity of urine may have
been somewhat greater in germfree animals, a reflection of the

greater amount of water ingested. Examination of the brain, spinal cord, and peripheral nerves indicates identity of the nervous system in the two groups of animals. No differences were seen in the sensory or endocrine systems by gross observation. The lymphatic system gave consistent differences which indicated gross underdevelopment of the lymphatic system of germfree animals when compared to that of conventional animals. The germfree animals represent a resting or normal state of these tissues, while the stimulation by bacteria leads to an excited state in conventional animals which is reflected in increased size and function. The lymph nodes were larger and more numerous and the concentration of lymphocytes in the nodes was generally greater in animals which harbored microorganisms. Plasma cells apparently were absent in germfree guinea pigs as were secondary reaction centers of lymph nodules. The spleen appeared to be the same by macroscopic observation but the relative size was greater in conventional than in germfree animals. There was little difference in the lymphocyte concentration in nodular tissue between the two groups. Plasma cells were found in the spleen of germfree chicks and mammals. In weight and general appearance of the thymus gland there were no consistent differences between animals with and without microorganisms.

Biochemistry

From the chemical viewpoint the liver and the bile were the least stable of the tissues, while very few biochemical differences were found between germfree and conventional animals in bone, kidney, and muscle tissue. The dry weight of heart, lungs, proventriculus, gizzard, intestinal wall, liver, gonads, kidney, brain, spleen, and thymus was the same in germfree and conventional conditions. Conventional animals had a greater dry weight in cecal contents and bile than was found in germfree animals. The cecum wall and pancreas in germfree Bantam chicks had more dry weight than was found in conventional Bantam chicks. Germfree rats had greater dry weight in the muscle than had conventional rats, this difference was definitely not seen in chicks.

The ash values were more variable than the dry weight. Variability was particularly great in the young rats, the conventional animals having more ash than the germfree rats in bone, spleen, liver, cecal contents, and kidney. In older rats, the ash in muscle, bone, spleen, liver and brain was similar in the presence or absence of microorganisms. In the liver, brain, cecal contents, and lung the quantities of ash were lower in conventional than in the germfree chicks. The kidney, muscle, bile, small intestine cecum, and bone showed no differences in ash content in the two categories of chicks.

The nitrogen content of the muscle and liver of young germfree rats was greater than that found for conventional rats. In neither of these organs did this difference persist with age. The nitrogen content of the small intestines in chicks was less in the conventional state than in the germfree state. Other chick tissues and organs had the same nitrogen content under both conditions.

The fat content of the brain and bone of young rats was greater in the germfree condition than in the conventional condition. Again, these rats were not typical of older rats where few differences in fat content of tissues were seen. The fat content of the lung of conventional chicks was less than that of germfree chicks. Kidney, liver, muscle, and brain had the same fat content in both germfree and conventional animals.

One difference in metabolism was indicated for each vitamin studied. No difference in the vitamin C content of the adrenal gland was noted but the liver and muscle of conventional White Leghorn chicks had a much higher vitamin C content than was found for germfree chicks. No differences were found in the riboflavin and biotin content of tissues with the exception that the bile of conventional chicks contained much less riboflavin and biotin than that of germfree chicks. The cecum of conventional chicks had much more niacin than was found in the cecum of germfree chicks; other tissues examined showed no difference in niacin. The pantothenic acid content of liver was less and that of brain was greater in conventional chicks than in germfree chicks. Other tissues showed the same pantothenic acid concentrations. Folic acid and vitamin B_{12} concentrations were low in livers of conventional chicks and showed no differences between the two groups for other tissues examined. Folic acid and pantothenic acid concentrations were low in the conventional rat liver also.

Immunology

The underdeveloped lymphatic system of germfree animals, noted in the section on morphology, was characteristic of the general state of the defense mechanisms. The paucity of leucocytes in germfree animals combined with poor phagocytic response makes these animals very susceptible to infection. Surprisingly, germfree animals were found to be very effective in clearing injected particles or dead

TABLE 5.31

SUMMARY OF THE DEVELOPMENT OF POTENTIAL
"ANTIMICROBIAL DEFENSE SYSTEMS" IN GERMFREE ANIMALS

Good	Intermediate	Little or none
Skin	Mucosa of gastrointestinal tract	Cilia and squamous epithelium in sinuses
Thymus	Liver	Sinus and nasal lymphatic tissue
Bursa Fabricius	Spleen lymphopoiesis	
Spleen	Spleen secondary reaction centers	Tissue secondary reaction centers
	Plasma cells	Guinea pig plasma cells
Tissue monocytes, basophils, eosinophils, and heterophils	Tissue reticuloendothelial cells	
Periodic vaginal exudation, inflammation, and neutrophil infiltration	Tissue exudation (in cuts)	
Lymphocytes production	Lymph nodes (number and size) Lymphocytes in lymph nodes Circulating lymphocytes	
Serum heterophils	Serum monocytes	
Serum α- and β-globulins	Serum γ- and α-globulins	
Heterohemagglutinins	Antibacterial agglutinins	Dietary protein antibodies
Antibody production system		
Complement	Properidin	Foreign tissue antibody production Serum bactericidal activity
Blood clearing mechanism		Phagocytosis
"Shock" defense system Defecation	Reparative processes	Blood vessel formation in new tissue

bacteria from the blood. The serum of germfree animals had very little germicidal activity and low globulin content; very few antibacterial agglutinins were found in germfree animals. This was particularly true with young animals; older animals developed antibodies from the small amounts of dead bacteria which were in the diet. Injection of bacterial or other antigens into germfree animals gave a prompt antibody response. Heterohemagglutinins, properdin, and complement were present in germfree animals. A summary of the potential antimicrobial defense system (Table 5.31) shows a wide spectrum of preparedness of individual components.

Pathology

A variety of noninfectious diseases have been found in germfree animals; these include malnutrition, mineral and vitamin deficiencies, and anoxia. Germfree mammals were found to have a variety of tooth and oral diseases, although dental caries were never seen. The distention of the cecum was the greatest pathological problem in germfree mammals; this syndrome never occurred in birds. The cecum size was reduced by the inclusion of fiber in the diet or by contamination with bacteria. Spontaneous tumors have not been seen in germfree animals with one possible exception. Tumors could be induced with carcinogens or certain viruses. Hemorrhagic and heat shock were equally harmful to germfree and conventional animals. Radiation sickness from high doses may be slightly less harmful in germfree animals: little difference was seen between conventional and germfree animals for most dosages. A variety of other abnormalities of form and function, such as anal blockage in chicks, has been found but few studies have been carried out on such diseases. Enough has been done to indicate that the germfree animal is an ideal tool for the study of physiologic diseases.

CHAPTER 6

Gnotophoric Animals

Introduction

Inoculation of germfree animals has shown them to be ideal culture media for fastidious microorganisms. Interactions between the micro and macro species may be studied with neither the participation of well developed defense mechanisms nor the competition from other microorganisms. Exploration of this concept demonstrates two major classes of gnotobiotic animals: germfree and gnotophoric. Inoculation of germfree organisms with one or more known species of microorganisms results in gnotobiotic systems which might be used to study the ways and means by which the microorganisms become established in the host, the effect of the microorganism on the host, the effect of the host upon the microorganism, or the *in vivo* cultivation of fastidious microorganisms. The limited work done to date gives a general view of the types and rates of reactions which were found when a microorganism came into intimate contact with a vertebrate. Most of the work performed involved only one or two species of microorganisms present in the gnotophore. More interest has focused on the effect of the micro species upon the macro species than *vice versa*.

The presence of microbial gnotobiotes in gnotophoresis complicates both the theory and the methods of detection of unwanted organisms. The problem changes from the relatively simple procedure of showing that no living microorganisms are present to the delicate task of showing that all the individual microorganisms present belong to the species known to be in the system. With gnotophoric systems one must consider the distinction between different species and strains of microorganisms, many of which change morphologic and physiologic character under environmental influences. The former type of change was exemplified by the work of Maggini (1942) who found that the inoculation of *Streptococcus* sp. into germfree guinea pigs allowed its development (dissociation) into rougher strains of the same microorganism. The theoretical problems associated with gnotophoric animals must be partially ignored by the present-day investigator who is concerned with the application of this new tool. In practice he must use the accepted methods of microbiology much as described previously.

Sometimes another difficult nuance must be considered with gnotophoric animals that could be ignored in germfree work; this is the distinction between the inoculation of known microorganisms into a germfree system and the identification of contaminants of a germfree experiment. In practice there is no difference between a dibiotic system in which germfree rats were contaminated and one in which they were contaminated with a single strain of S. *faecalis.* Accepted methods make the practical problem relatively simple. In theory the two operations are diametrically opposed: the addition of a known pure culture of microorganisms to a known germfree animal leaves no uncertainty, whereas the identification of contaminant of a germfree animal leaves many questions unanswered. Did other contaminants enter which did not survive long enough to be detected, which are latent, or which are not easily detected? Such questions indicate reasons for reluctance to work with contaminated gnotophoric animals.

Having germfree animals as a control for inoculated gnotobiotes is an acceptable system for precise experimental work. However, interpretation of the data is more difficult than would at first be apparent. As previously indicated, certain characteristics of life are carried in dead organisms. It is evident that the best interpretations of the effect of one or more microbial species upon gnotobiotic animals will require knowledge of the effect of the dead microbes and/or their cell parts as well as that of the living culture. It is necessary to learn whether the living microorganism can produce, in the host, reactions that are qualitatively and quantitatively different from those reactions attributable to dead cells, cell parts, or microbial products. All of the work to date has omitted one of the three groups mentioned in any one definitive experiment. Antigen-free animals will be needed for the true base line.

The amount of material reported with gnotophores is only a small fraction of that available for germfree animals, and only one systematic approach to the general field has been made. Where specific microorganisms were not used, the material will be presented at the end of this chapter under the heading of "conventionalization." The implication that specific microorganisms should have been used is clear: much of the work should be repeated to determine which species were responsible for the responses noted. Although most gnotobiotic work has been done using only one or two microbial species, there is no limit to the number involved. One gnotobiotic colony began with germfree rats contaminated with two species of bacteria. This colony was continued for about a year (Reyniers, 1957c) in a small building modified to admit sterile food, water, and bedding. The air was admitted after a good cleaning, and the caretaker entered through a series of locks after donning sterilized clothes. The variety of microorganism found in the animals quickly increased from 2 to 8, and finally 11 different species were carried. Since none of the microorganisms were pathogenic, this colony was the prototype for the gnotobiotic colonies used by commercial suppliers of laboratory mammals. The methods could be readily adapted for a source of laboratory eggs and chicks.

Material will be arranged in the order of bacteria, virus, protozoa, and invertebrate experiments with chicks, guinea pigs, rats, and other mammals. The index must be consulted to obtain a complete picture of the effects obtained by any species of microorganism.

Methods

A doleful, but historically important, method of obtaining gnotophoric animals was to find them. If a germfree experiment were found to be contaminated, identification of all species present might reveal biota useful for a dibiotic or a tribiotic experiment. Many times a single contaminant was the only species which entered a break in the germ barrier; or only one might have been present from the beginning of an experiment. Although some of the investigators used such chance gnotophores for certain experiments, it must be admitted that progress was slow and results were not systematically accumulated with such haphazard presentation of material. Other disadvantages were the chance presence of unnoted microbes, the appearance of different strains of a microorganism, or the appearance of the same strain when another important experimental variable, such as diet or age, had been altered. Nevertheless, it was occasionally practical to use this method which was available too frequently to all who did much germfree work.

Inoculation of germfree animals with known pure culture of microorganisms is certainly the method of choice. Small inocula of $10^3 - 10^4$ organisms were usually given in order that the microorganisms might not overwhelm the undeveloped defenses of the germfree animal. Routes varied from simply adding the organisms to the food, milk, or water to placing them directly in the mouth, crop, rectum, or cecum. Usually the pure culture of microorganisms is sealed in an ampoule which is taken into the germfree cage *via* a germicidal trap. The ampoule is broken and a swab used to inoculate the gnotobiote by touching the mouth. All animals need not be inoculated as any growth of microorganisms in one will usually be found in all.

A third method by which gnotobiotic animals may be obtained is *via* decontamination. This method has been used only in preliminary experiments to date; however, it might become the method of choice for certain experiments once easy routines are established. The major states of gnotobiosis have been obtained by this technique although no avenues have been fully explored. Conventional animals have been maintained in a sterile environment in such a manner that their total flora has been reduced to one or two detectable species. Animals having two known microorganisms have lost one, and on another occasion one of two has been purposely removed; and animals having one species have been reduced to germfree animals. Details were presented under methods of obtaining germfree animals, Chapter 3.

Gnotophoric animals demand the same maintenance and care required by germfree animals. The physical barrier, sterilization of air, food, water, and utensils, and bacteriological examination require the same strict attention to every detail. Routine microbiological examination becomes more exacting. More attention must be given to microscopic examination of all material, and special media may be needed to detect certain contaminants in the presence of the gnotobiotic microflora. Procedural details are not given since they vary depending upon the character and number of known microorganisms present.

When gnotophoric animals are used, the tests for gnotobiosis should include not only the usual search for host contaminants, but also an examination for contaminants parasitic to all species present. The exemplary problem is the question of phage in a dibiotic experiment involving bacteria. If a bacterium is one of the gnotobiotes, a virus carried by that organism would be a contaminant with little or no direct effect on the metazoan host, but its indirect effect *via* the bacterium might be great. If a known virus were present in a microorganism which was inoculated into a germfree animal, the system is theoretically gnotophoric, and both the microorganism and its host are gnotophores. Such a condition has not been studied at the present time, but phage virulence might be studied *in vivo* as well as *in vitro*.

Bacteria—Host Gnotobiotes

Most early investigators worked with dibiotic animals. Schottelius (1902) inoculated germfee chicks with different strains of *E. coli* and concluded that these organisms were essential to maintenance of life. Cohendy (1912a) found monocontaminated chicks grew less well than conventional chicks. Cohendy and Wollman (1922) inoculated germfree guinea pigs with *Staphylococcus mesentericus* before injecting *Vibrio cholerae* into them. The response was the same as in germfree animals—many vibrios survived and the guinea pigs died in 6–9 days. Balzam (1937) found chicks inoculated with *Bacillus coli* grew no faster and died at about the same time as germfree birds when both groups were fed a vitamin B deficient diet.

In Cohendy's 1910 experiment, the 25 day old sterile chicks were inoculated with *Escherichia coli*. Two days later respiratory difficulties were noted and the chicks grew slowly. Autopsy showed the intestine, lungs, and liver to be hyperemic. The heart blood was sterile. Pure culture of these coli administered orally to man, dogs, and the control chicks caused no disease. Apparently *E. coli* alone caused the disturbance in health, while *E. coli* in the presence of other bacteria was innocuous. In his experiment of 1911, Cohendy's chicks were contaminated with *Bacillus subtilis* at 28 days. They died 3 days later with infection.

Chickens which were contaminated with a single microorganism such as *B. subtilis, Alcaligenes faecalis,* or *Staphylococcus albus* after 1 month of germfree life showed granulation tissue development with valvular involvement. The heart became enlarged and the organism settled on a valve. The lesion was seen histologically (H. A. Gordon, personal communication) as a proliferation of connective tissue and clinically as valvular insufficiency. These loci in germfree chickens showed no leucocytic response. Reyniers (1948) stated ". . . here, at last, is a direct laboratory approach to certain types of heart disease."

Mycoplasma gallinarum, an avian pleuropneumonia-like organism, produced chronic respiratory disease when inoculated intratrachealy into germfree turkey poults by Smibert *et al.* (1959). Neither cell-free filtrates of the inoculum broth nor sinus exudates produced aerosaccitis when injected into germfree or conventional poults, nor could a viral agent be demonstrated by other means.

Analysis of the liver and cecal contents of dibiotic chicks harboring *Streptococcus faecalis,* an organism with a dietary requirement for

TABLE 6.1

CONCENTRATION OF B-VITAMINS IN THE LIVER AND CECAL CONTENTS OF GERMFREE AND MONOFLORA CHICKS FED DIET L-258

		Liver					Cecal contents				
		No.[a]	M[b]	Min–Max	σ	P[c]	No.[a]	M	Min–Max	σ	P
Thiamine	Gf[d]	4	4.53	3.91–4.98	0.342	—					
	Mf. S.f.	4	4.47	3.22–5.37	0.792	0.90					
	Cv	3	4.91	4.77–5.03	0.0103	0.46					
Riboflavin	Gf	4	19.0	13.8–23.6	4.55		3	1.73	0.34–3.3	1.21	
	Mf. S.f.	4	25.6	25.5–28.6	2.01	0.073	3	16.2	10.7–20.5	4.08	0.004
	Cv	4	19.4	14.0–26.6	4.74	0.086	2	10.5	9.5–11.4		
Niacin	Gf	4	117	100–129	10.8		3	24.2	20.3–28.5	3.37	
	Mf. S.f.	4	12.7	8.8–16.9	2.87	<0.001	3	2.5	1.6–3.4	0.74	<0.001
	Cv	4	83.7	43.0–143	51.72	0.84	4	9.9	1.5–21.7	7.75	0.25
Pantothenate	Gf	4	15.4	13.0–16.6	1.43		4	16.2	7.8–23.6	6.24	
	Mf. S.f.	4	26.2	15.6–47.3	12.0	0.89	3	18.8	16.7–20.8	1.67	0.58
	Cv	4	18.2	15.5–21.3	2.27	0.32	2	12.6	10.6–14.5		
Biotin	Gf	4	6.5	5.6–7.5	0.72		3	0.42	0.29–0.54	0.10	
	Mf. S.f.	3	4.6	4.5–4.7	0.007	0.012	3	0.48	0.44–0.51	0.03	0.46
	Cv	4	4.2	3.5–4.8	0.458	0.42	3	0.37	0.19–0.72	0.24	0.78
Folic acid	Gf	4	2.7	2.3–2.9	0.23		1	1.7			
	Mf. S.f.	4	1.3	1.2–1.4	0.007	0.001	3	2.6	1.4–4.3		
	Cv	4	1.4	1.1–2.0	0.352	0.65					

[a] No. = Number of chicks. The chicks were 36 ± 3 days of age.

[b] M = Mean value in gm on a wet weight basis.

[c] The top P value compares germfree and gnotophoric chicks; the bottom p compares conventional and gnotophoric chicks.

[d] Mf S.f. = Gnotophoric chicks with a monoflora of Streptococcus faecalis.

most of the B vitamins and those tissues of germfree chicks fed the same diet revealed no difference consistent with the idea that the microorganism was utilizing measurable quantities of the vitamins it required (Table 6.1). The cecal contents of the monocontaminated birds contained more riboflavin, less niacin and possibly folic acid, and about the same concentrations of pantothenic acid and biotin as were found in the cecal contents of germfree birds. The concentrations of all vitamins were similar to those in the two control (polycontaminated) birds tested at the same time. The niacin difference was reflected in the livers of these chicks. The livers of S. *faecalis* monoflora chicks were found to have lower concentrations of thiamin, riboflavin, and pantothenic acid. Monocontaminated chicks having a single species which produced B vitamins as the other member of the dibiotic system were also studied (Table 6.2). With the possible exception of the vitamin B_{12} and biotin concentrations of the cecal contents of chicks contaminated with *Aerobacter aerogenes*, the values were not higher than those found in germfree chicks. The general tendency seen was that microorganisms in dibiotic existence with chicks had little effect on liver B vitamins and that they lowered cecal vitamin concentrations more often than they raised it, regardless of the synthetic potential or nutritive requirement of the microorganism.

In one experiment where chicks were fed what was thought to be a complete purified diet, both the germfree and conventional chicks exhibited a thiamine deficiency at about 9 days. As shown in Fig. 6.1, thiamine was presented to both groups at 10 days and at 21 days. Thiamine was presented a third time to the germfree chicks at 30 days and to the conventional chicks at 50 days. At 53 days of age the germfree chicks were found to be contaminated with *Staphylococcus* sp. They grew very well thereafter with no added thiamine. The conventional chicks apparently used up the thiamine given to them within 20 days and began to lose weight. The different growth rates dramatically illustrate that staphylococci decreased the apparent thiamine requirement of the host.

In a study with a diet containing a suboptimum amount of folic acid (100 μg/kg), Miller (1962) reported the hemoglobin and hematocrit values for germfree chicks to be 4.0 gm/100 ml and 11.0%, respectively. These values obtained in dibiotic chicks with *Escherichia coli* (an organism which can synthesize this vitamin) were 9.5 gm/100 ml and 28%, respectively. When germfree chicks, fed 200 μg folic acid per kg diet, were inoculated with *Streptococcus faecalis*, they grew at a

TABLE 6.2

ANALYSIS OF MONOBIOTIC, DIBIOTIC, AND POLYBIOTIC (CONVENTIONAL) CHICKS

	No. of chicks	Liver			Cecal contents		
		Biotin	Folic acid	Vitamin B_{12}	Biotin	Folic acid	Vitamin B_{12}
Germfree[a]	7 to 13	5.14	4.41	0.32	0.24	2.29	0.015
43–32 Aerobacter aerogenes	2	4.01 3.89/4.14	3.80 3.50–4.09	0.33 0.33/0.33	0.436 0.457/0.478	— —	0.057 —
43–41 Pseudomonas jaegeri	3	5.64 5.08/6.06	4.66 2.88/8.18	0.15 0.13/0.16	0.15	2.12	0.019
Conventional	3	7.35 4.11/10.3	3.98 3.51/4.31	0.10 0.09/0.11	0.21	1.87[a]	0.017[a]

[a] These values taken from other experiments. All chicks on diet L-245. All data is $\mu g/gm$, wet weight.

significantly lower rate than control germfree chicks fed the same diet. The folic acid content of muscle and brain was the same in the two latter groups while the germfree birds had a higher concentration of liver folic acid than did the Gn *S.f.* chicks. The folic acid content of

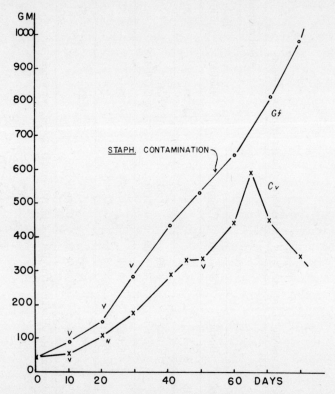

FIG. 6.1. Apparent thiamine requirement in germfree, monoflora, and conventional chicks. Thiamine added at each v.

feces of Gn *E. coli* chicks was 14 times greater than the average value obtained with Gn *S.f.* chicks. This provides further indirect evidence for the intestinal synthesis theory.

The presence of bacteria increased the serum cholesterol of chicks. At 10 weeks of age the serum cholesterol level was 136 ± 6 mg % in 8 germfree chicks fed diet L-289F and it was 152 ± 7 mg % in 7 conventional chicks (Wostmann *et al.*, 1960). *Clostridium perfringens* (*welchii*) monoflora chicks had 212 mg %, *Streptococcus faecalis* monoflora chicks had 206 and 216 ± 11 mg % in 2 experiments, and *Staphyl-*

ococcus aureus monoflora chicks had 203 mg cholesterol per 100 ml of serum. *Clostridium perfringens* monoflora chicks were found to have less liver monoamine oxidase activity than germfree chicks according to A. W. Phillips (1960). *Clostridium perfringens* monoflora chicks were found to have twice as many reticuloendothelial cells in the mucosa and submucosa of the ileum (Gordon *et al.*, 1959) as were found in germfree chicks. The lymphocyte content of the blood was as great as that of conventional chicks; the plasma cells were about two-thirds as plentiful while the Schollen leucocytes were only one-third as numerous as those of conventional chicks. Similar but less striking results were obtained with *Streptococcus faecalis* as the monoflora inoculum. It would be most interesting to see the results of feeding dead clostridia to these chicks; the cells might then be fractionated chemically to determine what compounds caused this stimulation. The *Streptococcus* stimulated the production of γ-globulin and specific agglutinin in the serum much more than did *Clostridium*.

Since germfree birds grew at a faster rate than conventional birds and did not respond to relative high levels of antibiotics, it was logical to determine if intestinal microorganisms which caused growth depression in conventional birds could be "counteracted" by feeding antibiotics to gnotophoric chicks. Coates *et al.* (1952) demonstrated that *Clostridium welchii* type A (*Cl. perfringens*) depressed growth in conventional chicks, and the growth depression was eliminated when antibiotics were fed. Forbes *et al.* (1959) and Lev and Forbes (1959) inoculated *Clostridium bifermentans,* or *E. coli* or a combination of *E. coli, Streptococcus liquefaciens,* and *Lactobacillus lactis* into germfree chicks. The resulting monoflora or triflora chicks showed no growth depression, and the presence of the microorganisms and 45 mg of procaine penicillin per kg of diet did not stimulate any increment in growth rate. When the toxin producing *Clostridium perfringens* type A was added to germfree chicks, a depression in growth rate was noted which could be prevented by feeding procain penicillin. This confirmed the work of Coates *et al.* (1952) with conventional chicks reared in "clean," "dirty" and "clean inoculated environments." Gordon (1961) confirmed this experience using *Cl. perfringens* or *Streptococcus faecalis* in monoflora chicks.

Penicillin virtually eliminated the population of clostridia in the intestine but had litttle effect on the total number of streptococci at 60 days. The number of *Cl. perfringens* present in monoflora chicks in the Forbes experiment (György, 1959) was found to be 9.7×10^6 in the duodenum, 3.7×10^6 in the ileum and 2.7×10^9 in the cecum per gram dry weight. Less than 1000 bacteria per gram were found when the monoflora chicks were fed 45 mg penicillin per kilogram diet. When *E. coli* and *L. lactis* were added for a tetrabiotic experiment, feeding antibiotic reduced *Cl. perfringens* 300-fold in the duodenum, 4-fold in the ileum, and 200-fold in the cecum while no decrease was found in the population of *E. coli* or *L. lactis*. Wostmann *et al.* (1960) found a similar pattern; in *Cl. perfringens* monoflora chicks, penicillin feeding resulted in 99.99+% reduction in the number of organisms in the ileum. When penicillin was fed to *Cl. perfringens* monoflora chicks, Wostmann *et al.* (1960) found a lower quantity of serum γ-globulin, decreased agglutinating antibody titer against *Cl. perfringens* to the point of questionable detection, no activity of the organism in the stimulation of the reticuloendothelial system, and a reduction in the lamina propria from that equivalent to the quantity found in conventional chicks to the decreased development found in germfree chicks. When penicillin was fed to *S. faecalis* monoflora chicks, it did not substantially reduce the number of organisms, change the γ-globulin level, or change the agglutinating antibody titers, and it had little effect on the reaction of the reticuloendothelial system. However, the quantity of lamina propria tissue in the mucosal wall was reduced to the quantity found in germfree chicks. Apparently all of the systems followed the activity of the microorganisms used, except the lamina propria tissue which was correlated inversely to the presence of the antibiotic.

Such data confirmed one possibility, proposed by Moore *et al.* (1946) and presented more fully by Coates *et al.* (1952), that one of the mechanisms of action of growth promotants was in the depression of activities of noxious microorganisms in the gastrointestinal tract. A review of this work and of other possible mechanisms was presented by Luckey (1959a). It was emphasized that this mechanism did not exclude the direct action of antibiotics upon animals, as found in germfree chicks, turkey poults, and plants (Nickell, 1958).

A systematic study of the effect of adding different bacteria to germfree chicks was proposed by Matsumura *et al.* (1929) and was started by his students Naito and Kobayash (1936) and Akazawa (1942) at Chiba University. Saito (1955) found that bacteria such as *E. coli, Cl. perfringens,* and *Cl. sporogenes* infected the germfree intestinal wall and caused injury, while the simultaneous administration of one of these microorganisms with *S. faecalis* or *L. acidophilus* pre-

vented injury to the digestive organs. This principle was confirmed by
the work of Hasegawa (1959), Nakamura (1959), Tomioka (1959),
and Tanami (1959) with guinea pigs. A guinea pig strain of *E. coli*
(M_1), which was innocuous when inoculated into conventional animals, produced necrotic and hemorrhagic enteritis in the intestine of
germfree guinea pigs; *E. coli* could be recovered from the blood. When

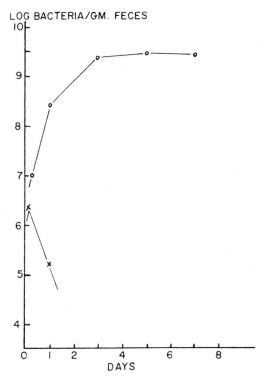

Fig. 6.2. *In vivo* antagonism of microorganisms; —o—o, *E. coli*, M_1; —x—x,
E. coli, F_6 (guinea pig strain) and F_6 (human strain) of *E. coli* inoculated in
equal quantities (7×10^4) in 3 germfree guinea pigs at 20 days of age. (Tanami,
1959).

E. coli F6, a human strain of the species, was introduced, it reached
the same concentration (10^9 organism per gram of feces) at 1 week.
The animals developed diarrhea, but no obvious tissue damage could
be seen. When the two strains were added in equal numbers, the
human strain disappeared rapidly (Fig. 6.2) and the guinea pigs died
showing the symptoms caused by *E. coli* M_1 alone. When *E. coli* M_1

was added at 2×10^3 organisms and *E. coli* F_6 (the human strain) was added at 7×10^5 organisms, the *E. coli* M_1 disappeared from the feces in 3–4 days (Fig. 6.3) and no histopathology was noted. The two strains were separated for identification by phage typing. When *L. acidophilus*, *L. bifidus*, or *S. faecalis* was introduced, the monoflora guinea pigs showed slight change in subepithelial tissue, the mesenteric lymph nodes developed slightly, and both germinal centers and Flemming's secondary nodes were found. An unknown bacillus

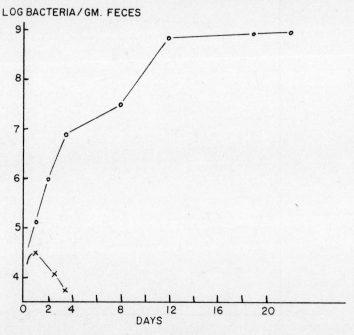

LOG BACTERIA / GM. FECES

DAYS

FIG. 6.3. *In vivo* antagonism of microorganisms; —o—o, *E. coli*, F_6; x—x—, *E. coli*, M_1. Average population changes of M_1 (2×10^3) and F_6 (7×10^5) strains of *E. coli* when injected in unequal numbers into 3 germfree guinea pigs at 20 days. (Tanami, 1959.)

gave greater stimulus to the lymphatic development than any of the above organisms without causing the damage seen by the *E. coli*. Tanami (1959) noted an increased growth rate in monoflora guinea pigs harboring *L. bifidus*.

When lactic acid bacteria were added prior to the addition of *E. coli* (M_1), no pathological effect from *E. coli* (M_1) was noted. *Streptococcus faecalis* did not inhibit the growth of the *E. coli* (Fig.

6.4). *Lactobacillus acidophilus* or *L. bifidus* caused a decrease in the number of *E. coli* found (Fig. 6.5). When a great excess of *L. bifidus* was added, *E. coli* could not establish itself (Fig. 6.6). This is experimental confirmation of a common clinical observation in colostrum-fed babies. These remarkable studies on antagonism of microorganisms indicated the lactic acid organisms either decreased the virulence of the *E. coli* or increased the effectiveness of the first

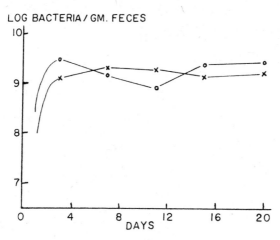

FIG. 6.4. *In vivo* antagonism of microorganisms; —o—o, *Strep. faecalis;* x—x—x, *E. coli*, M_1. Typical population changes of *S. faecalis* (3×10^7) and *E. coli* M_1 (3×10^3) inoculated in unequal numbers into 5 germfree guinea pigs at 21 days. These two organisms can live together, but the *S. faecalis* greatly reduces the effect of the *E. coli* upon the host. (Tanami, 1959.)

line of host defense mechanisms. Presumably, the first line of defense is a local reaction at the mucosal wall, since lactobacilli give little or no stimulus to lymphatic development, phagocyte education, or the production of immune γ-globulins.

The bactericidal power against *Salmonella typhus* of the serum of *E. coli* monoflora guinea pigs was almost as great as that of serum from conventional guinea pigs (Ootaka, 1959; Togano, 1958; Tanami, 1959) and that of germfree animals was very weak (Fig. 6.7). Surprisingly the bactericidal power of sera of *E. coli* + *L. bifidus* diflora guinea pigs was little greater than that of sera from germfree or *L. acidophilus* monoflora animals. Since Tanami (1959) had also shown that the presence of *L. bifidus* could greatly decrease the population of *E. coli*, it might be postulated that in the presence of

L. bifidus, E. coli never effectively penetrated the first defense barrier
and thus could not stimulate certain activities associated with the
bactericidal potency of the blood serum. His other studies had shown
that the phagocytic activity in the diflora guinea pigs was greater than
that of germfree animals; therefore this defense system had been
awakened by one or both of the microorganisms. Apparently, phagocytosis was activated more easily (or earlier) than the serum bactericidal activity.

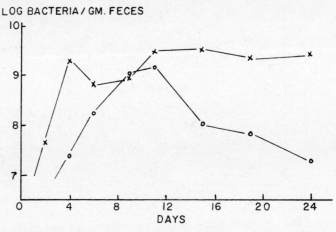

Fig. 6.5. *In vivo* antagonism of microorganisms; x—x—x, *L. bifidus;* o—o—o,
E. coli M₁. Typical population change of *L. acidophilus* (4×10^7) and *E. coli* M₁
(6×10^7) inoculated into 5 germfree guinea pigs at 20 days of age. (Tanami,
1959.)

Cohendy and Wollman (1922) showed that germfree and monoinoculated (or contaminated) guinea pigs were susceptible to *Vibrio
cholerae* infection. Inoculated animals died while conventional guinea
pigs showed no response. When germfree guinea pigs were inoculated
with *Shigella flexneri*-2a, ulcerative lesions were found in the colon
(Dammin, 1959). These animals showed eosinophils in the lamina
propria at some distance from the mucosal lesions. This work was
verified by György (1959) who reported also that *Shigella flexneri*
could not be established in monoflora guinea pigs carrying *E. coli*
(human strain). Neither heat killed *S. flexneri* nor live lactobacilli protected gnotophoric guinea pigs against live *S. flexneri:* (Formal *et al.*,
1961). Likewise no effect was seen when conventional guinea pigs
were inoculated with the bacillary dysenteric organism.

Wagner (1959c) reported that *Bacillus subtilis* was highly pathogenic and lethal to germfree guinea pigs, while conventional pigs
harbored it with no apparent disease. Miyakawa (1959b) inoculated
9 germfree guinea pigs with a spore forming bacillus and 10 with an
unidentified coccus. Five of the 19 died with a blood diarrhea.
Autopsy revealed emphysema, bleeding, and intestinal wall necrosis.

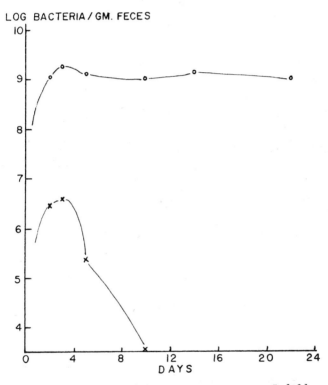

FIG. 6.6. *In vivo* antagonism of microorganisms; o—o—o, *L. bifidus;* x—x—x,
E. coli, M_1. Average population change of *L. bifidus* (6×10^7) inoculated at 20
days and *E. coli* (3×10^3) inoculated at 21 days into 5 germfree quinea pigs. No
E. coli could be found after 10–14 days. (Tanami, 1959.)

Peyer's patches were seen to break into numerous small pieces with
air vesicles isolating small pieces of tissue. Clear-centered, secondary
nodules were seen in those lymph nodes and in those of conventional
animals. These had not been found in germfree animals. Large cells
of unknown origin were also found.

Woolpert *et al.* (1936) found the fetal germfree guinea pigs to be

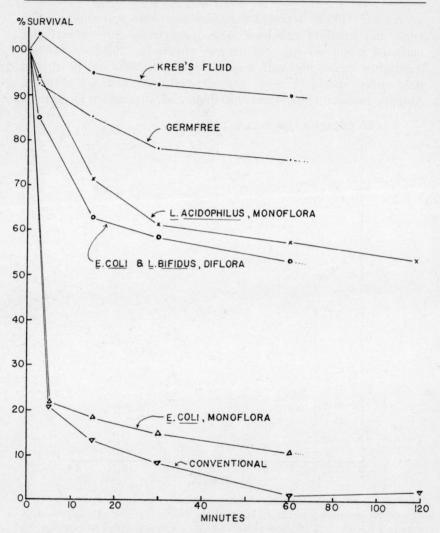

Fig. 6.7. Bactericidal power of sera of 40-day-old guinea pigs against *Salmonella typhi*. (Data of Tanami, 1959 and Ootaka, 1959.)

easily infected with small doses of bacteria and viruses. His experiments suggest that the susceptibility of the mammalian fetus *in utero* might be greater than that of the postnatal animal. Fitzgerald *et al.* (1958) found that human strains of the oral spirochete, *Treponema microdentium,* would not survive in germfree guinea pigs.

TABLE 6.3

COMPOSITION OF LIVER AND CECAL CONTENTS OF GERMFREE AND MONOFLORA RATS (DIET L-128) AT 153–163 DAYS

Material	Cat.	Liver (μg/gm, wet weight)					Cecal contents (μg/gm, wet weight)				
		No.	Mean	Min–Max	σ^b	P^c	No.	Mean	Min–Max	σ	P
Dry weight (%)	Gf	6	29.2	28.2–30.6	—	—	4	15.9	14.5–17.0	0.916	0.002
	GnL. a.[a]	6	29.5	29.0–30.4	—	0.9+	6	13.6	12.9–14.2	0.624	—
	Cv	2	27.5	27.3–28.6	—	—	4	22.3	20.7–23.4	1.10	<0.001
Ash (%)	Gf	6	4.50	4.34–4.96	0.108	0.004					
	GnL. a.	6	6.04	4.91–7.69	0.896	—					
	Cv	2	4.18	4.03–4.32	—	—					
Riboflavin (μg per gram)	Gf	6	16.3	10.7–22.6	4.90	0.9+	4	7.55	7.08–7.65	0.312	<0.001
	GnL. a.	4	16.2	15.1–17.8	1.05	<0.001	5	5.92	5.07–6.35	0.469	—
	Cv	6	10.3	7.8–12.6	1.69	—	5	1.80	0.60–3.34	1.19	<0.001
Niacin (μg per gram)	Gf	4	168	162–173	5.24	0.15	6	14.1	8.6–18.1	3.81	0.096
	GnL. a.	6	154	135–178	14.7	—	5	9.84	5.8–13.6	3.11	—
	Cv						4	53.2	47.7–58.3	4.46	<0.001
Pantothenate (μg per gram)	Gf	6	81	61–101	19.2	0.57	6	7.13	5.81–8.53	1.32	0.017
	GnL. a.	5	87	75–100	9.74	—	5	17.9	7.20–30.2	8.31	—
	Cv	4	47	43–52	3.74	<0.001	6	13.2	10.6–15.0	1.87	0.275
Biotin (μg per gram)	Gf	4	7.14	5.02–9.97	1.96	<0.001	6	0.412	0.368–0.541	0.066	<0.001
	GnL. a.	5	1.92	1.63–2.17	0.202	—	5	0.143	0.102–0.164	0.022	—
	Cv	6	5.34	2.15–6.96	2.19	0.12	3	0.690	0.118–1.84	0.812	0.22
Folic acid (μg per gram)	Gf	6	7.54	5.09–10.4	2.09	0.003	6	1.39	0.73–1.92	0.474	0.030
	GnL. a.	6	3.21	1.14–5.02	1.30	—	4	0.64	0.56–0.74	0.065	—
	Cv	5	2.95	2.34–3.66	0.481	0.61	4	1.66	0.99–2.72	0.648	0.11

[a] GnL. a. indicates Gnotophoric animals carrying only *Lactobacillus acidophilus*.

[b] This denotes the standard deviation.

[c] The top P compares Gf and GnL. a.; the lower P compares GnL. a. with Cv.

When germfree rats were inoculated with a species of *Lacto-bacillus acidophilus* taken from a human dental lesion, the strain established itself, and the dibiotic system was studied biochemically as shown in Table 6.3. The percentage dry weight of the liver of the gnotophoric rats was almost identical to the average found for germ-free rats fed a diet of the same composition. The ash content of the livers of the gnotophoric rats was definitely higher than that found for livers of germfree rats. The livers from both groups were found to have similar concentrations of riboflavin and pantothenic acid, while the livers of the germfree rats were found to have higher con-centrations of biotin and folic acid. The livers of these monoflora rats had a higher concentration of riboflavin and pantothenic acid than livers of conventional rats. *Lactobacillus* gnotophore rats aligned themselves closer to germfree than to conventional rats when the % dry weight of the cecal contents were considered (Table 6.3). They actually had more water in the cecal contents than had germfree rats. The cecal contents of monoflora rats were found to contain greater concentrations of niacin than those of conventional rats and less than those of germfree rats. Cecal concentrations of biotin and folic acid were lower in monoflora rats than in germfree animals and conven-tional rats had mean values which were the highest of the three categories. The vitamin requirements of this microorganism included most of the B vitamins (Peterson and Peterson, 1945). Therefore, one would have expected the concentration of B vitamins in the intestinal tract of *Lactobacillus* gnotophore rats to be consistently lower than that in germfree rats. The extent to which this was not found is an index of a less simple explanation.

Gustafsson (1959a) found that the cecal contents were about 4.5% of the body weight in germfree rats and about 1% in conventional rats. *Lactobacillus acidophilus* in monoflora rats did not decrease the size of the cecum. *Proteus vulgaris* and *E. coli* in monoflora rats were effective in reducing the size of the cecal wall. When germfree rats were inoculated with fecal material from conventional rats, the cecum and contents were found to be reduced 4 days later.

The pattern of serum proteins of germfree rats changed to that of conventional rats when bacteria were introduced (Wostmann and Gor-don, 1960). Two weeks after inoculation the α-2 fraction had developed to the extent of two-thirds of the conventional value, the β-fraction began to increase and the γ-value was not changed. Gustafsson and Laurell (1959) used both electrophoresis and immunologic titrations to study the γ-globulin response in germfree rats following contamination with a mold for 6 days and a full microbial flora thereafter. Young rats showed a 4 week lag period followed by a fast increase in globulin, while older rats responded slowly with no distinct lag period. The 4 week lag period was also found when 3 month old rats were contaminated with *Bacillus subtilis* for 3 days and full microbic contamination thereafter. Wagner and Wostmann (personal communication) found that the appearance of agglutinins for *E. coli* occurred about 2 weeks following inoculation of germfree rats. This was correlated with the production of β-globulins prior to the appearance of γ-globulins in the serum. Monoflora rats with *Cl. perfringens* A, *E. coli*, *Strep. faecalis*, or *L. casei* gave little change in serum α-, β- or γ-globulins but showed good agglutinin formation to the microorganism when compared to germfree rats. Inoculation of germfree chickens resulted in a marked response to each monoflora in the γ-globulin fraction and *Strep. faecalis* induced a good aggluination titer; however no agglutinin was found for *Cl. perfringens*. Nor could they find antibody against the α-toxin (lecithinase) of *Cl. perfringens*.

Wagner (1959b) and Wagner and Wostmann (1961) found no agglutinins to *L. casei* or *L. acidophilus* in dibiotic animals born by monoflora mothers carrying that organism. The mothers, which had been inoculated a short time after birth, or rats inoculated at 48 days had good titers against the organism. When the second generation dibiotic animals were challenged parenterally with the homologous lactobacilli, there was a dramatic increase in both γ-globulin and agglutinin production. Apparently the organism had never effectively penetrated the primary defense mechanism of the epidermal or mucosal surfaces and never had the opportunity to activate secondary defense mechanisms. When the experiment was repeated with *Strep. faecalis*, the results indicated that this organism had penetrated the first defenses because the second generation monoflora rats had a high titer (1 to 256–2048) before being challenged by parenteral injection. Injection of the homologous *S. faecalis* gave slightly higher titer of agglutinin and an unsteady rise in α-2- and γ-globulins. Injection of the lactobacilli into fourth generation *Lactobacillus* dibiotic rats (which had been born from mothers carrying only this bacterium) gave an increase in serum α-2 and γ-globulins and a dramatic rise in antibody titer.

Serum cholesterol levels were not changed when germfree rats were inoculated with *Clostridium perfringens*, but they were increased somewhat in *Strep. faecalis* monoflora rats (Wostmann and Wiech, 1960). Monoflora *Clostridium* (G62) rats produced urobilins in the feces, but neither this organism alone nor it plus *E. coli* gave values as high as were found in conventional rats (Gustafsson and Swenander Lanke, 1960).

Since dental caries were absent in germfree rats (Orland *et al.*, 1954; Fitzgerald *et al.*, 1960b) several different microorganisms have been inoculated into germfree rats in order to determine which species might initiate carious lesions. The work reported by Orland *et al.* (1955a) with inoculated rats excluded interesting data obtained while the author was actively engaged as the Lobund project coordinator in this collaboration. The first series of experiments comprised a thorough study of a colony of rats inoculated with *Lactobacillus* sp. (ND465) which was a human oral isolate recommended for the quantity of acid it could produce in culture. Work with this gnotophoric colony made it one of the best studied of monoflora animals. When fed a cariogenic diet for an experimental period of 150 days, a period which allowed virtually all of the conventional rats to develop dental caries, the monoflora (*Lactobacillus* ND465) rats showed microscopic lesions in about 30% of the rats and gross lesions in none. The teeth of the "lactobacillus rats" looked more like those of the germfree rats than those of conventional rats which usually had lesions readily observed upon gross observation. In a single experiment with 3 diflora rats in which *Micrococcus* sp. (acidogenic and proteolytic) was present for 157 days, no carious lesions were found. When *Streptococcus liquefaciens* monoflora rats were fed the cariogenic diet, such extensive lesions developed that the second and third molars were sometimes almost missing. The lesions were considered atypical and not worthy of further study. Subsequent work with enterococci was reported by Orland *et al.* (1955a); an organism resembling *Strep. faecalis* inoculated into rats harboring a slow growing, noncariogenic, pleomorphic contaminant resulted in dental caries in all 8 rats. Tribiotic rats with the enterococcus and a proteolytic bacillus were found to develop typical carious lesions. Fitzgerald *et al.* (1960b) reported that a nonproteolytic, homofermentive, α-type *Streptococcus* produced lesions in monoflora rats. The caries obtained included advanced cavitation involving dentine which occasionally penetrated the pulp cavity to produce intrapulpal abscesses.

When *Bacillus anthracis* (vollum 1B) was inoculated into rats 5 weeks of age, Taylor *et al.* (1960) found that the LD_{100} for germfree rats was less than 100 spores while the LD_{50} for conventional rats was 10^9 spores. Description of germfree rats following contamination with *Aerobacter aerogenes* and a gram positive bacterium was presented by Reyniers *et al.* (1946).

Shigella flexneri from human infections grew when inoculated into germfree rats and mice. Counts in the intestinal tract reached 10^9 without causing disease (Wagner, 1959c).

When germfree C3H mice were monocontaminated with *Micrococcus epidermis* the number of microorganisms in the intestinal tract were 10^{10}. These mice had enlarged spleens and cervical and inguinal lymph nodes and showed a general thickening of the intestinal wall (Reyniers, 1958). No general sickness or abnormalities developed within 2 weeks.

The first germfree monkey reared by J. A. Reyniers, J. Reback, and others (Reyniers and Trexler, 1943b) became contaminated at 31 days with *S. aureus, B. proteus,* and an aerobic spore former. When the animal died, 2 weeks later, these organisms were found in the intestinal tract but not in blood nor tissues. *Bacillus subtilis* as the only contaminant in one goat of Küster (1913b) gave no evidence of disease.

Virus—Host Gnotobiotes

Germfree animals were often defined as being free from symptomatic viruses, but they were not proven to be free from occult viruses. In spite of this handicap the germfree animal is one of the most exciting tools for virus research visualized to date. They are more standardized than conventional animals in having no microbial experience and undoubtedly have greatly reduced viral experience. The host sensitivity should be high since certain defense mechanisms have not been activated and others may have reduced activity. Germfree animals offer a good means to study phenomena such as latent virus, virus activation, origin of virus, host susceptibility to virus, and specific virus defense mechanisms.

There is good evidence that germfree animals are free from virus disease. In the experience of those who worked with germfree animals, symptomatic viruses were rarely suspected and no *de novo* viruses have never been isolated and transmitted as an infectious agent.

The work of T. G. Ward (1960) with occult viruses involved transfers into material from conventional hosts. He admitted (1960) that it would be preferable to use germfree tissue and animals in such work. No tumors were seen in 6 generations of germfree C3H mice by Reyniers and Sacksteder (1958a) while 98% of conventional control mice showed mammary carcinoma within 18 months. It was assumed that Cesarean birth and foster suckling to Swiss mice prohibited the transmission of a transmissible milk agent. Iijima (1950) assumed that virus caused some of the pneumonia seen in germfree guinea pigs.

J. A. Reyniers and J. Reback (personal communication) worked out methods to take virus into a germfree system, and they (Reyniers, 1959b) obtained tumors by injection of Rous sarcoma virus into chickens. When Rous sarcoma tissue ultrafiltrates were injected into germfree chickens, Reyniers and Sacksteder (1959b) found the incidence of tumors and the time required for the tumors to reach 1 cm in diameter was similar in germfree and conventional chicks. This similarity extended to the later growth of the tumor and death of the birds in both categories. Reyniers and Sacksteder (1958c) reported that when inoculated with human hepatitis serum, germfree white Leghorn chicks 30–60 days old developed a fatal disease which could be transmitted to other germfree chicks. No response was noted when this virus was inoculated into conventional chicks. Others (György, 1959; J. Reback, personal communication) could not induce serum hepatitis in germfree chicks despite repeated efforts. No published reports are known of a comprehensive study on any virus disease in bacteria-free animals.

It is presumptive to put material regarding transmissible tumors and "wasting disease" in this chapter. Although all Koch's postulates have not been met in the determination of an etiological factor in these studies, the presumptive evidence suggests a viral etiology as being closer to the truth than any other classic etiology. Gordon and Reyniers (personal communication) found that injection of methyl cholanthrene dissolved in benzene would induce tumor formation in germfree chicks. The data of Reyniers (1957b) with repeated passage of homogenates from such tumors tissue suggested that an increased pathogenicity was obtained. All attempts to pass methyl cholanthrene induced tumors of conventional chicks were negative unless the recipient chicks were fed 50 mg/kg diet of streptomycin or procaine penicillin. Injection of tumor ultrafine homogenate from germfree birds would produce both tumor and wasting disease in germfree chicks while it produced wasting disease but no tumor in conventional chicks (Reyniers and Sacksteder, 1959b). Taylor (1959) and A. R. Taylor *et al.* (1959) reported that the injection of pure methyl cholanthrene in benzene into germfree chicks resulted in the production of large quantities of 20 microsomal particles in the tumor tissue which were called "virus or viruslike." The particles and the tumor were transmissible by tissue homogenates. These fibrosarcomas grew to a large size and the chicks succumbed. Ultrafine filtrates of these tumor would not transmit tumors into other birds but would "cause a disease characterized by extreme muscular wasting of the breast muscle" (Reyniers, 1959a). This wasting disease was associated with a special microsomal fraction by Taylor *et al.* (1959). These experiments should be repeated with conventional control chicks.

A sporadic encephalo-meningeal syndrome affecting germfree chicks but not conventional chicks was reported by Gordon *et al.* (1959). Clinical symptoms were seen in all chicks within the cage whenever the disease appeared. Successful transmission of agent *via* cell free homogenates was attempted but was not accomplished. The meningeal proliferation seen in some of the afflicted chicks could not be classified as being either inflammatory or neoplastic in nature, but it displayed characteristics of both. The symptoms noted were (1) general weakness, (2) slight body tremors and an unsteady gait, (3) course tremors ("jitters"), and (4) death. Vitamin deficiencies were first suspected since thiamine, pyridoxine, or vitamin E deficiencies showed similar characteristics. Vitamin therapy failed. Evidently some change in metabolism, the presence or absence of some metabolite in abnormal quantity, allowed this manifestation to exert itself in the absence of microorganisms.

Several years of collaboration between the author and associates at the University of Notre Dame and Dr. G. E. Cottral, Dr. A. M. Lucas, and Dr. B. B. Burmester of the U. S. Regional Poultry Research Laboratory, East Lansing, Michigan, on the possible presence of lymphomatosis in germfree chicks revealed no positive evidence. Although few chicks were maintained long enough for thorough examination of the problem, it was evident that this agent was not rampant in germfree chicks obtained from the highly susceptible flock. The virologist of the Lobund group, Dr. J. Reback, reported (personal communication) that results with the filterable agent of lymphomatosis in germfree chickens were quite inconclusive in spite of the examination of several germfree birds from the highly susceptible flock which were maintained for 5 months.

Phillips and Wolfe (1961) suggested an "unvirus" as a possible causative agent in a pneumonia disease which was fatal to most germfree guinea pigs from 66 Cesarean operations in 1955. The first symptoms were respiratory difficulty with convulsions at 10–14 days. About 50% survived this first attack, which lasted from a few minutes to several hours. The recurrence of the convulsions within 36 hours was fatal to most guinea pigs. Red blood cell and white blood cell counts were normal for germfree guinea pigs. Histopathologic examination indicated the cause of death to be acute broncho-pneumonia. Patchy areas of the lungs showed consolidation with inflammation. No etiologic agent was isolated nor shown by tissue transfer experiments. Increasing the vitamins did not relieve or prevent the disease. Amazingly, the disease could be prevented in the germfree guinea pigs by feeding *autoclaved* cecal contents from conventional animals. The authors suggested this "may have provided a stimulus for the normal defenses."

Protozoa—Host Gnotobiotes

The gnotobiotic animal promises to be a most valuable tool in parasitic research. Studies to be followed include host specificity, host susceptibility, parasitic nutrition, mechanisms and kinetics of infection, mechanisms and kinetics of defense, and interrelationships between tissue parasites, intestinal microorganisms, intestinal parasites, and host. The early work in this field is being pioneered with guinea pigs by different groups of scientists at the U. S. Public Health Service.

In a study on amebiasis in guinea pigs, Phillips and Wolfe (1959) inoculated 73 germfree guinea pigs intracecally with *Endamoeba histolytica* which had been cultured with *Trypanosoma cruzi*. None of these animals had any gross lesions when autopsied 1 to 58 days following the inoculation. Microscopic examination revealed no ameba in the cecal tissues and no evidence of invasion. It was apparent that *E. histolytica* did not survive more than a few days in germfree guinea pigs. Ulcerative amebiasis was seen in 41 of 53 inoculated conventional guinea pigs. *T. cruzi* was found in the blood of three-quarters of "germfree" guinea pigs but not in conventional pigs

(Phillips *et al.*, 1955). No detectable lesions were seen in guinea pigs
inoculated with *T. cruzi* in the absence of the ameba. *T. cruzi* could
not be established in conventional guinea pigs by Phillips and Wolfe
(1959). However, *T. cruzi* was apparently present in the inoculum
each time *E. histolytica* was introduced into gnotobiotic guinea pigs.
The tribiotic guinea pigs, infected with both *Endamoeba histolytica*
and *Trypanosoma cruzi* were found to have blood characteristics
similar to those of conventional guinea pigs. The guinea pigs had
reduced hemoglobin and red blood cell values when compared to
germfree and conventional animals. The white blood cell and lymphocyte counts were within the lower range of counts found for conventional guinea pigs. In the next series of experiments a single species
of bacteria was established into germfree guinea pigs. Protozoa were
then inoculated into the monoflora guinea pigs. When the Shaffer-
Frye *Streptobacillus* sp. was the bacterial vector and *E. histolytica*
the protozoan, no lesions were produced. When the bacterium was
Escherichia coli, Aerobacter aerogenes, or *Bacillus subtilitis,* amebic
lesions were obtained in 80–100% of the animals. Details of the
pathology at autopsy showed some differences in the lesions obtained
in monofauna guinea pigs and conventional animals. In a summary
of their results Phillips and Wolfe (1959) reported no lesions were
seen when only *E. coli* was inoculated into germfree guinea pigs. This
result was somewhat surprising in view of the harmful effects of
E. coli and other gram-negative bacteria reported in detail under
bacterial infections in this chapter. Before *E. histolytica* could be
directly implicated in the production of the lesions, it should be used
in the absence of *T. cruzi*. Another control of interest would be one
with the bacterium plus *T. cruzi* injected into germfree guinea pigs.

When germfree guinea pigs were fed sterile cecal contents from
conventional guinea pigs and then inoculated with *E. histolytica,* the
parasite survived in the cecum and one-third to one-half of the
guinea pigs developed amebic lesions. When reducing compounds
such as cysteine or sodium thioglycollate were given with the inoculum, about one-half of the guinea pigs of Phillips *et al.* (1958) developed amebic lesions in the presence of the ameba without any
bacteria. When the cecal tissue was traumatized by repeated needle
puncture at the time of inoculation of *E. histolytica,* about one-third
of the guinea pigs developed amebic lesions and active ameba were
found in the lesions at autopsy. The lesions obtained in the absence
of bacteria were of nodular character and had little similarity to the

extensive ulceration which typifies the lesions obtained in the presence of bacteria.

Trichomonas vaginalis caused no gross reaction and did not survive when injected subcutaneously into conventional guinea pigs by Newton *et al.* (1960b). When injected into germfree guinea pigs, the trichomonads survived. The results ranged from no gross lesions to lesions, abscesses, and cysts up to 5 cm in diameter. Some of these were filled with gas, pus, and active trichomonads. The gas was found to contain up to 25% hydrogen. These workers observed that germfree animals are useful for fine differentiation between strains of protozoa.

Invertebrate—Host Gnotobiotes

The first work was that in which attempts to obtain germfree dogs resulted in a high percentage of dibiotic experiments in which a parasitic worm was the only species found in the pups. Such was the experience of Glimstedt (personal communication) and the group at Lobund as reveiwed by B. P. Phillips (1960). In 4 Lobund experiments only 1 pup in 6 attempted was found to be parasite free. *Toxocara canis* was found in all of the others and one was difaunated with *T. canis* and *Ancyclostoma canium.* Only in one experiment was an adult parasite seen. Landy (1961, personal communication) has obtained germfree, wormfree pups.

Subcutaneous injection of 2,000 to 20,000 infective larvae of the rat nematode, *Nippostrongylus muris,* into 6 germfree and 6 conventional guinea pigs by Newton *et al.* (1959) revealed no parasites in the conventional guinea pigs at 3 and 10 days. One of the 6 dibiotic guinea pigs harbored fourth stage worms; a second contained adults with fertile eggs; the others contained no parasites. The tissues of the guinea pigs reacted to encyst the unnatural parasite. When 1,500 to 3,000 infective third stage larvae of the mouse nematode *Nematosperoides dubius* were given *per os* to germfree and conventional guinea pigs, no parasites were recovered from the conventional animal at 17 days post-inoculation. Significant numbers of worms, including females with eggs were found in the 2 dibiotic guinea pigs, and embryonated eggs were found in the feces. Similar results were obtained in a confirmatory experiment in which 2 of 3 Cesarean born and 3 of 4 normal born germfree guinea pigs were found to harbor worms following inoculation. In a third experiment Newton *et al.* showed that from 1 week to 4 weeks the age of inoculation of the germfree guinea pigs gave no marked difference in the number of worms recovered. *Hymenolopis nana* was also found in some of the germfree guinea pigs. The eggs of this mouse tapeworm were given inadvertently with the larvae of *N. dubius.* Wright *et al.* (1959) reported that infective eggs of *Ascaris lumbricoides* produced larvae which had no difference in migratory capability in germfree and conventional guinea pigs.

The trematode, *Schistosoma mansoni,* was injurious to germfree snails fed yeast and formalin-killed *E. coli,* but not to conventional snails (Chernin, 1960).

Conventionalization

Changes observed following the inoculation of germfree animals with specific microroganisms have been presented in this chapter. These changes are placed in good perspective by observing the changes which occur during the conventionalization of germfree animals. The over-all effect of placing germfree animals into a stock colony of conventional animals was presented previously (see characteristics of germfree animals). No change was seen in the general appearance of germfree chicks, chickens, or turkey poults when they were taken from the germfree cage and placed in brooder with conventional birds.

The situation was less clear with mammals. Küster (1915) maintained a germfree kid following his last germfree experiment. The first day it feared its keeper and for a short period its growth was interrupted. Reyniers *et al.* (personal communication) reminisced that when one of the germfree monkeys was taken from the cage it exhibited kenophobia and was tremendously upset until it was placed back in the cage. The monkey died with generalized infection. Germfree rats routinely died in 5–7 days after being placed in a conventional rat colony. When placed in an area with fewer potential "pathogenic" (qualified for germfree animals) microorganisms (i.e. in a cage on the author's desk) for 5–7 days before being introduced to conventional rats, they survived. The reaction of germfree guinea pigs and mice is probably similar to that of rats: the author had less experience with these species and little has been published on their conventionalization.

A preliminary study of the transition of the germfree rat to the conventional state was made by Gordon and Wostmann (1959).

Germfree rats were inoculated with a suspension prepared from cecal contents of conventional rats into both the stomach and the cecum. Immediately thereafter the rats were taken from the germfree cages. The survival of the animals was good and the animals gave the impression of good health. Signs of severe stress were absent. Examina-

TABLE 6.4

TRANSITION OF GERMFREE TO CONVENTIONAL ALBINO RATS[a]

		Time after inoculation				
	Germ-free	5–7 hr	1 week	2 weeks	4 weeks	Conventional state
Small intestine (mg/100 gm)	100	102	147	151	—	136
Small intestine (% dry)	100	94	86	85	—	87
Cecum empty (mg/100 gm)	100	101	87	67	—	39
Cecum contents (mg/100 gm)	100	76	10	12	—	15
Submandibular nodes (mg/100 gm)	100	111	165	302	—	361
Peyers patches (mg/100 gm)	100	126	213	275	—	260
Ileocecal nodes (mg/100 gm)	100	107	482	410	—	242
Ileocecal lymphocytes	100	70	139	155	—	108
Thymus (mg/100 gm)	100	101	117	105	—	126
Thymocytes	100	106	109	109	—	121
Adrenal gland (mg/100 gm)	100	90	88	84	—	75
Adrenal ascorbic	100	84	104	91	—	89
α-2 Serum globulins	100	—	100+	100+	100+	100+
β-Serum globulins	100	—	100	100+	100+	100+
γ-Serum globulins	100	—	100	100	100+	100+

[a] From Gordon and Wostmann (1959). The values given are based upon Gf = 100. The (mg/100 gm) simply indicates the basis of measurement.

tion of the cecal contents, 5 to 7 hours after inoculation showed that the total bacterial count and the quantity of the more common bacterial groups found in the cecum were comparable to the quantities found in the cecum of conventional rats. The data were presented for 12 to 19 rats in each category. The rate of change might be compared with the germfree values equated to 100 (Table 6.4). A dramatic change was noted in the total contents of the cecum which dropped very rapidly to a value one-tenth of that found in a germfree rat within the first week. Gustafsson (1959a) reported a similar condition for cecal contents while the weight of the empty cecum changed more slowly. Apparently the intestinal microflora or compounds associated with it were responsible for a remarkable change in the muscle tonus of the cecum. Interpretation of the data indicated that the cecum has contracted under the influence of the inoculation. The weight of the small intestine, in milligrams per 100 gm of body weight, changed within the first week to approximately that of conventional rats. The increase in size of the small intestines was accompanied by a decrease in the dry weight as the transition period progressed. The adrenal gland tended to decrease in size; the rate was certainly less fast than those of the changes seen in the intestine. No remarkable change was seen in the ascorbic acid concentration of the adrenal gland. The ileocecal lymph nodes gradually increased and by the end of a week they were double the size of those seen in conventional rats per 100 gm body weight. This overcompensation was greater than was seen in the other parameters measured. At the same time there was an increase above normal in the lymphocyte count of the ileocecal lymph tissue. The quantity of Peyer's patches in the intestine increased rapidly to the conventional value within 2 weeks. The change in the submandibular lymph nodes was similar to that seen for Peyer's patches. No remarkable change was seen in thymus weight and the thymocytes in thymus tissue remained relatively constant. This would be expected since there was no basic difference in the thymocyte count between germfree and conventional animals.

Although quantitative data were not given for the serum proteins, the authors did state that the α-globulin increased above the germfree value at 1 week while at 2 weeks both the α- and the β-globulin fractions were higher than the germfree but neither was as high as was found for conventional animals. The γ-globulin fraction was not increased at 2 weeks but it did begin to increase by 4 weeks. It would be most interesting to see if the increased γ-globulin production could be correlated to the appearance of plasma cells.

It is difficult to interpret these data without the germfree control animal being inoculated with autoclaved cecal contents containing dead bacteria. Presumably future studies will have this control and will present the capability of specific microorganisms in effecting the changes noted. Since some of the changes were quite rapid, it would be helpful to have data at 1 and 2 days. In order to study the slow changes and the overcompensation of the animals this fine study should be repeated with a longer period of conventionalization.

Summary

Characteristics are presented of a second class of gnotobiotic animals, those of which *bear known forms* of living organisms, or gnotophoric animals. Gnotophoric animals include monoinoculated germfree animals which have a monoflora and are therefore dibiotic, or more microorganisms can be inoculated to give tribiotes, tetrabiotes, etc. The methods involved in maintaining gnotophoric animals are very similar to those required for germfree research. The added burden to the microbiological testing is that there is always expected to be one or more known microorganisms present and the test must differentiate these from possible contaminants. Gnotophoric animals are ideal as experimental animals with germfree animals as the true control. The difference between the two can be attributable directly or indirectly to the inoculated organism. Contaminants accidentally introduced into germfree animals can be identified and the animals used in gnotobiotic studies. This is not the ideal procedure, but it has been done. Decontamination has given both gnotophoric animals and germfree animals. Preliminary work with decontamination was presented in the chapter on methods.

Some microorganisms which are considered to be innocuous for conventional animals are quite harmful to germfree animals. Thus, heart disease was seen in chickens contaminated with *B. subtilis* and many "innocuous" gram-negative bacteria are harmful when injected into germfree guinea pigs. Chemical changes in germfree animals have been studied following the inoculation or contamination with a single microorganism. The data are presented as preliminary experiments in a fascinating field. The work with antibiotics fed to monoflora chicks gave evidence that *one* mechanism of action of antibiotics is to counteract certain microorganisms which inhibited growth. *Clostridium perfringens* depressed growth of monoflora animals and stimulated increased cellular defense systems more than other microorganisms. When penicillin was added, the *Clostridium* was dramatically reduced in number and the chickens grew at a faster rate. It was emphasized that this did not exclude other mechanisms of antibiotic action.

Lactobacilli generally did not stimulate defense mechanisms in germfree animals while *Streptococcus faecalis* generally stimulated both humoral and cellular systems of defense including increased white blood cell count, proliferation of lymphatic tissue, phagocytosis, serum γ-globulins, and the appearance of specific agglutinins. Most of the gram-negative microorganisms studied also stimulated defense mechanisms. Studies on the interrelation of two different micro-organisms in germfree guinea pigs showed *E. coli* could be rendered innocuous by the presence of lactic acid organisms.

In the study of dental caries in monoflora rats it was found that while germfree rats had no dental caries, *L. acidophilus* produced microscopic lesions, enterococci produced typical lesions, and *S. liquefaciens* give such large lesions that the crowns of teeth were missing.

Exhaustive virus studies have not been made with germfree animals. Most workers agreed that germfree animals were free from symptomatic virus, and thus far pathology attributable to virus has never had clear evidence with Koch's postulates to prove that a virus was the causative agent. Three virus-like diseases found in germfree animals are detailed.

Work with parasites indicated that monofauna parasitic infections were not always easily obtained. On the other hand some parasites could be established in germfree animals which could not be estab-lished in conventional animals. The work with *Endamoeba histolytica* in experimental amebic dysentery was reviewed in detail; the proto-zoan was implicated but further work is needed. Protozoa have not been found to be good stimulants for the development of defense mechanisms. Less work has been reported for invertebrate parasites.

Studies on the conventionalization of germfree animals indicated that most of the differences between germfree and conventional animals could be nullified rapidly. Some time between 1 and 14 days of contamination remarkable changes would occur in germfree animals which had been conventionalized.

References

Abrams, G. D., J. E. Bishop, H. D. Appelman, and A. J. French. 1960. Development of a laboratory for germfree research in the department of pathology. *Univ. Mich. Med. Bull.*, **26:** 165–175.

Ahmadjian, V., and J. T. Reynolds. 1961. Production of biologically active compounds by isolated lichenized Fungi. *Science*, **133:** 700–701.

Akazawa, K. 1942. Growth of germfree reared chicks and intestinal bacterial flora. *J. Chiba. Med. Soc.*, **20:** 1884–1920.

Albanese, A. A., L. E. Holt, Jr., V. I. Davis, S. E. Snyderman, M. Lein, and E. M. Smetak. 1948. Synthetic milk studies in the infant. *J. Nutrition*, **36:** 133–138.

Allen, M. B. 1952. The cultivation of Myxophyceae. *Arch. Mikrobiol.*, **17:** 34–53.

Allison, F. E., S. R. Hoover, and H. J. Morris. 1937. Physiological studies with the nitrogen fixing alga, *Nostoc Muscorum. Botan. Gaz.*, **98:** 433–463.

Andrewes, C. H. 1959. Latent and masked virus infections. *In* "Recent Progress in Microbiology" (G. Tunevall, ed.), pp. 210. Almquist and Wiksell, Stockholm.

Angula, A. W., and Y. Gonzales. 1932. The prenatal growth of the albino rat. *Anat. Record*, **52:** 117–138.

Arnold, J. 1887. Über Theilungsvorgänge an den Wanderzellen, ihre progressiven und regressiven Metamorphosen. *Arch. Mikroskop. Anat.*, **30:** 205–310.

Atwater, W. O. 1885. On the acquisition of atmospheric nitrogen by plants. *J. Am. Chem. Soc.* **6**: 365–388; **8**: 398–420.

Atwater, W. O. 1886. III. On the liberation of nitrogen from its compounds and the acquisition of atmospheric nitrogen by plants. *Am. J. Chem.* **8**: 398–420.

Babes, V. 1882. No bacteria in blood or tissues of healthy men. *Biol. Zentr.,* **II**: 97–101.

Bach, F. W. 1913. Über die "Microfilarienculturen" von Wellman und Johns, nebst Bemerkungen über die Messung der Mikrofilarien. *Centr. Bakteriol. Parasitenk. Abt. I, Orig.,* **70**: 50–60.

Bacot, A. W., and A. Hardin. 1922. Vitamin requirements of *Drosophila*. I. Vitamins B and C. *Biochem. J.,* **16**: 148–152.

Baer, P. N., and W. L. Newton. 1959. The occurrence of periodontal disease in germfree mice. *J. Dental Research,* **38**: 1238.

Baer, P. N., and W. L. Newton, 1960. Studies on periodontal disease in the mouse. The germfree mouse and its conventional control. *Oral Surg. Oral Med. Oral Pathol.,* **13**: 1134–1144.

Baer, W. S. 1931. The treatment of chronic osteomyelitis with the maggot (larva of the blow fly). *J. Bone and Joint Surg.,* **13**: 438–475.

Baker, J. A., and M. S. Ferguson. 1942. Growth of platyfish (Platypoecilus maculatus) free from bacteria and other microorganisms. *Proc. Soc. Exptl. Biol. Med.,* **51**: 116–119.

Balzam, N. 1937a. Destin de la flore bactérienne pendant la métamorphose de la mouche à viande (*Calliphora erythrocephala*). (Bacterial change in development of the meat fly.) *Ann. inst. Pasteur,* **58**: 181–211.

Balzam, N. 1937b. Aseptische Zucht von Tieren. I. Apparatus and Methods. II. Aseptische Zucht von Hakenworm mit vitaminhaltigem und vitaminfreiem Futter, *Acta Biol. Exptl. (Warsaw)* **11**: 43–56; *Ber. Biol.,* **48**: 545.

Barnes, R. H., and G. Fiala. 1959. Effects of the prevention of coprophagy in the rat. VI. Vitamin K. *J. Nutrition,* **68**: 603–614.

Barrett, J. P. 1959. Sterilizing agents for Lobund flexible film apparatus. *Proc. Animal Care Panel,* **9**: 127–133.

Baumberger, J. P. 1919. A nutritional study of insects, with special reference to microorganisms and their substrates. *J. Exptl. Zool.,* **28**: 1–81.

Bausor, S. C., T. G. Yerasimides, and J. J. Landy. 1960. Germ-free plants used as a supplement in the nutrition of the germfree guinea pig. *Abstr. 5th Intern. Congr. Nutrition, Washington, D.C., 1960,* p. 26.

Beaver, D. L. 1960. The hormonal induction of a vaginal leukocytic exudate in the germ-free mouse. *Am. J. Pathol.,* **37**: 769–773.

Beaver, D. L. 1961. Vitamin A deficiency in the germ-free rat. *Am. J. Pathol.,* **38**: 335–357.

Beaver, D. L., and L. L. Ashburn. 1960. Lipid deposits in the lungs of germfree rats—a preliminary report. *Abstr. 5th Intern. Congr. Nutrition, Washington, D.C., 1960,* p. 14.

Beck, S. D. 1950. Nutrition of the European corn borer, Pyrausta nubilalis (Hbn.) II. Some effects of diet on larval growth characteristics. *Physiol. Zoöl.,* **23**: 353–361.

Beck, S. D., and J. F. Stauffer. 1950. An aseptic method for rearing European corn borer larvae. *J. Econ. Entomol.,* **43**: 4–6.

Belser, W. L. 1959. Where is science taking us? *Saturday Rev.*, Dec. 12, p. 58.

Berthelot, M. 1876. Sur l'absorption de l'azote libré par les principes immediats des végétaux, sous l'influence de l'électricité atmosphérique. *Compt. rend. acad. sci.*, 83: 677–682.

Berthelot, M. 1877. Fixation de l'azote sur les matières organiques et formation de l'ozone sous l'influence des faibles tensions électriques. *Compt. rend. acad. sci.*, 85: 173–178.

Berthelot, M. 1885. Fixation directe de l'azote atmosphérique libre par certains terrains argileux. *Compt. rend. acad. sci.*, 101: 775–784.

Berthelot, M. 1887. Sur la fixation direct de l'azote gazeux de l'atmosphère par les terres végétales. *Compt. rend. acad. sci.*, 104: 205–209.

Berthelot, M. 1888. Sur quelques conditions générales de la fixation de l'azote par la terre végétale. *Compt. rend. acad. sci.*, 106: 569–574.

Beyerinck, M. W. 1890. Culturversuche mit Zoochlorellen, Lichengonidien und anderen niederen Algen. *Botan. Tidsskr.*, 48: 725–785.

Bisset, K. A. 1947. The effect of temperature on immunity of amphibia. Use streptomycin to produce sterile amphibia embryo. *J. Pathol. Bacteriol.*, 59: 301–306.

Blayney, J. R. 1952. Germ-free life and dental research. *In* "Science and Society." Symposium, 1950 (R. F. Ervin, ed.). Univ. Notre Dame Press, Notre Dame, Indiana.

Bloch, H. 1960. How specific is immunity. *Experientia*, 16: 255–258.

Bogdanow, E. A. 1906. Über das Zuchten der Larven der gewöhnlichen Fleischfliege (*Calliphora vomitoria*) in sterilisierten Nährmitteln. (Germfree larva reared to pupa stage.) *Arch. ges. Physiol. Pflügers*, 113: 97–105.

Bogdanow, E. A. 1908. Über die Abhängigkeit des Wachstums der Fliegenlarven von Bakterien und Fermenten und über Variabilität bei den Fleischfliegen. Germfree rearing of fly-larvae. *Arch. ges. Physiol. Pflüger's* (*Englemann*), Suppl. 173–199.

Bold, H. C. 1942. The cultivation of algae. *Botan. Rev.*, 8: 69–138.

Bonner, J. T. 1959. The cellular slime molds. 150 pp. Princeton Univ. Press, Princeton, New Jersey.

Borgstrom, B., A. Dahlquist, B. E. Gustafsson, G. Lundh, and J. Malmquist. 1959. Trypsin, invertase and amylase content of feces of germfree rats. *Proc. Soc. Exptl. Biol. Med.*, 102: 154–155.

Boussingault, J. B. 1838a. Recherches chimiques sur la végétation, entreprises dans le but d'examiner si les plantes prennent de l'azote à l'atmosphère. *Ann. chim. et phys.* (2), 67: 5–54.

Boussingault, J. B. 1838b. Recherches chimiques sur la végétation, entreprises dans le but d'examiner si les plantes prennent de l'azote à l'atmosphère. *Compt. rend. acad. sci.*, 7: 889–891; 1149–1155.

Boussingault, J. B. 1855. Recherches sur la végétation, entreprises dans le but d'examiner si les plantes fixent dans leur organisme l'azote qui est à l'état gazeux dans l'atmosphère. *Ann. chim. et phys.* (3), 43: 149–228.

Bowman, R. O., and F. W. Thomae. 1961. Long-term non toxic support of animal life with algae. *Science*, 134: 55–56.

Brambel, C. E. 1960. Vitamin K deficiency in germfree rats. *Abstr. 5th Intern. Congr. Nutrition, Washington, D.C., 1960* p. 25.

Briggs, G. M., T. D. Luckey, C. A. Elvehjem, and E. B. Hart. 1944. Effect of ascorbic acid on chick growth when added to highly purified rations. *Proc. Soc. Exptl. Biol. Med.*, **55**: 130–134.

Briggs, G. M., T. D. Luckey, C. A. Elvehjem, and E. B. Hart. 1944b. Further studies on vitamin B_{10} and B_{11} and their relation to "folic acid" activity. *J. Biol. Chem.*, **153**: 423–434.

Briggs, G. M., T. D. Luckey, C. A. Elvehjem, and E. B. Hart. 1944c. Studies on methods of increasing folic acid activity in liver preparations and in yeast. *J. Biol. Chem.*, **155**: 687.

Briggs, G. M., T. D. Luckey, C. A. Elvehjem, and E. B. Hart. 1945. Studies on vitamin B_{10} and B_{11} and related substances in chick nutrition. *J. Biol. Chem.*, **158**: 303.

Brody, S. 1945. "Bioenergetics and Growth," 1019 pp. Reinhold, New York.

Brody, S., and R. Nisbet. 1938. Growth and development XLVII. A comparison of the amounts and energetic efficiencies of milk production in rat and dairy cow. *Mo. Agr. Expt. Sta. Research Bull.*, **285**: 5–30.

Brookes, V. J. 1956. The nutrition of the larvae of the house fly, *Musca domestica* L. (Muscidae, Diptera). Ph.D. Thesis, University of Illinois, Urbana, Illinois.

Brooks, M. A., and A. G. Richards. 1955. Intracellular symbiosis in cockroaches: II. Mitotic division of mycetocytes. *Science*, **122**: 242.

Brust, M., and G. Fraenkel. 1958. The nutritional requirements of the larvae of a blowfly, *Phormia regina* (Meig.) *Physiol. Zoöl.*, **28**: 186–204.

Buchanan, C. M. 1895. "Antisepsis and Antiseptics," 352 pp. The Terhune Co., Newark, New Jersey.

Buchman, J., and J. E. Blair. 1932. Maggots and their use in the treatment of chronic osteomyelitis. *Sur. Gynecol. Obstet.*, **55**: 177–190.

Buchner, P. 1930. "Tier und Pflanze in Symbiose," p. 336. Bornträger, Berlin.

Buchner, P. 1955. Endosymbio sestudien an schildläusen. II. *Stictococcus diversiseta*. *Z. Morphol. Ökol. Tiere*, **43**: 397–424.

Buddington, A. R. 1941. The nutrition of mosquito larvae. *J. Econ. Entomol.*, **34**: 275–281.

Bulloch, W. 1938. "The History of Bacteriology," p. 422. Oxford Univ. Press, London and New York.

Bunt, J. S. 1955. A note on the faecal flora of some Antarctic birds and mammals at Macquarie Island. *Proc. Linnean Soc., N.S. Wales*, **80**: 44–46.

Burlew, J. S. 1953. Algal culture: From laboratory to pilot plant. *Carnegie Inst. Wash. Publ. No.* **600**.

Burmester, B. R. 1957. Routes of natural infection in avian lymphomatosis. *Ann. N. Y. Acad. Sci.*, **68**: 487–495.

Burrows, M. T. 1910. The cultivation of tissues of the chick embryo outside the body. *J. Am. Med. Assoc.*, **55**: 2057–2058.

Calaby, J. H. 1958. Studies on marsupial nutrition. II. The rate of passage of food residues and digestibility of crude fiber and protein by the quokha, *Setonix brachyurus* (Quoy and Gaimard). *Australian J. Biol. Sci.*, **11**: 572–580.

Calvin, M. 1961. The chemistry of life. *Chem. Eng. News*, **39**: 96–104.

Caplin, S. M. 1947. Growth and morphology of tobacco tissue cultures *in vitro*. *Botan. Gaz.*, **108**: 379–393.

Carlson, G. 1961. The grasshopper neuroblast culture technique and its value in radiobiological studies. *Ann. N. Y. Acad. Sci.*, **95**: 932–941.

Carrel, A. 1911. Rejuvenation of cultures of tissues. *J. Am. Med. Assoc.*, **57**: 1611.

Carrel, A. 1912. Pure cultures of cells. *J. Exptl. Med.* **16**: 165–168.

Carrel, A. 1924. Tissue culture and cell physiology. *Physiol Revs.*, **4**: 1–20.

Carrel, A., and C. A. Lindbergh. 1938. "The Culture of Organs." Hoeber, New York.

Catron, D. V. 1959. Trends in swine nutrition. *Proc. 14th Distillers Feed Conf. Cincinnati, Ohio, 1958* pp. 70–87.

Chamberland, M. C. 1884. Sur un filtre donnant de l'eau physiologiquement pure. *Compt. rend. acad. sci.*, **99**: 247–248.

Cheever, A. W., and T. H. Weller. 1958. Observations on the growth and nutritional requirements of *Schistosoma mansoni in vitro. Am. J. Hyg.* **68**: 322–339.

Cheldelin, V. H., and E. Hodgson. 1959. Studies of choline and related methyl donors in the nutrition of the blowfly, *Phormia regina. Federation Proc.* **18**: 521.

Cheldelin, V. H., and R. W. Newburgh. 1959. Nutritional studies on the blowfly. *Ann. N. Y. Acad. Sci.* **77**: 373–383.

Chernin, E. 1957. A method of securing bacteriologically sterile snails. (*Australorbis glabratus*). *Proc. Soc. Exptl. Biol. Med.*, **96**: 204–210.

Chernin, E. 1959. Cultivation of the snail, *Australorbis glabratus*, under axenic conditions. *Ann. N. Y. Acad. Sci.* **77**: 237–245.

Chernin, E. 1960. Infection of *Australorbis glabratus* with *Schistosoma Mansoni* under bacteriologically sterile conditions. *Proc. Soc. Exptl. Biol. Med.*, **105**: 292–296.

Cherrington, E. H. 1926. "Standard Encyclopedia of the Alcohol Problems," 6 vols. American Issue Publ. Co., Westerville, Ohio.

Chienne, J., and J. C. Ewart. 1878. Do bacteria or their germs exist in the organs of healthy living animals? *J. Anat. Physiol.*, **12**: 448.

Chick, H. 1903. A study of a unicellular alga occurring in polluted water with special reference to its nitrogenous metabolism. *Proc. Roy. Soc.*, **71**: 458–476.

Claff, C. L. 1940. A migration-dilution apparatus for the sterilization of protozoa. *Physiol. Zoöl.* **13**: 334–341.

Coates, M. E., C. D. Dickinson, G. F. Harrison, S. K. Kon, J. W. G. Porter, S. H. Cummins, and W. F. J. Cuthbertson. 1952. A mode of action of antibiotics in chick nutrition. *J. Sci. Food Agr.*, **1**: 43–49.

Cohendy, M. 1912a. Expériences sur la vie sans microbes. *Ann. inst. Pasteur*, **26**: 106–137.

Cohendy, M. 1912b. Presentée par M. E. Roux. Bacteriologie. Expériences sur la vie sans microbes. *Compt. rend. acad. sci.*, **154**: 533–536.

Cohendy, M., and E. Wollman. 1914. Présentée par M. Roux. Bacteriologie. Expériences sur la vie sans microbes. Elevage aseptique de cobayes. *Compt. rend. acad. sci.*, **158**: 1283–1284.

Cohendy, M., and E. Wollman. 1922. Quelques resultats acquis par la méthode des élevages aseptiques: I. Scorbut expérimental; II. Infection cholérique du cobaye aseptique. *Compt. rend. acad. sci.*, **174**: 1082–1084.

Conner, R. L., W. J. Van Wagtendonk, and C. A. Miller. 1953. The isolation from lemon juice of a growth factor of steroid nature required for the growth of a strain of *Paramecium aurelia. J. Gen. Microbiol.*, 9: 434–439.

Conrad, H. E., W. R. Watts, J. M. Iacono, H. F. Kraybill, and T. E. Friedemann. 1958. Digestibility of uniformly labeled carbon-14 soybean cellulose in the rat. *Science*, 127: 1293.

Constantin, V., J. Fosset and C. Meynadier. 1961. Culture de tissue à partir d'insectes élevés aseptiquement. *Compt. rend. acad. sci.*, 252: 2759–2761.

Cools, A., and C. Jeuniaux. 1961. Fermentation de la cellulose et absorption d'acides gras volatils au niveau du caecum du lapin. *Arch. intern. physiol. et biochem.*, 69: 1–8.

Cooper, P. D., J. N. Wilson, and A. M. Burt. 1959. The bulk growth of animal cells in continuous suspension culture. *J. Gen. Microbiol.*, 21: 702–720.

Cordaro, J. T. 1937. "Studies of the infection technique. I. Critical investigation of certain phases of the Reyniers technique for raising biological specimens germfree," 82 pp., M. S. Thesis. Univ. of Notre Dame, Notre Dame, Indiana.

Corliss, J. O. 1954. The literature on *Tetrahymena;* its history, growth and recent trends. *J. Protozool.*, 1: 156.

Corliss, J. O. 1957. Concerning the "Cellularity" or acellularity of the protozoa. *Science*, 125: 988.

Coutelen, F. R. 1927. Essai de culture *in vitro* des scolex et d'hydatides echinococciques (*Echinococcus granulasis*). *Ann. parasitol. humaine et comparee*, 5: 1–19.

Coutelen, F. R. 1928. Contribution aux essais de culture *in vitro* d'embryons de filaires. *Bull. Soc. pathol. exotique*, 21: 316–322.

Coutelen, F. R. 1929a. Essai de culture *in vitro* du Cenure serial, vesiculation des scolex. *Compt. rend. soc. biol.* 100: 619–621.

Coutelen, F. R. 1929b. Essai de culture *in vitro* de microfilaires de Bancroft. *Ann. parasitol. humaine et comparée*, 7: 399–409.

Couvreur, M. E. 1906. Sur la destinée des microbes normaux du tube digestif chez les insectes à métamorphose (Ex. B. mori). *Compt. rend. soc. biol.*, 61: 422–423.

Cox, W. M., Jr., and A. J. Mueller. 1937. The composition of milk from stock rats and an apparatus for milking small laboratory animals. *J. Nutrition*, 13: 249–261.

Coze, L., and V. Feltz. 1866. *Gaz. méd Strasbourg*, 26: 61–115.

Currier, A., W. D. Kitts, and I. M. Cowan. 1960. Cellulose digestion in the beaver (*Castor canadensis*). *Can. J. Zool.*, 38: 1109–1116.

Cuthbertson, D. P., and A. T. Phillipson. 1953. Microbiology of digestion. *In* "Biochemistry and Physiology of Nutrition" (G. H. Bourne and G. W. Kidder, eds.), Vol. II, pp. 130–131. Academic Press, New York.

Daft, F. S. 1959. Introduction and discussion leader. Symposium V: Germfree Animals. *In* "Recent Progress in Microbiology" (G. Tunevall, ed.), pp. 260 and 366–368. Almquist & Wiksell, Stockholm.

Daft, F. S. 1960. Role of bacteria in prevention of pantothenic acid deficiency in rats fed penicillin or ascorbic acid. *Abstr. 5th Intern. Congr. Nutrition, Washington, D.C., 1960* p. 13.

Dammin, G. J. 1959. Panel discussion. *Ann. N. Y. Acad. Sci.*, 78: 381.

Daniel, L. J., M. Gardiner, and L. J. Ottey. 1953. Effect of vitamin B_{12} in the diet of the rat and on the vitamin B_{12} contents of milk and livers of young. *J. Nutrition,* **50:** 275–289.

Danielsson, H., and B. Gustafsson. 1959. On serum-cholesterol levels and neutral fecal sterol in germfree rats. *Arch. Biochem. Biophys.,* **83:** 482–485.

Devaine, C. 1870. Études sur la contagion du chardon chez les animaux domestiques. *Bull. acad. méd. (Paris),* **35:** 215–235.

Davis, H. L. 1951. A study of the mechanisms and evaluation of antiseptic action. *J. Soc. Cosmetic Chemists,* **2:** 296–303.

Davy, H. 1813. "Elements of Agricultural Chemistry," p. 323. Longmans, London.

Delcourt, A., and E. Guyenot. 1911. Génétique et milieu. Nécessité de la détermination des conditions. Sa possibilité chez les Drosophiles. Technique. *Bull. sci. France et Belg.,* **45:** 249–337.

DeMent, J. 1960. Sterilization of interplanetary vehicles. *Science,* **132:** 1569.

de Somer, P., and H. Eyssen. 1961. Personal communication.

Deve, F. 1928. Scoliculture hydatique en sac de collodion et *in vitro. Compt. rend. soc. biol.,* **98:** 1176–1177.

Dewey, V. C., and G. W. Kidder. 1960. Antimetabolites of acetate in *Tetrahymena. Arch. Biochem. Biophys.,* **88:** 78–82.

Diamond, L. S. 1960. The axenic cultivation of two reptilian parasites, *Entamoeba terrapinae,* Sanders and Cleveland, 1930, and *Entamoeba invadens,* Rodhain, 1934. *J. Parasitol.,* **46:** 484.

Dmochowski, L. 1961. Viruses and Tumors. *Science* **133:** 551–561.

Dolley, C. S. 1891. "The Technology of Bacteria Investigation," p. 263. Bradlee Whidden, Boston.

Dougherty, E. C. 1949. Pure-culturing of a free-living rhabditid nematode. *Comp. rend. 13e congr. intern. zool., Paris, 1948,* pp. 447–448.

Dougherty, E. C. 1950a. Sterile pieces of chick embryo as a medium for the indefinite axenic cultivation of *Rhabditis briggsae,* Dougherty and Nigon, 1949 (Nematoda: Rhabditidae). *Science,* **111:** 258.

Dougherty, E. C. 1950b. Some sources and characteristics of the heat-labile nutritional requirement(s) of the nematode, *Rhabditis briggsae. Anat. Record* **108**(3): 514.

Dougherty, E. C. 1951a. Factor Rb activity in human plasma. *Nature,* **168:** 880.

Dougherty, E. C. 1951b. The axenic cultivation of *Rhabditis briggsae,* Dougherty and Nigon, 1949 (Nematoda: Rhabditidae). II. Some sources and characteristics of "factor Rb." *Exptl. Parasitol.,* **1**(1): 34–45.

Dougherty, E. C. 1953a. Axenizing and monoxenizing soil nematodes. *J. Parasitol.,* **39** (4, Sect. 2): 33.

Dougherty, E. C. 1953b. Problems of nomenclature for the growth of organisms of one species with and without associated organisms of other species. *Parasitology* **42:** 259–261.

Dougherty, E. C. 1953c. Some observations on the axenic cultivation and attempted cultivation of certain rhabditid nematodes. *J. Parasitol.,* **39:** 32–33.

Dougherty, E. C. 1953d. Some observations on the monoxenic cultivation of certain rhabditid nematodes. *J. Parasitol.,* **39** (4, Sect. 2): 32.

Dougherty, E. C. 1954. Some effects of urea on the liver protein used in the nutrition of *Caenorhabditis briggsae* (Nematoda: Rhabditidae). *Anat. Record,* **120**(3): 804–805.

Dougherty, E. C. 1959. Introduction to *Axenic Culture of Invertebrate Metazoa:* a Goal. *Ann. N. Y. Acad. Sci.,* **77**(2): 27–54.

Dougherty, E. C. 1960. Cultivation of aschelminths; especially rhabditid nematodes. *In* "Nematology, Fundamental and Recent Advances with Emphasis on Plant Parasitic and Soil Forms" (J. N. Sasser and W. R. Jenkins, eds.), 336 pp. Univ. North Carolina Press, Chapel Hill, North Carolina.

Dougherty, E. C., and H. G. Calhoun. 1948a. Experiences in culturing *Rhabditis pellio,* Schneider, 1866, Butschli, 1873 (Nematoda: Rhabditidae), and related soil nematodes. *Proc. Helminthol. Soc., Washington, D.C.,* **15**(2): 55–68.

Dougherty, E. C., and H. G. Calhoun. 1948b. Techniques for temporarily freeing soil nematodes from bacteria by the use of antibiotics and merthiolate. *Anat. Record,* **100**(3): 395.

Dougherty, E. C., and E. L. Hansen. 1956a. A synthetic basal complement to liver medium for axenic cultivation of the nematode *Caenorhabditis briggsae.* *J. Parasitol.,* **42** (4, Sect. 2): 17.

Dougherty, E. C., and E. L. Hansen. 1956b. Axenic cultivation of *Caenorhabditis briggsae* (Nematoda: Rhabditidae). V. Maturation on synthetic media. *Proc. Soc. Exptl. Biol. Med.,* **93**(2): 223–227.

Dougherty, E. C., and E. L. Hansen. 1956c. Further studies on the axenic cultivation of the nematode *Caenorhabditis briggsae* (Rhabditidae): *Anat. Record,* **125**(3): 638–639.

Dougherty, E. C., and E. L. Hansen. 1957a. The folic acid requirement and its antagonism by aminopterin in the nematode *Caenorhabditis briggsae* (Rhabditidae). *Anat. Record,* **128**: 541–542.

Dougherty, E. C., and E. L. Hansen. 1957b. Unidentified factors required by *Caenorhabditis briggsae* (Nematoda). I. Factors Rb and Cb. *J. Parasitol.,* **43** (5, Sect. 2): 46–47.

Dougherty, E. C., and E. L. Hansen. 1957c. Unidentified factors required by *Caenorhabditis briggsae.* II. An assay system for Factor Cb. *J. Parasitol.,* **43** (5, Sect. 2): 47.

Dougherty, E. C., and E. L. Hansen. 1959. Test procedures used in nutritional studies of *Caenorhabditis briggsae.* Appendix to Nicholas, W. L. The cultural and nutritional requirements of free-living nematodes of the genus *Rhabditis* and related genora. *Tech. Bull. Ministry Agr. (London)* **7**: 169–170.

Dougherty, E. C., and D. F. Keith. 1951. The axenic cultivation of *Rhabditis briggsae* on a dialysed liver protein fraction with known supplementation. *Anat. Record* **111**(3): 571.

Dougherty, E. C., and D. F. Keith. 1953. The axenic cultivation of *Rhabditis briggsae* Dougherty and Nigon, 1949 (Nematoda: Rhabditidae). IV. Plasma protein fractions with various supplementation. *J. Parasitol.,* **39** (4, Sect. 1): 381–384.

Dougherty, E. C., and H. K. Mitchell. 1948. A quantitative measure of growth for axenic cultures of the nematode, *Rhabditis pellio. Anat. Record,* **101**(4): 742–743.

Dougherty, E. C., and V. Nigon. 1949. A new species of the free-living nematode genus *Rhabditis* of interest in comparative physiology and genetics. *J. Parasitol.,* **35** (6, Sect. 2): 11.

Dougherty, E. C., and B. Solberg. 1959a. Laboratory culture of rotifers and gastrotrichs. I. Xenic cultures. *Anat. Record,* 134(3): 555.

Dougherty, E. C., and B. Solberg. 1959b. Laboratory culture of rotifers and gastrotrichs. II. Dixenic, monoxenic and attempted axenic cultures. *Anat. Record,* 134(3): 555–556.

Dougherty, E. C., and B. Solberg. 1959c. Male-producing (normal) lines and a maleless (aberrant) line in the rotifer *Brachionus variabilis. Genetics,* 44 (4, Pt. 1): 536–537.

Dougherty, E. C., and B. Solberg. 1960. Monoxenic cultivation of an enchytraeid annelid. *Nature,* 186: 1067–1068.

Dougherty, E. C., and B. Solberg. 1961. Axenic cultivation of an enchytraeid annelid. *Nature,* 192: 184–185.

Dougherty, E. C., J. C. Raphael, Jr., and C. H. Alton. 1949. Improved axenic cultivation of *Rhabditis briggsae* Dougherty and Nigon, 1949 (Nematoda). *Anat. Record,* 105(3): 532.

Dougherty, E. C., J. C. Raphael, Jr., and C. H. Alton. 1950. The axenic culture of *Rhabditis briggsae* Dougherty and Nigon, 1949 (Nematoda: Rhabditidae). I. Experiments with chick embryo juice and chemically defined media. *Proc. Helminthol. Soc. Washington, D.C.,* 17(1): 1–10.

Dougherty, E. C., E. L. Hansen, W. L. Nicholas, J. A. Mollett, and E. A. Yarwood. 1959. Axenic cultivation of *Caenorhabditis briggsae* (Nematoda: Rhabditidae) with unsupplemented and supplemented chemically defined media. *Ann. N. Y. Acad. Sci.,* 77: 176–217.

Dougherty, E. C., B. G. Chitwood, and A. R. Maggenti. 1960a. Observations on Antarctic fresh water Micrometazoa. *Anat. Record,* 137: 350.

Dougherty, E. C., B. Solberg, and L. G. Harris. 1960b. Synxenic and attempted axenic cultivation of rotifers. *Anat. Record,* 137(3): 350–351.

Dougherty, E. C., B. Solberg, and L. G. Harris. 1960c. Synxenic and attempted axenic cultivation of rotifers. *Science,* 132: 416–417.

Dougherty, E. C., B. Solberg, and D. J. Ferral. 1961. The first axenic cultivation of a Rotifer species. *Experientia,* 17: 131–133.

Dowdeswell, G. F. 1884. On some appearances in the blood of vertebrated animals, with reference to the occurrence of bacteria therein. *J. Roy. Microscop. Soc.,* pp. 525–529.

Dubos, R. J. 1960. Germfree nurture of test animals induces health but susceptibility. *Scope,* 5: 9.

Duclaux, E. 1885. Presentée par M. Pasteur, Physiologie végétale. Sur la germination dans un sol riche en matières organiques, mais exempt de microbes. *Compt. rend. acad. sci.,* 100: 66–68.

du Vigneaud, V., C. Ressler, and J. R. Rachele. 1950. The biological synthesis of labile methyl groups. *Science,* 112: 267–271.

du Vigneaud, V., C. Ressler, J. R. Rachele, J. A. Reyniers, and T. D. Luckey. 1951. The synthesis of "biologically labile" methyl groups in the germfree rat. *J. Nutrition,* 45: 361–376.

Eagle, H. 1955. Nutritional needs of mammalian cells in tissue culture. *Science,* 122: 501–504.

Eagle, H., V. I. Oyama, M. Levy, C. L. Horton, and R. Fleischman. 1956. The growth response of mammalian cells in tissue culture to L-glutamine and L-glutamic acid. *J. Biol. Chem.,* 218: 607–616.

Earl, P. R. 1959. Filariae from the dog *in vitro*. *Ann. N. Y. Acad. Sci.*, **77**: 163–175.

Egorova, A. A. 1940. Microflora of intestine of arctic animals. *Mikrobiologiya*, **1**: 59–64. (*Arctic Biblio.* **8**: 50709.)

Ehret, C. F. 1960. Organelle systems and biological organization. *Science*, **132**: 115–123.

Ekelof, E. 1908. Bakteriologische Studien wahrend der schwedischen Südpolar Expedition 1901–1903. *Botanik* (*Stockholm*) 1.

Ells, H., and C. P. Read. 1952. The cultivation of *Turbatrix aceti* (Rhabditoidea: Nematoda) in the absence of microorganisms. *J. Parasitol.*, **38**: 21.

Ervin, R. F. 1938. "Studies of the infection technique. II. A critical study of the bacteriological methods used in the Reyniers germfree technique," M. S. Thesis. Univ. Notre Dame, Notre Dame, Indiana.

Ervin, R. F. 1946. Lobund, Notre Dame's contribution to bacteriology. *Notre Dame Scholastic*, **88**: pp. 32–48.

Ervin, R. F. 1949. Germ-free life. *Notre Dame* (magazine of the University of Notre Dame) UND2(3).

Ervin, R. F., P. C. Trexler, and J. A. Reyniers. 1944. History of bacteriology at the University of Notre Dame. *Proc. Indiana Acad. Sci.* **53**: 62–65.

Ferguson, M. S. 1940. Encystment and sterilization of metacercariae of the avian strigeid trematode, *Posthodiplostomum minimum,* and their development into adult worms in sterile culture. *J. Parasitol.*, **26**: 359–372.

Ferguson, M. S. 1943. *In vitro* cultivation of trematode metacercariae free from microorganisms. *J. Parasitol.*, **29**: 319–323.

Fisher, R. A., and F. Yates. 1943. "Statistical Tables for Biological Agricultural and Medical Research," p. 98. Oliver & Boyd, Edinburgh and London.

Fitzgerald, R. J., and K. Habel. 1959. Discussion to Symposium V. Germfree Animals. *In* "Recent Progress in Microbiology" (G. Tunevall, ed.), pp. 352–353. Almquist and Wiksell, Stockholm.

Fitzgerald, R. J., and P. H. Keyes. 1960. Demonstration of the etiologic role of streptococci in experimental caries in the hamster. *J. Am. Dental Assoc.*, **61**: 9–19.

Fitzgerald, R. J., and E. G. McDaniel. 1960. Dental calculus in the germ-free rat. *Arch. Oral Biol.*, **2**: 239–240.

Fitzgerald, R. J., E. G. Hampp, and W. L. Newton. 1958. Infectivity of oral spirochetes in cortisone-treated and germ-free guinea pigs. *J. Dental Research*, **37**: 11.

Fitzgerald, R. J., H. V. Jordan, D. B. Scott, and H. G. McCann. 1960. Dental calculus and antibiotics in the white rat. *Arch. Oral. Biol.* **2**: 85–86.

Fitzgerald, R. J., E. G. Hampp, and H. R. Stanley. 1960a. Studies on the survival of parenterally inoculated oral treponemes in the guinea pig. *Oral Surg., Oral Med. Oral Pathol.*, **13**: 883–890.

Fitzgerald, R. J., H. V. Jordan, and H. R. Stanley. 1960b. Experimental caries and gingival pathologic changes in the gnotobiotic rat. *J. Dental Research*, **39**: 923–935.

Fleming, A. 1929. On the antibacterial action of cultures of a *Penicillium,* with special reference to their use in the isolation of *B. influenzae*. *Brit. J. Exptl. Pathol.*, **10**: 226–236.

Flood, R. E., and T. J. Kelly. 1937. "Artificial feeding of the new-born guinea pig and rabbit," B.S. Thesis (under Fr. Wenninger). Univ. of Notre Dame, Notre Dame, Indiana.

Forbes, M., and J. T. Park. 1959. Growth of germ-free and conventional chicks: effect of diet, dietary penicillin and bacterial environment. *J. Nutrition,* **67:** 69–84.

Forbes, M., R. M. Guttmacher, R. R. Kolman, and D. Kritchevsky. 1958a. Serum cholesterol levels in germfree chickens. *Experientia,* **15:** 441–444.

Forbes, M., F. Zilliken, G. Roberts, and P. Gyorgy. 1958b. A new antioxidant from yeast. Isolation and chemical studies. *J. Am. Chem. Soc.,* **80:** 385–389.

Forbes, M., W. C. Supplee, and G. F. Combs. 1958c. Response of germfree and conventionally reared turkey poults to dietary supplementation with penicillin and oleandomycin. *Proc. Soc. Extl. Biol. Med.* **99:** 110–113.

Forbes, M., J. T. Park, and M. Lev. 1959. Role of the intestinal flora in the growth response of chicks to dietary penicillin. *Ann. N. Y. Acad. Sci.,* **78:** 321–327.

Ford, W. W. 1939. "Bacteriology," 207 pp. Hoeber, New York.

Formal, S. B., G. Dammin, H. Sprinz, D. Kundel, H. Schneider, R. E. Horowitz, and M. Forbes. 1961. Experimental *Shigella* infections. V. Studies with germfree guinea pigs. *J. Bacteriol.,* **82:** 284–287.

Forsythe, R. H., J. C. Ayres, and J. L. Radlo. 1953. Factors affecting the microbiological populations of shell eggs. *Food Technol.,* **7:** 49–56.

Foster, H. L. 1959. A procedure for obtaining nucleus stock for a pathogen-free animal colony. *Proc. Animal Care Panel,* **9:** 135–142.

Foster, H. L. 1960. Commercial production of disease-free animals. *Proc. 2nd Symposium on Gnotobiotic Technol., 1959,* pp. 145–155. Univ. Notre Dame Press, Notre Dame, Indiana.

Foyn, B. 1934. Lebenszyklus, Cytologie und Sexualität der Chlorophycee *Clapophora suhriand Kutzing. Arch. Protistenk.,* **83:** 1–56.

Fracastorius, G. H. 1546. "De sympathia et antipathia verum," Liber I; "De contagione et contagiosis et curatione," Liber III venetics.

Fraenkel, G. 1952. The role of symbionts as sources of vitamins and other growth factors for their insect hosts. *Tijdschr. Entomol. (Amsterdam),* **95:** 183–195.

Fraenkel, G. 1954. The distribution of vitamin B_t (carnitine) throughout the animal kingdom. *Arch. Biochem. Biophys.,* **50:** 486–495.

Fraenkel, G. 1959. A historical and comparative survey of the dietary requirements of insects. *Ann. N. Y. Acad. Sci.,* **77:** 267–274.

Fred, E. B., I. L. Baldwin, and E. McCoy. 1932. "Root Nodule Bacteria and Leguminous Plants," 145 pp. Univ. Wisconsin Press, Madison, Wisconsin.

Friedmann, E. W., and J. Kern. 1956. The problem of cerophagy or wax-eating in the honey guides. *Quart. Rev. Biol.,* **31:** 19–30.

Friedman, E. W., F. B. Schweinburg, J. Yushar, and J. Fine. 1957. Bacterial factor in traumatic shock in the rat. *Am. J. Physiol.,* **189:** 197–202.

Friend, W. G., and R. L. Patton. 1956. Studies on vitamin requirements of larvae of the onion maggot, *Hylemya antiqua* (Meig.) under aseptic conditions. *Can. J. Zool.,* **34:** 152–154.

Friend, W. G., E. H. Salkeld, and I. L. Stevenson. 1959. Nutrition of onion maggots, larvae of *Hylemya antiqua* (Meig.) with reference to other members of the genus *Hylemya. Ann. N. Y. Acad. Sci.,* **77:** 384–393.

Frost, F. M., W. B. Herms, and W. M. Hoskins. 1936. The nutritional requirement of the larvae of the mosquito. *Theobaldia incidens* (Thom.) *J. Exptl. Zool.*, **73**: 461–479.

Fukushima, S. 1957. A study on physioloical significance of *L. acidophilus* in intestine. *J. Chiba Med. Soc.*, **33**: 495–511.

Gard, S. 1959. Discussion of Symposium V: Germfree Animals. *In* "Recent Progress in Microbiology" (G. Tunevall, ed.), p. 351. Almquist & Wiksell, Stockholm.

Garrison, W. M., D. C. Morrison, J. G. Hamilton, A. A. Benson, and M. Calvin. 1951. Reduction of carbon dioxide in aqueous solutions by ionizing radiation. *Science*, **114**: 416–418.

Gaumann, E., and H. Kern. 1959. "Uber chemische Abwehreaktionen bei Orchideen. *Phytopathol. Z.*, **36**(1): 1–26.

Gaumann, E., J. Nuesch, and R. H. Rimpau. 1960. Weitere Untersuchungen über die chemischen Abwehrreaktionen der Orchideen. *Phytopathol. Z.*, **38**: 274–308.

Gautheret, R. J. 1939. Physiologie végétale. Sur la possibilité de réaliser la culture indéfinie des tissus de tubercules de carotte. *Compt. rend. acad. sci.*, **208**: 118–120.

Gautheret, R. J. 1959. "La culture des tissues végétaux," 863 pp. Masson, Paris.

Gerloff, G. C., G. P. Fitzgerald, and F. Skoog. 1950. The isolation, purification, and culture of blue-green algae. *Am. J. Botany*, **37**: 216–218.

Glaser, R. W. 1918. A new bacterial disease of gipsy-moth caterpillars. *J. Agr. Research*, **13**: 515–522.

Glaser, R. W. 1920. Biological studies on intracellular bacteria. *Biol. Bull.*, **39**: 133–145.

Glaser, R. W. 1921. *Herpetomonas muscae-domesticae,* its behavior and effect in laboratory animals. *J. Parasitol.*, **8**: 99–108.

Glaser, R. W. 1924a. A bacterial disease of adult house flies. *Am. J. Hyg.*, **4**: 411–415.

Glaser, R. W. 1924b. A bacterial disease of silkworms. *J. Bacteriol.*, **9**: 339–355.

Glaser, R. W. 1926. The isolation and cultivation of *Herpetomonas muscae-domesticae. Am. J. Trop. Med.*, **6**: 205–219.

Glaser, R. W. 1928. Note on the cultivation of *Metarrhizium anisopliae* (Metsch.) Sorokin from the vegetative form in silkworms. *Ann. Entomol. Soc. Am.*, **21**: 202.

Glaser, R. W. 1930a. The intracellular "symbionts" and the "rickettsiae." *A.M.A. Arch. Pathol.*, **9**: 71–96, 557–576.

Glaser, R. W. 1930b. On the isolation, cultivation and classification of the so-called intracellular "symbiont" or "Rickettsia" of *Periplaneta americana. J. Exptl. Med.* **51**: 59–82.

Glaser, R. W. 1930c. Cultivation and classification of "bacteroides," "symbionts," or "Rickettsiae" of *Blattella germanica. J. Exptl. Med.* **51**: 903–907.

Glaser, R. W. 1931. The "Rickettsiae" and the intracellular "symbionts." *Science*, **74**: 243.

Glaser, R. W. 1938. A method for the sterile culture of houseflies. *J. Parasitol.*, **24**: 177–179.

Glaser, R. W. 1940. The bacteria-free culture of a nematode parasite. *Proc. Soc. Exptl. Biol. Med.,* 43: 512–514.

Glaser, R. W. 1943. The germ-free culture of certain invertebrates. *In* "Micrurgical and Germfree Methods" (J. A. Reyniers, ed.), pp. 164–187. Thomas, Springfield, Illinois.

Glaser, R. W. 1946. The intracellular bacteria of the cockroach in relation to symbiosis. *J. Parasitol.,* 32: 483–489.

Glaser, R. W., and N. A. Coria. 1930. Methods for the pure culture of certain protozoa. *J. Exptl. Med.,* 51: 787–806.

Glaser, R. W., and N. A. Coria. 1933. The culture of *Paramecium caudatum* free from living microorganisms. *J. Parasitol.,* 20: 33–37.

Glaser, R. W., and N. A. Coria. 1935a. The culture and reactions of purified protozoa. *Am. J. Hyg.,* 21: 111–120.

Glaser, R. W., and N. A. Coria. 1935b. The partial purification of *Balantidium coli* from swine. *J. Parasitol.,* 21: 190–193.

Glaser, R. W., and N. A. Coria. 1935c. Purification and culture of *Tritrichomonas foetus* (Riedmuller) from cows. *Am. J. Hyg.,* 22: 221–226.

Glaser, R. W., and N. R. Stoll. 1938a. Development under sterile conditions of the sheep stomach worm *Haemonchus contortus* (Nematoda). *Science,* 87: 259–260.

Glaser, R. W., and N. R. Stoll. 1938b. Sterile culture of the free-living and parasitic larval stages of *Haemonchus contortus. J. Parasitol.,* 24 (Dec. Suppl.): 16.

Glaser, R. W., and N. R. Stoll. 1938c. Sterile culture of the free-living stages of the sheep stomach worm, *Haemonchus contortus. Parasitology,* 30: 324–332.

Glaser, R. W., and N. R. Stoll. 1940. Exsheathing and sterilizing infective nematode larvae. *J. Parasitol.* 26: 87–94.

Glaser, R. W., E. E. McCoy, and H. B. Girth. 1942. The biology and culture of *Neoaplectana chresima,* a new nematode parasitic in insects. *J. Parasitol.,* 28: 123–126.

Glimstedt, G. 1932. Das Leben ohne Bakterien. Sterile Aufziehung von Meerschweinchen. (Verhandl. anat. Ges. Jena) *Anat. Anz.* 75: 79–89.

Glimstedt, G. 1933. Nagra nya ron baserade pa jamforelser mellan sterilt uppfodda djur och kontrolldjur. *Med. Foren. Tidsckr.,* 11: 271–277.

Glimstedt, G. 1936a. Bakterienfreie Meerschweinchen. *Acta Pathol. Microbiol. Scand., Suppl. No.* 30, 1–295.

Glimstedt, G. 1936b. Der Stoffwechsel bakterienfreier Tiere. I. Allgemeine Methodik. *Skand. Arch. Physiol.,* 73: 48–62.

Glimstedt, G. 1937. Sekund arfellsklarns i den lymfatiska varnaden funktion och denna varnads byggnad hos bakteriefria marsyin. (Function of secondary follicles in lymphatic tissue and structure of this tissue in guinea pigs free of bacteria.) *Nord. Med. Tidskr.* (*Stockholm*), 14: 1269–1272.

Glimstedt, G. 1959. The germfree animal as a research tool. *Ann. N. Y. Acad. Sci.,* 78: 281–284.

Glimstedt, G., H. A. Moberg, and E. M. P. Widmark. 1937. Der Stoffwechsel bakterienfreier Tiere. III. Die Gewinnung von Meerschweinchenmilch. *Skand. Arch. Physiol.,* 76: 148–157.

Goldberg, H. S. 1959. Antibiotics in the isolation and cultivation of microorganisms. *In* "Antibiotics: Their Chemistry and Non-Medical Uses" (H. S. Goldberg, ed.), pp. 528–560. Van Nostrand, Princeton, New Jersey.

Gordon, H. A. 1952. *In* "Studies on the Growth Effect of Antibiotics in Germ-free Animals," a Colloquium. 4: A morphological and biochemical approach. Univ. of Notre Dame, Notre Dame, Indiana.

Gordon, H. A. 1955. Germfree research: a basic study in host-contaminant relationship. III. Morphologic characterization of germfree life. *Bull. N. Y. Acad. Med.*, **31**: 239–242.

Gordon, H. A. 1958. El animal sin germenes: su uso en biologia experimental y en medicina. *Anales inst. farmacol. españ.*, **7**: 107–152.

Gordon, H. A. 1959a. The use of germ-free vertebrates in the study of "physiological" effects of the normal microbial flora. *Gerontologia*, **3**: 104–111.

Gordon, H. A. 1959b. Morphological and physiological characterization of germfree life. *Ann. N. Y. Acad. Sci.*, **78**: 208–220.

Gordon, H. A. 1960a. Historical aspects of germfree experimentation. *Proc. 2nd Symposium of Gnotobiotic Technol.*, *1959*, pp. 9–18. Univ. Notre Dame Press, Notre Dame, Indiana.

Gordon, H. A. 1960b. The germ-free animal: Its use in the study of "physiologic" effects of the normal microbial flora on the animal host. *Am. J. Digest. Diseases*, **5**: 841–867.

Gordon, H. A. 1961. Personal communication.

Gordon, H. A., and E. Bruckner-Kardoss. 1959. The distribution of reticuloendothelial elements in the intestinal mucosa and submucosa of germfree, monocontaminated and conventional chicks orally treated with penicillin. *Antibiotics Ann.*, **1958/59**, 1012–1019.

Gordon, H. A., and E. Bruckner-Kardoss. 1961a. Effects of the normal microbial flora on various tissue elements of the small intestine. *Acta Anat.* **4**: 210–225.

Gordon, H. A., and E. Bruckner-Kardoss. 1961b. Effect of the microbial flora on the intestinal surface area. Personal communication.

Gordon, H. A., and B. S. Wostmann. 1959. Responses of the animal host to changes in the bacterial environment: transition of the albino rat from the germfree to the conventional state. Symposium V. *In* "Recent Progress in Microbiology" (G. Tunevall, ed.), pp. 336–339. Almquist & Wiksell, Stockholm.

Gordon, H. A., and B. S. Wostmann. 1960. Morphological studies on the germfree albino rat. *Anat. Record*, **137**: 65–70.

Gordon, H. A., J. P. Doll, and B. S. Wostmann. 1958a. Effects of the "normal" bacterial flora on various morphological characteristics of the animal host: a comparative study of germfree and normal stock chickens, rats and mice. *Anat. Record*, **130**: 307–308.

Gordon, H. A., M. Wagner, and B. S. Wostmann. 1958b. Studies on conventional and germ-free chickens treated orally with antibiotics. *Antibiotics Ann.*, **1957/58**: 248–255.

Gordon, H. A., M. Wagner, T. D. Luckey, and J. A. Reyniers. 1959. An encephalomeningeal syndrome selectively affecting newly hatched germfree and monocontaminated chickens. *J. Infectious Diseases*, **105**: 31–37.

Gordon, H. A., E. Bruckner-Kardoss, and D. Kan. 1960a. Effects of normal microbiol flora on structural and absorptive characteristics of the intestine. *Abstr. 5th Intern. Cong. Nutrition, Washington, D.C., 1960*, p. 13.

Gordon, H. A., B. S. Wostmann, and M. Wagner. 1960b. Effects of the normal microbial flora on morphological and functional standards of higher vertebrates, Abstr. VII. International Anatomy, p. 199.

Grace, T. D. C. 1959. Prolonged survival and growth of insect ovarian tissue under *in vitro* conditions. *Ann. N. Y. Acad. Sci.*, **77**: 275–282.

Greenspan, F. P., M. A. Johnson, and P. C. Trexler. 1955. Peracetic aerosols. *Chem. Specialties Mfrs. Assoc., Proc. 42nd Ann. Meeting, 1952*, pp. 59–64.

Greenstein, J. P., S. M. Birnbaum, M. Winitz, and M. C. Otey. 1957. Quantitative nutritional studies with water-soluble, chemically defined diets. *Arch. Biochem. Biophys.*, **72**: 396–416.

Gremillion, G. G. 1960. The use of bacteria-tight cabinets in the infectious disease laboratory. *Proc. 2nd Symposium on Gnotobiotic Technol., 1959*, pp. 171–182. Univ. Notre Dame Press, Notre Dame, Indiana.

Gustafsson, B. E. 1946. Nagra erfarenheter fran bakteriefri uppfodning av rattor. (Med. dem. av forsoksanlaggningen.) (Some experiences in germfree rearing of rats.) *Nord. Med.*, **32**: 2665.

Gustafsson, B. E. 1947. Germ-free rearing of rats. Preliminary report. *Acta Anat.*, **2**: 376–391.

Gustafsson, B. E. 1948. Germ-free rearing of rats. General technique. *Acta Pathol. Microbiol. Scand., Suppl. No.* **73**: 1–130.

Gustafsson, B. E. 1957. Bakteriefri uppfodning av forsoksdjur. Nuvarande teknik och fragestallninger. (Germ-free rearing of laboratory animals. Present technique and problems.) *Nord. Med.*, **58**: 1515.

Gustafsson, B. E. 1959a. Germfree research at the Institute of Histology, University of Lund. Symposium V. *In* "Recent Progress in Microbiology (G. Tunevall, ed.), pp. 327–335. Almquist & Wiksell, Stockholm.

Gustafsson, B. E. 1959b. Lightweight stainless steel systems for rearing germfree animals. *Ann. N. Y. Acad. Sci.*, **78**: 17–28.

Gustafsson, B. E. 1959c. Aktuella resultat inom sterildjursforskningen. (Recent progress in germfree research.) *Nord. Med.*, **61**: 734.

Gustafsson, B. E. 1959d. Vitamin K deficiency in germfree rats. *Ann. N. Y. Acad. Sci.*, **78**: 166–173.

Gustafsson, B. E. 1960. Vitamin K deficiency in germfree rats and the curative effects of vitamin K active compounds on bacterial contamination. *Abstr. 5th Intern. Cong. Nutrition, Washington, D.C., 1960*, p. 13.

Gustafsson, B. E., and R. J. Fitzgerald. 1960. Alteration in intestinal microbial flora of rats with tail cups to prevent coprophagy. *Proc. Soc. Exptl. Biol. Med.*, **104**: 319–322.

Gustafsson, B. E., and C. B. Laurell. 1958. Gamma globulins in germfree rats. *J. Exptl. Med.*, **108**: 251–258.

Gustafsson, B. E., and C. B. Laurell. 1959. Gamma globulin production in germfree rats after bacterial contamination. *J. Exptl. Med.*, **110**: 675–684.

Gustafsson, B. E., and C. B. Laurell. 1960. Properdin titers in sera from germfree rats. *Proc. Soc. Exptl. Biol. Med.*, **105**: 598–600.

Gustafsson, B. E., and L. Swenander Lanke. 1960. Bilirubin and urobilins in germfree, ex-germfree and conventional rats. *J. Exptl. Med.*, **112**: 975–979.

Gustafsson, B. E., S. Bergstrom, S. Lindstedt, and A. Norman. 1956. On the metabolism of bile acids in germfree rats. *Acta Chem. Scand.,* **10**: 1052.

Gustafsson, B. E., S. Bergstrom, S. Lindstedt, and A. Norman. 1957a. Turnover and nature of fecal bile acids in germfree and infected rats fed cholic acid-24-^{14}C. Bile acids and steroids. *Proc. Soc. Exptl. Biol. Med.,* **94**: 467–471.

Gustafsson, B. E., G. Kahlson, and E. Rosengren. 1957b. Biogenesis of histamine studied by its distribution and urinary excretion in germ free reared and not germ free rats fed a histamine free diet. *Acta Physiol. Scand.,* **41**: 217–228.

Gustafsson, B. E., A. Norman, and J. Sjovall. 1960. Influence of *E. coli* infection on turnover and metabolism of cholic acid in germfree rats. *Arch. Biochem. Biophys.,* **91**: 93–100.

Guyenot, E. 1913a. Etudes biologiques sur une mouche, *Drosophila ampelophila.* Low. I—Possibilité de vie aseptique pour l'individu et la lignée. *Compt. rend. soc. biol.,* **74**: 97–99.

Guyenot, E. 1913b. Etudes biologique sur une mouche, *Drosophila ampelophila.* Low. II—Role des levures dans l'alimentation. *Compt. rend. soc. biol.,* **74**: 178–180.

Guyenot, E. 1913c. Etudes biologiques sur une mouche, *Drosophila ampelophila.* Low. IV—Nutrition des larves et fécondité. *Compt. rend. soc. biol.,* **74**: 270–272.

Guyenot, E. 1913d. Etudes biologiques sur une mouche, *Drosophila ampelophila.* V—Nutrition des adultes et fécondité. *Compt. rend. soc. biol.,* **74**: 332–334.

Guyenot, E. 1914. Etudes biologiques sur une mouche *Drosophila ampelophila* Low. Nécessité de réaliser un milieu nutritif défini. *Compt. rend. soc. biol.,* **76**: 483–485.

Guyenot, E. 1917. Recherches expérimentales sur la vie aseptique d'un organisme en fonction du milieu. *Bull. biol. France et Belg.,* **51**: 1–330.

György, P. 1959. Observations on germfree animals at the Walter Reed Army Institute of Research, Washington, D.C. Symposium V. *In* "Recent Progress in Microbiology," (G. Tunevall, ed.), pp. 288–298. Almquist & Wiksell, Stockholm.

György, P., and M. Forbes. 1958. Germfree animal studies (Univ. of Pennsylvania). Personal communication.

Haberlandt, G. 1902. Kulturversuche mit isolierten Pflanzenzellen. Sitzungsber. *Akad. Wiss. Wien., Math.-naturw. Kl.,* **III**: 69–92.

Haines, R. B. 1939. "Microbiology in the preservation of the hen's eggs," Food Investigation Special Report No. 47 (Dept. Sci. and Ind. Research), pp. 1–65. H.M.S.O., London.

Hall, A. D. 1905. The Book of the Rothamsted Experiments. John Murray, London.

Hamilton, B., and M. Bewar. 1938. Water and dry substance in the rat. *Growth,* **2**: 16–18.

Hansen, E. L., and E. C. Dougherty. 1957. Folic acid in axenic cultivation of nematode *Caenorhabditis briggsae. Federation Proc.,* **16**(1, Pt. 1): 304–305.

Harrison, R. G. 1907. Observations on the living developing nerve fiber. *Proc. Soc. Exptl. Biol. Med.,* **4**: 140–143.

Hartmann, H. T., and D. E. Kester. 1959. "Plant Propagation Principles and Practices." Prentice-Hall, Englewood Cliffs, New Jersey.

Hartmann, J. F., and L. J. Wells. 1948. Fate of food introduced directly into the fetal stomach. *Proc. Soc. Exptl. Biol. Med.,* **68:** 327–330.

Hasegawa, H. 1959. Physiologic significance of *Cl. welchii.* A study on anaerobic bacteria in the intestines of animals. *J. Chiba Med. Soc.,* **34:** 1470–1481.

Hawk, H. A., and O. Mickelson. 1955. Nutritional changes in diets exposed to ethylene oxide. *Science,* **121:** 442–444.

Hayes, M., and T. D. Luckey. 1957. Effect of incubation upon folic acid content of eggs. *Proc. Soc. Exptl. Biol. Med.,* **94:** 777–778.

Heggeness, F. W. 1959. Effect of antibiotics on the gastrointestinal absorption of calcium and magnesium in the rat. *J. Nutrition,* **68:** 573–582.

Hellriegel, H. 1887. Welche Stickstoffquellen stehen der Pflanze zu gebote. *Landwirtsch. Vers. Sta.,* **33:** 464–465.

Hellriegel, H., and H. Wilforth. 1888. Untersuchungen über die Stickstoffnahrung der Gramineen und Leguminosen. Beilageheft. *Z. Ver. Rübenzucker-Ind. deut. Reich.* (*Beren*), 234 pp.

Hendricks, S. B., and F. W. Went. 1958. Controlled climate facilities for biologists. *Science,* **128:** 510–512.

Heneghan, J. 1961. "Transfer of water and ions across the intestinal wall," M.S. Thesis. Univ. of Notre Dame, Notre Dame, Indiana.

Henthorne, R. D., and W. O. Kester. 1959. Disease-free laboratory animals as related to germfree life. *Ann. N. Y. Acad. Sci.,* **78:** 276–280.

Hesse, E. 1914. Bakteriologische Untersuchungen auf einer Fahrt nach Island, Spitzbergen und Norwegen im Juli 1913. *Centr. Bakteriol., Parasitenk., Abt. I, Orig.,* **72:** 454–477.

Hickey, J. L. S. 1960. A comparison of current types of germfree research apparatus. *Proc. 2nd Symposium on Gnotobiotic Technol.,* pp. 61–82. Univ. Notre Dame Press, Notre Dame, Indiana.

Hickey, J. L. S., and D. L. Snow. 1960. Irradiation sterilization of diets for germfree animals. *Public Works,* July, pp. 108, 109 and 188.

Hilchey, J. D. 1953. Studies on the qualitative requirements of *Blattella germanica* (L.) for amino acids under aseptic conditions. *Contribs. Boyce Thompson Inst.,* **17:** 203.

Hildebrand, E. M., 1938. Techniques for the isolation of single microorganisms. *Botan. Rev.,* **4:** 627–664.

Hildebrandt, A. C., and A. J. Riker. 1949. The influence of various carbon compounds on the growth of marigold, Paris-daisy, periwinkle, sunflower and tobacco tissue *in vitro. Am. J. Botany,* **36:** 74–85.

Hildebrandt, A. C., and A. J. Riker. 1953. Influence of concentrations of sugars and polysaccharides on callus tissue growth *in vitro. Am. J. Botany,* **40:** 66–76.

Hildebrandt, A. C., A. J. Riker, and B. M. Duggar. 1946. The influence of the composition of the medium on growth *in vitro* of excised tobacco and sunflower tissue cultures. *Am. J. Botany,* **33:** 591–597.

Hill, D. L., V. A. Bell, and L. E. Chadwick. 1947. Rearing of the blowfly, *Phormia regina* Meigen, on a sterile diet. *Ann. Entomol. Soc. Am.,* **40:** 213–216.

Hinton, T. 1959. Miscellaneous nutritional variations, environmental and genetic, in *Drosophila. Ann. N. Y. Acad. Sci.,* **77:** 366–372.

Hinton, T., J. Ellis, and D. T. Noyes. 1951. An adenine requirement in a strain of *Drosophila. Proc. Natl. Acad. Sci., U.S.,* **37:** 293–299.

Hmuriek, J. P., and L. T. Gabriel. 1936. "Determination of the efficiency of glass wool filters used in the germfree guinea pigs cage," B.S. Thesis. Univ. of Notre Dame, Notre Dame, Indiana.

Hodgson, B., V. H. Cheldelin, and R. W. Newburgh. 1960. Nutrition and metabolism of methyl donors and related compounds in the blowfly, *Phormia regina* (Meigen). *Arch. Biochem. Biophys.*, **87**: 48–54.

Hopkins, W. E., P. W. Wilson, and E. B. Fred. 1931. A method for the growth of leguminous plants under bacteriologically controlled conditions. *J. Am. Agron. Soc.*, **23**: 32–40.

Horowitz, R. E., S. M. Levenson, O. J. Malm, and V. M. Butler. 1960. The germfree laboratory at the Walter Reed Army Institute of Research. *Proc. 2nd Symposium on Gnotobiotic Technol. 1959*, pp. 29–48. Univ. Notre Dame Press, Notre Dame, Indiana.

Horsfall, F. L., and J. H. Bauer. 1940. Individual isolation of infected animals in a single room. *J. Bacteriol.*, **40**: 569–580.

Horton, R. E., and J. L. S. Hickey. 1961. Irradiated diets for rearing germfree guinea pigs. *Proc. Animal Care Panel*, **11**: 93–106.

House, H. L. 1949a. Nutritional studies with *Blattella germanica* (L.) reared under aseptic conditions. II. A chemically defined diet. *Can. Entomologist*, **81**: 105–112.

House, H. L. 1949b. Nutritional studies with *Blattella germanica* (L.) reared under aseptic conditions. III. Five essential amino acids. *Can. Entomologist*, **81**: 133–139.

House, H. L. 1954a. Nutritional studies with *Pseudosarcophaga affinis* (Fall.), a dipterous parasite of the spruce budworm, *Choristoneura fumiferana* (Clem.). I. A chemically defined medium and aseptic-culture technique. *Can. J. Zool.*, **32**: 331–341.

House, H. L. 1954b. Nutritional studies with *Pseudosarcophaga affinis* (Fall.), a dipterous parasite of the spruce budworm, *Choristoneura fumiferana* (Clem.). II. Effects of eleven vitamins on growth. *Can. J. Zool.*, **32**: 342–350.

House, H. L. 1954c. Nutritional studies with *Pseudosarcophaga affinis* (Fall.), a dipterous parasite of the spruce budworm, *Choristoneura fumiferana* (Clem.). III. Effects of nineteen amino acids on growth. *Can. J. Zool.*, **32**: 351–357.

House, H. L. 1954d. Nutritional studies with *Pseudosarcophaga affinis* (Fall.), a dipterous parasite of the spruce budworm, *Choristoneura fumiferana* (Clem.). IV. Effects of ribonucleic acid, glutathione, dextrose, a salt mixture, cholesterol, and fats. *Can. J. Zool.*, **32**: 358–365.

House, H. L. 1956. Nutritional requirements and artificial diets for insects. *Ann. Rept. Entomol. Soc. Ontario, 1955*, **86**: 5–9 and 21–23.

House, H. L. 1958a. The nutrition of insects with particular reference to entomophagous parasites. *Proc. Intern. Congr. Entomol., 10th Congr., Montreal, 1956*, **2**: 139–143.

House, H. L. 1958b. Nutritional requirements of insects associated with animal parasitism. *Exptl. Parasitol.*, **7**: 555–609.

House, H. L. 1959. Nutrition of the parasitoid *Pseudosarcophaga affinis* (Fall.) and of other insects. *Ann. N. Y. Acad. Sci.*, **77**: 394–405.

House, H. L. 1961. Insect nutrition. *Ann. Rev. Entomol.*, **6**: 13–26.

House, H. L. 1962. Insect nutrition. *Ann. Rev. Biochem.*, **31**: 653–672.

House, H. L., and J. S. Barlow. 1956. Nutritional studies with *Pseudosarcophaga affinis* (Fall.), a dipterous parasite of the srpuce budworm, *Choristoneura fumiferana* (Clem.). V. Effects of various concentrations of the amino acid mixture, dextrose, potassium ion, the salt mixture, and lard on growth and development; and a substitute for lard. *Can. J. Zool.*, 34: 182–189.

House, H. L., and J. S. Barlow. 1957a. Effects of nucleic acid on larval growth, pupation and adult emergence of *Pseudosarcophaga affinis* (Fall.). Nature, 180: 44.

House, H. L., and J. S. Barlow. 1957b. New equipment for rearing small numbers of *Pseudosarcophaga affinis* (Fall.) (Diptera: Sarcophagidae) for experimental purposes. *Can. Entomologist,* 89: 145–150.

House, H. L., and J. S. Barlow. 1958. Vitamin requirements of the housefly, *Musca domestica* L. (Diptera: muscidae). *Ann. Entomol. Soc. Am.,* 51: 299–302.

House, H. L., and J. S. Barlow. 1960. Effects of oleic and other fatty acids on the growth of *Agria affinis* (Fall.) (Diptera: Sarcophagidae). *J. Nutrition,* 72: 409–414.

House, H. L., and R. L. Patton. 1949. Nutritional studies with *Blattella germanica* (L.) reared under aseptic conditions. I. Equipment and technique. *Can. Entomologist,* 81: 94–100.

Hughes, A. 1959. "A History of Cytology," 128 pp. Abelard-Schuman, New York.

Hurel-Py, G. 1950. Recherches préliminaries sur la culture aseptique des prothalles de filicinées: *Rev. gen. botan.,* 57: 637–735.

Hutchinson, F. 1961. Molecular basis for action of ionizing radiations, *Science,* 134: 533–538.

Hutner, S. H., and W. Trager. 1953. Growth of protozoa. *Ann. N. Y. Acad. Sci.,* 56: 815–1094.

Iijima, S. 1950. Investigation relating to aseptic aspiration pneumonia. *Trans. Soc. Pathol. Japon.,* 39: 169.

Iijima, S. 1953. Some colloidochemical observations on autolytic liver cell nucleus. II. Postmortem changes of the liver under germ-free conditions. *Trans. Soc. Pathol. Japon.* 42: 210–212 (in Japanese).

Iijima, S. 1955. Morphological structure of the cell nucleus, and its autolytic decomposition in the germfree condition. I. II. *J. Nagoya Med. Assoc.,* 69(4): 294–323 and 413–436.

Iinoya, K. 1961. Cleaner rids air of fine particles. *Chem. Eng. News,* 39: 50.

Ishii, S., and C. Hirano. 1955. Qualitative studies on the essential amino acid requirements for the growth of the larvae of the rice stem borer, *Chilo simplex* Butler, under aseptic conditions. *Bull. Natl. Inst. Agr. Sci.* (*Japan*), C5: 35–48.

Itaya, J. 1958. Some fundamental studies on the inflammation of germfree animals. Especially on the inflammatory initial reaction and Menkin's factors. *Trans. Soc. Pathol. Japon.,* 47: 1257–1276.

Jenkins, D. W. 1960. Laboratory animal standards. *Proc. 2nd Symposium on Gnotobiotic Technol. 1959,* pp. 19–24. Univ. Notre Dame Press, Notre Dame, Indiana.

Joblot, L. 1718. "Descriptions et usages de plusieurs nouveaux microscopes," Vol. 1, p. 101. J. Collombat, Paris.

Jodin, M. 1862. Du role physiologique de l'azote. *Compt. rend. acad. sci.,* **55:** 612–615.

Johns, F. M., and P. L. Querens. 1914. Further note on the growth of filarial embryos *in vitro. Am. J. Trop. Diseases and Prev. Med.,* **1:** 620–624.

Johnson, L. F. 1957. Effect of antibiotics on the numbers of bacteria and fungi isolated from soil by the dilution-plate method. *Phytopathology,* **47:** 630–631.

Johnson, R. B., D. A. Peterson, and B. M. Tolbert. 1960. Cellulose metabolism in the rat. *J. Nutrition,* **72:** 353–356.

Johnson, W. H. 1952. Further studies on the sterile culture of *Paramecium. Physiol. Zoöl.,* **25:** 10–15.

Johnson, W. H., and E. G. S Baker. 1942. The sterile culture of *Paramecium multimicronucleata. Science,* **95:** 333–334.

Johnson, W. H., and C. A. Miller. 1957. The nitrogen requirements of *Paramecium multimicronucleatum. Physiol. Zoöl.,* **30:** 106–113.

Johnson, W. H., and E. L. Tatum. 1945. The heat labile growth factor for *Paramecium* in pressed yeast juice. *Arch. Biochem.,* **8:** 163–168.

Johnson, W. H., L. C. Franklin, and C. A. Miller. 1959. The complete loss of pigment is planarians in a solution of fungichromin. *Anat. Record,* **134:** 588–589.

Johnstone, J. F. W. 1844. "Elements of Agricultural Chemistry and Geology," 3rd ed., 228 pp. W. Blackwood & Sons, Edinburgh.

Jolly, M. J. 1903. Sur la durée de la vie et de la multiplication des cellules animales en dehors de l'organisme. *Compt. rend. soc. biol.,* **55:** 1266–1268.

Jones, M. F., and P. P. Weinstein. 1957. The axenic cultivation of *Nematospiroides dubius. J. Parasitol.,* **43:** 46.

Just, T. 1959. The ecological approach to germfree life studies. *Ann. N. Y. Acad. Sci.,* **78:** 371–374 and 389–393.

Kaiho, T. 1958. Studies on the phystiologic significance of aerobic bacteria in intestines. *J. Chiba Med. Soc.,* **34:** 406–421.

Kapterev, P. N. 1947. Anabioses in the eternal ice. *Deut. Gesundheitsw.,* **2:** 517. (*Arctic Biblio.* **4:** 2317.)

Kassel, R., and A. Rottino. 1955. Significance of diptheroids in malignant disease studied by germ-free techniques. *A.M.A. Arch. Internal Med.,* **96:** 804–808.

Kawai, M. 1955. Studies on physiological functions of *Enterococcus* and B. *sporogenes* germs in the intestine. *J. Chiba Med. Soc.,* **31:** 169–179.

Kawai, M., and S. Saito. 1955. Studies on germfree rearing of chicks. *J. Chiba. Med. Soc.,* **30:** 750–765.

Kelemen, G. 1960. Germfree reared animals in otolaryngic experimentation. *Proc. 2nd Symposium on Gnotobiotic Technol. 1959,* pp. 183–186. Univ. Notre Dame Press, Notre Dame, Indiana.

Kidder, G. W. 1953. The nutrition of invertebrate animals. *In* "Biochemistry and Physiology of Nutrition." (G. H. Bourne and G. W. Kidder, eds.), pp. 162–195. Academic Press, New York.

Kidder, G. W., and V. L. Dewey. 1951. The biochemistry of ciliates in pure culture. *In* "Biochemistry and Physiology of Protozoa" (S. H. Hutner and and A. Lwoff, eds.), pp. 323–400. Academic Press, New York.

Kijanizin, J. 1894a. Influence de l'air sterilisé sur l'assimilation de l'azote et l'excrétion d'acide carbonique chez les animaux. *Arch. biol.* (*Paris*), **13**: 339–388.

Kijanizin, J. 1894b. *J. hyg.* (*Paris*), **10** (in Russian).

Kijanizin, J. 1895. Influence de l'air sterilisé sur l'assimilation, la désassimilation de l'azote et l'excrétion de l' acide carbonique ches les animaux. *Arch. biol.* (*Liége*), **13**: 339–388.

Kijanizin, J. 1900a. Weiter Untersuchungen über den Einfluss sterilisierter Luft auf Tiere. *Virchows Arch.*, **16**(II): 515.

Kijanizin, J. 1900b. Nouvelles expériences sur l'influence de l'air stérilisé sur les animaux. *Arch. biol.* (*Paris*), **16**: 663–684.

Kijanizin, J. 1916. The effect on higher animals of the sterilisation of the inhabited medium, the air and the food. *J. Physiol.*, **50**: 391–396.

Kircher, A. 1658. "Scrutinium physico-medium." Romae.

Kishimoto, H. 1957. Some morphological characteristics in the lungs of germfree animals. *Nagoya Igakkai Zasshi*, **73**(3): 429–438.

Klebs, E. 1873. Beiträge zur Kenntniss der Micrococcen. *Ark. exptl. pathol. u. Pharmakol.* **1**: 31–64.

Klein, R. M., and A. C. Braun. 1960. On the presumed sterile induction of plant tumors. *Science*, **131**: 1612.

Knight, P. L. 1960. Microbial synthesis of thiamine in the rat. *Abstr. 5th Intern. Congr. Nutrition, Washington, D.C., 1960*, 13–14.

Knudson, L. 1933. Non-symbiotic development of seedlings of *Calluna vulgaris*. *New Phytologist*, **32**: 115–127.

Kobayashi, R. 1954. Nutritional pathology of guinea pigs reared on synthetic diets. I. Synthetic diets of germfree guinea pigs and their development. *Trans. Soc. Pathol. Japon.*, **43**: 438–449 (in Japanese); *Acta Pathol. Japon.*, **4**(3): 182 (in English).

Kobayashi, R. 1955. Nutritional pathology of guinea pigs reared on synthetic diets. II. Pregnancy, parturition of germ-free artificial diet reared guinea pigs and growth in successive generations. *Acta Pathol. Japon.*, **5**(3): 183 (in English).

Koch, A. 1954. Symbioten als Vitaminquelle der Insekten. *Forsch. u. Fortschr.*, **28**: 33–37.

Koch, R. 1881. Über Desinfektion. *Mitt. Gesundh. Amt.*, **1**: 1–48.

Komiya, Y., K. Yasuraoka, and A. Sato. 1956. Survival of ancylostoma canium *in vitro* (I). *Japan. J. Med. Sci. & Biol.*, **9**: 283–292.

Kossowitch, P. 1894. Untersuchungen uber die Frage, ob die Algen freien Stickstoffe fixiren. *Botan. Zentr.* **52**: 76–116.

Kratz, W. A., and J. Meyers. 1955. Nutrition and growth of several blue-green algae. *Am. J. Botany*, **42**: 282–287.

Krauss, R. M. 1958. Physiology of the fresh-water algae. *Ann. Rev. Plant Physiol.*, **9**: 207–244.

Kritchevsky, D., R. R. Kolman, R. M. Guttmacher, and M. Forbes. 1959. Influence of dietary carbohydrate and protein on serum and liver cholesterol in germfree chickens. *Arch. Biochem. Biophys.*, **85**: 444–451.

Küster, E. 1912. Die keimfreie Züchtung von Säugetieren und ihre Bedeutung fur die Erforschung der Körperfunktionen. *Zentr. Bakteriol. Parasitenk.*, **54**: 55–58.

Küster, E. 1913a. Die Bedeutung der normalen Darmbakterien für den gesunden

Menschen. *In* "Handbuch des pathogenen Mikroorganism," (W. Kolle and A. von Wasserman, eds.), 2nd ed., Vol. 6, pp. 468–482.

Küster, E. 1913b. Die Gewinnung und Züchtung keimfreier Säugetiere. *Deut. med. Wochschr.*, **39**: 1586–1588.

Küster, E. 1915a. Die Gewinnung, Haltung und Aufzucht keimfreier Tiere und ihre Bedeutung fur die Erforschung natürliecher Lebensvorgänge. *Arb. kaiserl. Gesundh.*, **48**: 412–424.

Küster, E. 1915b. Die keimfreie Züchtung von Säugetieren, *Handb. biochem. Arbeitsmethoden*, **8**: 311–323.

Küster, E. 1915c. Die Gewinnung, Haltung und Aufzucht keimfreier Tiere und ihre Bedeutung für die Erforschung natürlicher Lebersvorgänge. *Arb. Kaiserl, Gesundh.*, **48**: 1–79.

Küster, E. 1925. Aufzucht keimfreier Säugetiere. *Handb. biol. Arbeitsmethoden*, **4**(9): 419–436.

Kuhn, R. 1955. Darmflora und Ernährung. "Die Grundlagen unserer Ernährung," pp. 87–95. A. Kronerverlag, Stuttgart.

Lakey, B. E. 1945. "A method for raising bacteria-free chickens." M.S. Thesis, Univ. of Wisconsin, Madison, Wisconsin.

Landy, J. J. 1961. Sterile operative technique. *J. Arkansas Med. Soc.* **57**: 503–506.

Landy, J. J., and R. L. Sandberg. 1961. Delivery of the germfree pig. *Federation Proc.*, **20**: 369.

Landy, J. J., T. G. Yerasimides, J. H. Growdon, and S. C. Bausor. 1960. Germfree guinea pig delivery by hysterectomy. *Surg. Forum*, **11**: 425–426.

Landy, J. J., L. R. Powers, S. C. Bausor, and I. Havens. 1961. Germfree sprouts of *Phaseolus aureus* by peracetic acid sterilization. *Bacteriol. Proc.* (*Soc. Am. Bacteriologists*), **1961**: 61.

Landy, M., J. L. Whitby, J. G. Michael, M. W. Woods, and W. L. Newton. 1962. Effect of bacterial endotoxin in germfree mice. *Proc. Soc. Exptl. Biol. Med.*, **109**: 352–356.

Lane, C. E. 1959. The nutrition of *Teredo*. *Ann. N. Y. Acad. Sci.*, **77**: 246–249.

Larner, J., and R. E. Gillespie. 1957. Gastrointestinal digestion of starch. III. Intestinal carbohydrase activities in germ-free and non-germ-free animals. *J. Biol. Chem.*, **225**: 279–285.

Latimer, H. B. 1924. Postnatal growth of the body, systems, and organs of the single-comb White Leghorn chicken. *J. Agr. Research*, **29**: 363–397.

Lawes, J. B., and J. H. Gilbert. 1889. On the present position of the question of the sources of nitrogen of vegetation, with some new results, and preliminary notice of new lines of investigation. *Phil. Trans. Roy. Soc. London*, **180B**: 1–107.

Lawes, J. B., and J. H. Gilbert. 1890. New experiments on the question of the fixation of free nitrogen. *Proc. Roy. Soc.*, **47**: 85–118.

Lawes, J. B., and J. H. Gilbert. 1891. The sources of the nitrogen of our leguminous crops. *J. Roy. Agr. Soc. Engl.* [3] **2**: 657–702.

Lawes, J. B., and J. H. Gilbert. 1893. "Rothamsted Memoirs on Agricultural Chemistry and Physiology," Vol. 1, 111 pp. Dunn and Chidgey, London.

Lawes, J. B., J. H. Gilbert, and E. Pugh. 1861. On the sources of the nitrogen of vegetation; with special reference to the question whether plants assimilate free or uncombined nitrogen. *Phil. Trans. Roy. Soc. London,* **151:** 431–577.

Lawrence, J. J. 1948. The cultivation of the free-living stages of the hookworm, *Ancylostoma Braziliense* de faria, under aseptic conditions. *Australian J. Exptl. Biol. Med. Sci.,* **26:** 1–8.

Leeuwenhoek, A. 1677. Letter of October 9, 1676. *Phil. Trans. Roy. Soc. London,* **A133:** 821; see also A. Schierbeek and J. J. Swart: "The Collected Letters of Antoine van Leeuwenhoek," 5 vols. Swets and Zeitlinger, Amsterdam, 1939.

Lennox, F. G. 1939. Studies on the physiology and toxicology of blowflies. I. The development of a synthetic medium for the aseptic cultivation of *Lucilia cuprina* larvae. *Council Sci. Ind. Research (Australia),* **90:** 1–20.

Lepkovsky, S., E. Bingham, and R. Pencharz. 1959. The fate of the proteolytic enzymes from the pancreatic juice of chicks fed raw and heated soybeans. *Poultry Sci.,* **38:** 1289–1295.

Lev, M. 1961. Germfree animals and their uses in elucidating the action of the gut flora on the host. *J. Appl. Bacteriol.,* **24:** 307–315.

Lev, M. 1962. An autoclavable plastic unit for rearing animals under germfree conditions. *J. Appl. Bacteriol.,* **25:** 30–34.

Lev, M., and M. Forbes. 1959. Growth response to dietary penicillin of germfree chicks and chicks with a defined intestinal flora. *Brit. J. Nutrition,* **13:** 78–84.

Levenson, S. M., R. P. Mason, T. E. Huber, O. J. Malm, R. E. Horowitz, and A. Einheber. 1959. Germfree animals and surgical research. *Ann. Surg.,* **150:** 713–730.

Levenson, S. M., L. V. Crowley, R. E. Horowitz, and O. J. Malm. 1959. The metabolism of carbon-labeled urea in the germfree rat. *J. Biol. Chem.,* **234:** 2061–2062.

Levenson, S. M., N. Brown, and R. E. Horowitz. 1960a. Dietary cirrhosis of the liver in the germfree rat. *Abstr. 5th Intern. Cong. Nutrition, Washington, D.C., 1960,* p. 14.

Levenson, S. M., P. C. Trexler, O. J. Malm, R. E. Horowitz, and W. H. Moncrief. 1960b. A disposable plastic isolator for operating in a sterile environment. *Surg. Forum,* **11:** 306–308.

Levin. 1899. Les microbes dans les régions arctiques. *Ann. inst. Pasteur,* **13:** 558–567.

Lewis, K. H., and E. McCoy. 1933. Root nodule formation on the garden bean, studied by a technique of tissue culture. *Botan. Gaz.,* **95:** 316–329.

Lewis, M. R., and W. H. Lewis. 1911. The growth of embryonic chick tissues in artificial media, agar and bouillon. *Johns Hopkins Hosp. Bull.,* **22:** 126–127.

Lichtenstein, E. P. 1948. Growth of *Culex molestus* under sterile conditions. *Nature,* **162:** 227.

Liebig, J. 1843. Die Chemie in ihrer Anwendung auf Agricultur und Physiologie. Vieweg, Braunschweig.

Lisbonne, M. 1931. Microbes et actions microbiennes dans le tube digestif, *Traité physiol. norm. pathol.* **2:** 445–484.

Lister, J. 1878. On the lactic fermentation and its bearings on pathology. *Trans. Pathol. Soc. London,* **29:** 425–467.

Ljunggren, C. A. 1897–1898. Von der Fähigkeit des Hautepithels, ausserhalb des

Organismus sein Leben zu behalten, mit Berücksichtigung der Transplantation. *Deut. Z. Chir.,* **47:** 608–615.

Loeb, J., and J. H. Northrop. 1916. Nutrition and evolution. *J. Biol. Chem.,* **27:** 309–312.

Luckey, T. D. 1946–1954. Unpublished reports, University of Notre Dame.

Luckey, T. D. 1952. Effect of feeding antibiotics upon the growth rate of germ-free birds. *In* "Studies on the Growth Effect of Antibiotics in Germ-free Animals," a Colloquium. Univ. of Notre Dame, Notre Dame, Indiana.

Luckey, T. D. 1954a. A single diet for all living organisms. *Science,* **120:** 396–398.

Luckey, T. D. 1954b. Daily nutrient allowances: Germ-free rat, chicken. *In* "Standard Values in Nutrition and Metabolism" (E. A. Albrittion, ed.), p. 68. Saunders, Philadelphia, Pennsylvania.

Luckey, T. D. 1956a. Metabolism in germfree animals. *Texas Repts. Biol. and Med.,* **14:** 482–505.

Luckey, T. D. 1956b. Mode of action of antibiotics—evidence from germfree birds. *Intern. Conf. on Use of Antibiotics in Agr., 1st, Washington, D.C., 1956,* pp. 135–145 (Natl. Acad. Sci. Natl. Research Council).

Luckey, T. D. 1957. A comparative nutrition study. *Federation Proc.,* **16:** 390 (Abstr.).

Luckey, T. D. 1958. Modes of action of antibiotics in growth stimulation. *In* "Recent Progress in Microbiology," (G. Tunevall, ed.), pp. 340–349. Almquist & Wiksell, Stockholm.

Luckey, T. D. 1959a. Antibiotics in Nutrition. *In* "Antibiotics, Their Chemistry and Non-Medical Uses" (H. S. Goldberg), pp. 174–321. Van Nostrand, Princeton, New Jersey.

Luckey, T. D. 1959b. Modes of action of antibiotics in growth stimulation. Symposium V. *In* "Recent Progress in Microbiology" (G. Tunevall, ed.), pp. 340–349. Almquist & Wiksells, Stockholm.

Luckey, T. D. 1959c. Nutrition and biochemistry of germ-free chicks. *Ann. N. Y. Acad. Sci.,* **78:** 127–165.

Luckey, T. D. 1960. Germfree lamb nutrition. *Abstr. 5th Intern. Congr. Nutrition, Washington, D.C., 1960,* p. 25.

Luckey, T. D. 1961a. A study in comparative nutrition. *J. Comp. Biochem. Physiol.,* **2:** 100–124.

Luckey, T. D. 1961b. Vitamin metabolism in germfree and dibiotic rats. *Abstr. Intern. Congr. Biochem., 5th Congr., Moscow, 1961,* p. 235. (Pergamon Press, London).

Luckey, T. D., and H. Hittson. 1952. Lion feeding of the future. Parks and Recreation, May, 21 pp.

Luckey, T. D., and J. A. Reyniers. 1954. Biosynthesis of folic acid and citrovorum factor in the germfree rat. *Federation Proc.,* **13:** 466.

Luckey, T. D., G. M. Briggs, C. A. Elvehjem, and E. B. Hart. 1943. The activity of pyridoxine derivatives in chick nutrition. *Proc. Soc. Exptl. Biol. Med.,* **58:** 340–344.

Luckey, T. D., G. M. Briggs, and C. A. Elvehjem. 1944. The use of *Streptococcus lactis* R for the measurement of folic acid. *J. Biol. Chem.,* **153:** 157–167.

Luckey, T. D., G. M. Briggs, P. R. Moore, C. A. Elvehjem, and E. B. Hart. 1945.

Studies on the liberation of compounds in the folic acid group. *J. Biol. Chem.*, **161**: 395–403.

Luckey, T. D., P. R. Moore, C. A. Elvehjem, and E. B. Hart. 1946a. The activity of synthetic folic acid in purified rations for the chick. *Science,* **103**: 682–684.

Luckey, T. D., P. R. Moore, C. A. Elvehjem, and E. B. Hart. 1946b. Effect of diet on the response of chicks to folic acid. *Proc. Soc. Exptl. Biol. Med.*, **62**: 307–312.

Luckey, T. D., P. R. Moore, C. A. Elvehjem, and E. B. Hart. 1947. Growth of chicks on purified and synthetic diets containing amino acids. *Proc. Soc. Exptl. Biol. Med.*, **64**: 348–351.

Luckey, T. D., J. A. Reyniers, R. F. Ervin, M. Wagner, and H. A. Gordon. 1948. The use of Bantam chicks in nutritional and germ-free research. *Poultry Sci.*, **27**: 672–673.

Luckey, T. D., J. A. Reyniers, P. Gyorgy, and M. Forbes. 1954a. Germfree animals and liver necrosis. *Ann. N. Y. Acad. Sci.*, **57**: 932–935.

Luckey, T. D., T. J. Mende, and J. Pleasants. 1954b. The physical and chemical characterization of rat's milk. *J. Nutrition,* **54**: 345–359.

Luckey, T. D., J. R. Pleasants, and J. A. Reyniers. 1954c. Vitamin interrelationships in germfree chicks. *Poultry Sci.*, **33**: 1068.

Luckey, T. D., J. R. Pleasants, and J. A. Reyniers. 1955a. Germfree chicken nutrition. II. Vitamin interrelationships. *J. Nutrition,* **55**: 105–118.

Luckey, T. D., J. R. Pleasants, M. Wagner, H. A. Gordon, and J. A. Reyniers. 1955b. Some observations on vitamin metabolism in germ-free rats. *J. Nutrition,* **57**: 169–182.

Luckey, T. D., M. Wagner, J. A. Reyniers, and F. L. Foster, Jr. 1955c. Nutritional adequacy of a semi-synthetic diet sterilized by steam or by cathode rays. *Food Research,* **20**: 180–185.

Luckey, T. D., H. A. Gordon, M. Wagner, and J. A. Reyniers. 1956. Growth of germ-free birds fed antibiotics. *Antibiotics & Chemotherapy,* **6**: 36–40.

Luckey, T. D., M. Wagner, H. A. Gordon, and J. A. Reyniers. 1960. Rearing germfree turkeys. *Lob. Rept.,* **3**: 176–182.

Lwoff, A. 1923. Sur la nutrition des infusoires. *Compt. rend. acad. sci.,* **176**: 928–930.

McCullock, E. C. 1945. "Disinfection and Sterilization." 892 pp. Lea and Febiger, Philadelphia.

McDaniel, E. G. 1960. Folic acid deficiency in germfree rats. *Abstr. 5th Intern. Congr. Nutrition, Washington, D.C., 1960,* **13**: 24.

McDaniel, E. G., and F. S. Daft. 1961. Techniques in care and feeding of germfree animals. *Proc. Animal Care Panel,* **11**: 107–110.

McGinnis, A. J., R. W. Newburgh, and V. H. Cheldelin. 1956. Nutritional studies on the blowfly, *Phormia regina* (Meig.). *J. Nutrition,* **58**: 309–316.

MacHattie, L., and H. Rahn. 1960. Survival of mice in absence of inert gas. *Proc. Soc. Exptl. Biol. Med.,* **104**: 772–775.

McLaughlin, J. J. A., and P. A. Zahl. 1959. Axenic zooxanthellae from various invertebrate hosts. *Ann. N. Y. Acad. Sci.* **77**: 55–72.

McLaughlin, M. M., M. P. Dacquisto, D. P. Jacobus, M. Forbes, and P. E. Parks. 1958. The effect of the germfree state on survival of the ten-day old chick after x-radiation. *Radiation Research,* **9**: 147.

Maggini, A. 1942. "Dissociation in a type C *Streptococcus* infecting guinea pigs," M.S. Thesis. Univ. of Notre Dame, Notre Dame, Indiana.

Malyath, G., H. W. Stein, E. Herman, and R. S. Schuler. 1953. Paper chromatography investigations of human, bovine and rat milk. *Experientia*, 9: 70–71.

Martin, B. 1722. "A New Theory of Consumptions," 2nd ed. London.

Matsumura, S., G. Kakinuma, K. Kawashima, K. Tanikawa, S. Ochiai, R. Miyata, K. Fujisaki, R. Kanao, K. Noguch, L. Aoki, T. Sato, K. Itoe, and M. Suzuki. 1929. The etiology of beriberi. *J. Am. Med. Assoc.*, 92: 1325–1327.

Meeks, R. 1950. "Identification, distribution and metabolism of a vitamin C-like substance in brain," M.S. Thesis. Univ. of Notre Dame, Notre Dame, Indiana.

Meister, A. 1960. Deamination of amino acids: specificity and biological significance. (Quoted unpublished data from S. Scott and A. Meister.) In "Biochimie comparée des acides amines basiques," p. 22. Editions du centre national de la recherche scientifique.

Meleney, H. E. 1957. Some unsolved problems in amebiasis. *Am. J. Trop. Med. Hyg.*, 6: 487–498.

Melville, D. B., and W. H. Horner. 1953. Blood ergothionine in the germ-free chicken. *J. Biol. Chem.*, 202: 187–191.

Merkenschlager, M. 1962. Antibiotika in der Tierernährung—Studien über antibiotika-verteilung und- ruckstandsbildung im Tierkörper sowie ihren Einfluss auf Darmflora und Bakteriensensitivität. Thesis in Veterinary Science, Universität München.

Metchnikoff, E. 1901. The Wilde Lecture. Sur la flore du corps humain. *Mem. Proc. Manchester Lit. Phil. Soc.* 45(5): 1–38.

Metchnikoff, E. 1903. Les microbes intestinaux. *Bull. inst. Pasteur*, 1: 265–282.

Metchnikoff, E. 1909. Rousettes et microbes. Introduction. *Ann. inst. Pasteur*, 23: 937–941.

Metchnikoff, E., W. Weinberg, E. Pozerski, A. Distaso, and A. Berthelot. 1909. Roussettes et microbes. *Ann. inst. Pasteur*, 23: 937–978.

Metchnikoff, O. 1901. Note sur l'influence des microbes, dans le dévelopment des têtards. *Ann. inst. Pasteur*, 15(5): 631–634.

Metchnikoff, O. 1921. "Life of Elie Metchnikoff." Houghton, Mifflin, Boston, Massachusetts.

Michelbacher, A. E.. W. M. Hoskins, and W. B. Herms. 1932. The nutrition of flesh fly larvae, *Lucilia sericata* (Meig.). I. The adequacy of sterile synthetic diets. *J. Exptl. Zool.*, 64: 109–131.

Mickelsen, O. 1962. Nutrition—germfree animal research. *Ann. Rev. Biochem.*, 31: 515–548.

Miller, C. A., and W. H. Johnson. 1957. A purine and pyrimidine requirement for *Paramecium multimicronucleatum. J. Protozool.*, 4: 200–204.

Miller, C. A., and W. H. Johnson. 1959. Preliminary studies on the axenic cultivation of a planarian (*Dugesia*). *Ann. N. Y. Acad. Sci.*, 77: 87–92.

Miller, C. A., and W. H. Johnson. 1960. Nutrition of *Paramecium:* A fatty acid requirement. *J. Protozool.*, 7: 297–301.

Miller, C. A., W. H. Johnson, and S. C. Miller. 1955. The sterilization and preliminary attempts in the axenic cultivation of the black planarian, *Dugesia dorotocephalia. Proc. Indiana Acad. Sci.*, 65: 27.

Miller, H. 1962. "Gnotobiotic techniques and intestinal synthesis of folic acid in the chick." Ph.D. Thesis. Univ. of Missouri, Columbia, Missouri.

Miller, H. T., and T. D. Luckey. 1962. A new germfree chicken cage—Characteristics and use. *J. Appl. Microbiol.*, **10**: 52–54.

Miller, H. T., and T. D. Luckey. 1962. Germfree research: Indirect evidence for the intestinal synthesis of folic acid by monoinfected chicks. *Federation Proc.*, **21**: 476.

Mills, R. C., G. M. Briggs, T. D. Luckey, and C. A. Elvehjem. 1944. Production of unidentified vitamins by a strain of *Mycobacterium tuberculosis* grown on a medium with *p*-aminobenzoic acid. *Proc. Soc. Exptl. Biol. Med.*, **56**: 240–242.

Miner, R. W. (ed.) 1953. Growth of Protozoa. *Ann. N. Y. Acad. Sci.*, **77**: 815–1094.

Miquel, P. 1892. De la culture artificielle des Diatomes. *Le Diatomiste*, **8**: 9–12.

Miyakawa, M. 1951. Studies on germfree breeding of animals. *Trans. Soc. Pathol. Japon.*, **40**: 227.

Miyakawa, M. 1952. Germfree rearing of animals. *Igaku no Ayumi.*, **16**: 137–146.

Miyakawa, M. 1954a. Long term germ-free rearing of guinea pigs. *Trans. Soc. Pathol. Japon.*, **43**: 450–452 (in Japanese); *Acta Pathol. Japon.*, **4**(3): 182 (in English).

Miyakawa, M. 1954b. The apparatus of germ-free animals. *Trans. Soc. Pathol. Japon.*, **43**: 450–453 (in Japanese); *Acta Pathol. Japon.*, **4**(3): 182 (in English).

Miyakawa, M. 1955a. Rearing germfree experimental animals. *Nisshin Igaku*, **42**: 553–566.

Miyakawa, M. 1955b. The blood forming tissue of germ-free animals. XIV. *Jap. Med. Congr.*, **2**: 86–87.

Miyakawa, M. 1955c. The lymphatic tissue of germ-free animals. *Acta Haematol. Japon.*, **18**(5): 406–424 (in Japanese and English); *Acta Pathol. Japon.*, **5**(3): 182–183 (in English).

Miyakawa, M. 1956a. On the oral cavity of the germfree guinea pig. *J. Japan. Oral Sci.*, **5**: 263–271.

Miyakawa, M. 1956b. Sterility of animals reared under aseptic conditions. *Japan. Med. J.*, **1674**: 26–33.

Miyakawa, M. 1957a. Experimental studies on the transplantation of Yoshida sarcoma, human cancer, and human leukemic cells to germ-free guinea pigs. *Acta Pathol. Japon.*, **7**: 725–736.

Miyakawa, M. 1957b. Fundamental behavior of the inflammatory reaction. *Nihonrinsho.*, **15**: 14–25.

Miyakawa, M. 1957c. Le tissu lymphoide du cobaye bactériologiquement stérile. *Le Sang*, **28**(8): 698–717.

Miyakawa, M. 1958a. Rearing germ-free animals. *Kagaku (Tokyo)*, **28**: 292–295.

Miyakawa, M. 1958b. Studies on inflammation. (Using germfree guinea pigs.) *Saishin Igaku*, **13**: 38–50.

Miyakawa, M. 1959a. Report on germfree research at the Department of Pathology, University of Nagoya, Japan, and some observations on wound healing, transplantation and foreign body inflammation in the germfree guinea pig. Symposium V. *In* "Recent Progress in Microbiology" (G. Tune-vall, ed.), pp. 299–313. Almquist & Wiksell, Stockholm.

Miyakawa, M. 1959b. The lymphatic system of germfree guinea pigs. *Ann. N. Y. Acad. Sci.,* **78:** 221–236.

Miyakawa, M. 1959c. The Miyakawa remote-control germfree rearing unit. *Ann. N. Y. Acad. Sci.,* **78:** 37–46.

Miyakawa, M. 1960. Observations on the vitamin B_{12} and pteroylglutamic acid deficient germ-free guinea pigs. *Abstr. 5th Intern. Congr. Nutrition, Washington, D.C., 1960,* p. 13.

Miyakawa, M., S. Iijima, H. Kishimoto, R. Kobayashi, and M. Tajima. 1951a. Germ-free apparatus and germ-free rearing methods. *Acta Pathol. Japon.,* **40:** 227–229.

Miyakawa, M., S. Iijima, H. Kishimoto, R. Kobayashi, and M. Tajima. 1951b. Studies on germfree breeding of animals. *Trans. Soc. Pathol. Japon.,* **40:** 227–229.

Miyakawa, M., Iijima, R. Kobayashi, M. Tajima, and N. Isomura. 1953. Studies on argentaffine fibers of postnatally formed lymphatic apparatus of intestinal and nasal mucosa. VII. Studies on inflammation using germ-free animals. *Trans. Soc. Pathol. Japon.* **42:** 107–108 (in Japanese).

Miyakawa, M., S. Iijima, R. Kobayashi, M. Tajima, N. Isomura, T. Shimizu, I. Kobayashi, and M. Asano. 1954. Report on success of long duration rearing of germfree guinea pigs. *Trans. Soc. Pathol. Japon.,* **43:** 450–452.

Miyakawa, M., S. Iijima, R. Kobayashi, and M. Tajima. 1957a. Observation on the lymphoid tissue of the germ-free guinea pig. *Acta Pathol. Japon.,* **7:** 183–210.

Miyakawa, M., H. Kishimoto, J. Itaya, Y. Uei, Y. Uno, and M. Miyazu. 1957b. On the heterotransplantation of *yoshida sarcoma,* human cancer and human leukemic cells into germ-free guinea pigs. *Gann.,* **48**(4): 530–532.

Miyakawa, M., N. Isomura, H. Shirasawa, and K. Yokoi. 1958a. Wound healing in germ-free animals. *Acta Pathol. Japon.,* **8:** 79–97.

Miyakawa, M., H. Kishimoto, J. Itaya, Y. Uei, and T. Kashio. 1958b. Homo-transplantation experiment in germ-free animals. *Acta Pathol. Japon.,* **8:** 177–187.

Miyakawa, M., S. Iijima, H. Kishimoto, R. Kobayashi, M. Tajima, N. Isomura, M. Asano, and S. C. Hong. 1958c. Rearing germ-free guinea pigs. *Acta Pathol. Japon.,* **8:** 55–78.

Moir, R. F., M. Somers, and H. Waring. 1956. Studies on marsupial nutrition. I. Ruminant-like digestion in a herbivorous marsupial (*Setonix brachyurus* Quoy and Gaimard). *Australian J. Biol. Sci.,* **9:** 293–304.

Moore, P. R., T. D. Luckey, A. Evenson, E. McCoy, C. A. Elvehjem, and E. B. Hart. 1946. Use of sulfasuxidine, streptothricin and streptomycin in nutritional studies with the chick. *J. Biol. Chem.,* **165:** 437–441.

Moore, P. R., A. Lepp, T. D. Luckey, C. A. Elvehjem, and E. B. Hart. 1947. Storage, retention, and distribution of folic acid in the chick. *Proc. Soc. Exptl. Biol. Med.,* **64:** 316–319.

Morgan, J. F. 1958. Tissue culture nutrition. *Bacteriol. Revs.,* **22:** 20–45.

Morgan, J. F., H. J. Morton, and R. C. Parker. 1950. Nutrition of animal cells in tissue culture. I. Initial studies on a synthetic medium. *Proc. Soc. Exptl. Biol. Med.,* **73:** 1–8.

Moro, E. 1905. Morphologische und biologische Untersuchungen über die Darmbakterien des Säuglings. IV. Der Schottelius' sche Versuch am Kaltblütler. *Jahrb. Kinderheilk.* **62:** 467–478.

Moscona, A. A. 1959. Tissues from dissociated cells *Sci. American,* **200:** 132–144.

Moscona, A. A. 1961. How cells associate. *Sci. American,* **205:** 142–162.

Mueller, J. F. 1958. *In vitro* cultivation of the sporogonium of *Spirometra* mansonoides to the infective stage. *J. Parasitol.,* **44:** 14–15.

Müller, O. F. 1786. Animacula infusoria fluratilia et marina. Haunide, Copenhagen, pp. 376.

Muir, W. H., A. C. Hildebrandt, and A. J. Riker, 1958. The preparation, isolation and growth in culture of single cells from higher plants. *Am. J. Botany,* **45:** 589–597.

Murdock, F. F., and T. L. Smart. 1913. A method of producing sterile blowfly larvae for surgical use. *U. S. Naval Med. Bull.,* **29:** 406.

Murray, M. R., and G. Kopech. 1953. A bibliography of the research in tissue culture. 1741 pp. Academic Press, New York.

Nagando, K. 1923. Beitrag zur "Kultur" der Mikrofilarien ausserhalb des Wirtskörpers. *Arch. Schiffs u. Tropen-Hyg.,* **27:** 178–185.

Naito, R. 1937. Zur Frage der Bakteriophagenentstehung im tierischen Orgasmaus. *Zentr. Bakteriol. Parasitenk. Abt. I, Orig.,* **138:** 34–43.

Naito, R., and M. Kobayash. 1936. On the germfree rearing of chicks. *J. Japan. Microbiol.,* **30:** 1867–1868.

Nakahara, T. 1959. Studies on construction of germfree rearing apparatus. *J. Chiba Med. Soc.,* **35:** 791–802.

Nakamura, J. 1959. Administration of intestinal bacteria to germfree guinea pigs and pathologic findings on intestinal mucosa. *J. Chiba Med. Soc.,* **35:** 803–812.

Nathan, H. A., and A. D. Laderman. 1959. Rotifers as biological tools. *Ann. N. Y. Acad. Sci.,* **77:** 96–101.

Nelson, J. B. 1951. Studies on endemic pneumonia of the albino rat. IV. Development of a rat colony free from respiratory infections. *J. Exptl. Med.,* **94:** 377–386.

Nelson, R. C. 1941. "Progressive changes in the flora of the intestinal tract of guinea pigs from birth to maturity," M.A. Thesis. Univ. of Notre Dame, Notre Dame, Indiana.

Nencki, M. 1886. Bemerkungen zu einer Bemerkung Pasteur's. *Arch. expt. Pathol. u. Pharmakol. Naunyn-Schmiedeberg's,* **20:** 385–388.

Nencki, M., and P. Giacosa. 1880. Giebt es Bakterien und deren Keime in den organer gesunder lebender Tiere. Beitrage zur Biologic der Saltpilze, Leipzig.

Newton, W. L. 1960. Some effects of germ-free environment and diet on serum protein levels in the germ-free guinea pig. *Abstr. 5th Intern. Congr. Nutrition, Washington, D.C., 1960,* p. 25.

Newton, W. L., and W. B. DeWitt. 1961. Nutrition and serum protein levels in germfree guinea pigs. *J. Nutrition* **75:** 145–151.

Newton, W. L., P. P. Weinstein, and M. F. Jones. 1959. A comparison of the development of some rat and mouse helminths in germfree and conventional guinea pigs. *Ann. N. Y. Acad. Sci.,* **78:** 290–307.

Newton, W. L., R. M. Pennington, and J. E. Lieberman. 1960a. Comparative hemolytic complement activities of germfree and conventional guinea pig serum. *Proc. Soc. Exptl. Biol. Med.,* **104:** 486–488.

Newton, W. L., L. V. Reardon, and A. M. DeLeva. 1960b. A comparative study of the subcutaneous inoculation of germfree and conventional guinea pigs with two strains of *Trichomonas vaginalis. Am. J. Trop. Med. Hyg.,* **9:** 56–61.

Nicholas, W. L. 1956. The axenic culture of *Turbatrix aceti* (the vinegar eelworm). *Nematologica,* **1:** 337–340.

Nicholas, W. L., and M. G. McEntegart. 1955. The establishment of cultures of free-living nematodes in media free from micro-organisms. *Trans. Roy. Soc. Trop. Med. Hyg.,* **49:** 301–302.

Nicholas, W. L., and M. G. McEntegart. 1957. A technique for obtaining axenic cultures of rhabditid nematodes. *J. Helminthol.,* **31:** 135–144.

Nicholas, W. L., E. C. Dougherty, and E. L. Hansen. 1959. Axenic cultivation of *Caenorhabditis briggsae* (Nematoda: Rhabditidae) with chemically undefined supplements; comparative studies with related nematodes. *Ann. N. Y. Acad. Sci.,* **77:** 218–236.

Nicholas, W. L., E. C. Dougherty, and E. L. Hansen. 1960. The incorporation of ^{14}C from sodium acetate-2-^{14}C into the amino acids of the soil-inhabiting nematode, *Caenorhabditis briggsae. J. Exptl. Biol.,* **37:** 435–443.

Nickell, L. G. 1953. Antibiotics in the growth of plants. *Antibiotics & Chemotherapy,* **3:** 449–459.

Nickell, L. G. 1954. Nutritional aspects of virus tumor growth. Abnormal and pathological plant growth. *Brookhaven Symposia Biol.,* No. **6:** 174–186.

Nickell, L. G. 1955. Effects of antigrowth substances in normal and atypical plant growth. *In* "Antimetabolites and Cancer" (C. P. Rhoads, ed.), 312 pp. Am. Assoc. Advance Sci. Washington, D.C.

Nickell, L. G. 1956. The continuous submerged cultivation of plant tissue as single cells. *Proc. Natl. Acad. Sci. U. S.,* **42:** 848–850.

Nickell, L. G. 1958. Gibberellin and the growth of plant tissue cultures. *Nature,* **181:** 499–500.

Nickell, L. G., and W. Tulecke. 1959. Production of large amounts of plant tissue by submerged culture. *Science,* **130:** 863–864.

Nickell, L. G., and A. R. English. 1953. Effect of maleic hydrazide on soil bacteria and other microorganisms. *Weeds,* **2:** 190–195.

Nickell, L. G., and W. Tulecke. 1960. Submerged growth of cells of higher plants. *J. Biochem. Microbiol. Technol. Eng.,* **2:** 287–297.

Niss, H. 1945. Personal communication.

Nobecourt, P. 1939. Sur la pérennité et l'augmentation de volume des cultures de tissus végétaux. *Compt. rend. soc. biol.,* **130:** 1270–1271.

Nonnenmacher, J. 1961. Autoradiographic studies with tritiated thymidine in a nematode (*Caenorhabditis briggsae*) *Record Genet. Soc. Am.,* **30:** 97–98.

Noronha, J. M., and A. Sreenivasan. 1959. Metabolism of folic acid in folic acid and biotin deficient rat. *Proc. Soc. Exptl. Biol. Med.,* **101:** 803–807.

Nuttall, G. H. F. 1888. Experimente über die bakterienfeindlichen Einflüsse des thierischen Körpers. *Z. Hyg.,* **4:** 353–354.

Nuttall, G. H. F. 1899. On the role of insects, arachnids and myriapods, as carriers in the spread of bacterial and parasitic diseases of man and animals. A critical and historical study. *Johns Hopkins Hosp. Repts.*, **8**: 1–154.

Nuttall, G. H. F., and H. Thierfelder. 1895–1896. Thierisches Leben ohne Bakterien im Verdauungskanal. *Z. physiol. Chem. Hoppe-Seyler's*, **21**: 109–121.

Nuttall, G. H. F., and H. Thierfelder. 1896a. Weitere Untersuchungen über bakterienfreie Thiere. *Arch. Physiol.* (*Leipzig*), pp. 363–364.

Nuttall, G. H. F., and H. Thierfelder. 1896b. Thierisches Leben ohne Bakterien im Verdauungskanal (II. Mittheilung). *Z. physiol. Chem. Hoppe-Seyler's*, **22**: 62–73.

Nuttall, G. H. F., and H. Thierfelder. 1897. Thierisches Leben ohne Bakterien im Verdauungskanal. (III. Mittheilung). Versuche an Hühnern. *Z. physiol. Chem. Hoppe-Seyler's*, **23**: 231–235.

Ootaka, S. 1959. Studies on power of sera, phagocytic power of leucocytes and titer of hemolytic comlement in germfree guinea pigs. *J. Chiba Med. Soc.*, **35**: 1838–1849.

Oparin, A. I. 1957. "Origin of Life on the Earth." 3rd ed., 495 pp. Academic Press, New York.

Oppenheimer, C. H., and A. L. Keely. 1952. *Escherichia coli* in the intestine of a wild sea lion. *Science*, **115**: 527–528.

Orland, F. J. 1955a. Experimental tooth decay in gnotobiotic rats. *Office Naval Research, Research Revs.* pp. 10–14.

Orland, F. J. 1955b. Oral/environmental factors in experimental caries research. *In* "Advances in Experimental Caries Research." Am. Assoc. Advance Sci., Washington, D.C.

Orland, F. J. 1959. A review of dental research using germfree animals. *Ann. N. Y. Acad. Sci.*, **78**: 285–289.

Orland, F. J., J. R. Blayney, R. W. Harrison, J. A. Reyniers, P. C. Trexler, M. Wagner, H. A. Gordon, and T. D. Luckey. 1954. Use of the germfree animal technic in the study of experimental dental caries. *J. Dental Research*, **33**: 147–174.

Orland, F. J., J. R. Blayney, R. W. Harrison, J. A. Reyniers, P. C. Trexler, R. F. Ervin, H. A. Gordon, and M. Wagner. 1955a. Experimental caries in germfree rats inoculated with enterococci. *J. Am. Dental Assoc.*, **50**: 259–272.

Orland, F. J., J. R. Blayney, R. W. Harrison, J. A. Reyniers, P. C. Trexler, M. Wagner, H. A. Gordon, and T. D. Luckey. 1955b. El uso de animales libres de germenes en el estudio experimental de la caries dental. I. Observationes basicas en rates cridas libres de todo microorganisms. (Use of germ-free animals in experimental study of dental caries. I. Basic study in rats kept free from all microorganisms. *Rev. asoc. odont. arg.*, **43**(6): 224–232.

Orskov, J. 1922. Method for the isolation of bacteria in pure culture from single cells and procedure for the direct tracing of bacterial growth on a solid medium. *J. Bacteriol.*, **7**: 537–549.

Osawa, E., and L. H. Muschel. 1960. The bactericidal action of normal serum and the properdin system. *J. Immunol.*, **84**: 203–212.

Park, J. T., and M. Forbes. 1957. The present status of germ-free animal research. *The Capital Chemist*, **1**: 102–105.

Parport, A. K. 1928. The bacteriological sterilization of paramecium. *Biol. Bull.*, **55**: 113–120.

Pasteur, L. 1885. Observations relatives à la Note précédente de M. Duclaux. *Compt. rend. acad. sci.*, **100**: 68.

Paul, J. 1959. "Cell and Tissue Culture," 269 pp. Livingstone, Edinburgh and London.

Penniston, V. A., and L. R. Hedrick. 1947. The reduction of bacterial count in egg pulp by use of germicides in washing dirty eggs. *Food Technol.*, **1**: 240–244.

Perry, J. F., B. Herman, P. J. Odenbrett, and A. J. Kremen. 1955. Bacteriologic studies of the human liver. *Surgery* **37**: 533–535.

Peterson, W. H., and M. S. Peterson. 1945. Relation of bacteria to vitamins and other growth factors. *Bacteriol. Rev.*, **9**: 49–110.

Phillips, A. W. 1939. A study of glass wool air filters for sterilizing air. B.S. Thesis. Univ. of Notre Dame, Notre Dame, Indiana.

Phillips, A. W. 1941a. "Studies on air-borne infection," M.S. Thesis. Univ. Notre Dame, Notre Dame, Indiana.

Phillips, A. W. 1941b. Efficiency of glass wool filters in removing bacteria from air. *J. Bacteriol.*, **41**: 270.

Phillips, A. W. 1960. Microbial effects on liver monoamine oxidase in the chick. *Abstr. 5th Intern. Congr. Nutrition, Washington, D.C., 1960*, p. 26.

Phillips, A. W., and J. E. Smith. 1959. Germfree animal techniques and their applications. *Advances in Appl. Microbiol.*, **1**: 141–174.

Phillips, A. W., F. A. Rupp, J. E. Smith, and H. R. Newcomb. 1960. A plexiglas isolator for germfree animal research. *Proc. 2nd Symposium on Gnotobiotic Technol., 1959*, pp. 49–54. Univ. Notre Dame Press, Notre Dame, Indiana.

Phillips, B. P. 1957. The pathogenic mechanisms in amebiasis. *Am. J. Proctol.*, **8**: 445–450.

Phillips, B. P. 1960. Parasitological survey of Lobund germ-free animals. *Lobund Rept.*, **3**: 172–175.

Phillips, B. P., and P. A. Wolfe. 1959. The use of germfree guinea pigs in studies on the microbial interrelationships in Amoebiasis. *Ann. N. Y. Acad. Sci.*, **78**: 308–314.

Phillips, B. P., and P. A. Wolfe. 1961. Pneumonic disease in germfree animals. *J. Infectious Diseases*, **108**: 12–18.

Phillips, B. P., P. A. Wolfe, C. W. Rees, H. A. Gordon, W. H. Wright, and J. A. Reyniers. 1955. Studies on the ameba-bacteria relationship in amebiasis. Comparative results of the intracecal inoculation of germfree, monocontaminated, and conventional guinea pigs with *Entamoeba histolytica*. *Am. J. Trop. Med. Hyg.*, **4**: 675–692.

Phillips, B. P., P. A. Wolfe, and I. L. Bartgis. 1958. Studies on the ameba-bacteria relationship in amebiasis. II. Some concepts on the etiology of the disease. *Am. J. Trop. Med. Hyg.*, **7**: 392–399.

Phillips, B. P., P. A. Wolfe, and H. A. Gordon. 1959. Studies on rearing the guinea pig germfree. *Ann. N. Y. Acad. Sci.*, **78**: 183–207.

Phillips, C. R., and R. K. Hoffman. 1960. Sterilization of interplanetary vehicles. *Science*, **132**: 991–995.

Phillips, G. B., F. E. Novak, and R. L. Alg. 1955. Portable inexpensive plastic safety hood for bacteriologists. *Appl. Microbiol.,* 3: 216–217.

Phillips, G. B., M. Reitman, C. L. Mullican, and G. D. Gardner, Jr. 1957. Applications of germicidal ultraviolet in infectious disease laboratories. III. The use of ultraviolet barriers on animal cage racks. *Proc. Animal Care Panel,* 7: 235–244.

Pillemer, L. 1956. The nature of the properdin system and its interactions with polysaccharide complexes. *Ann. N. Y. Acad. Sci.,* 66: 233–243.

Pincher, C. 1952. A germ-free laboratory. *Discovery (Brit.),* February.

Pitts, T. D., and G. H. Ball. 1955. Further studies on the *in vitro* culture of the larvae of *Ascaris lumbricoides suum. J. Parasitol.,* 41: 47–48.

Pleasants, J. R. 1959. Rearing germfree cesarean-born rats, mice, and rabbits through weaning. *Ann. N. Y. Acad. Sci.,* 78: 116–126.

Pomerat, C. M. 1951. Tissue culture methods. *Methods in Med. Research* 4: 198–291.

Pomerat, C. M. 1961. The use of animal cell, tissue and organ cultures in radiobiology. *Ann. N. Y. Acad. Sci.,* 95: 741–1020.

Portier, M. P. 1905. La vie dans la nature a l'abri des microbes. *Compt. rend. soc. biol.,* 58: 605–607.

Poulson, D. F., and B. Sakaguchi. 1961. Nature of "sex-ratio" agent in *Drosophila. Science,* 133: 1489–1490.

Pra, Dal L. 1960. Germfree animals. *Ann. medicina navole e trop.,* 65: 277–284.

Prentiss, P. C., H. Rosen, and O. J. Malm. 1960. The metabolism of choline by the germ-free rat. *Abstr. 5th Intern. Congr. Nutrition, Washington, D.C., 1960,* p. 25.

Priestley, J. 1796. "Considerations on the Doctrine of Phlogiston and the Decomposition of Water." 142 pp. Thomas Dobson, Philadelphia, Pennsylvania.

Pringsheim, E. G. 1926. Kulturversuche mit chlorophyllführenden Mikroorganismen. V. Methoden und Erfahrungen. *Beitr. Biol. Pflanz.,* 14: 283–312.

Provasoli, L., and K. Shiraishi. 1959. Brine shrimps reared axenically. *Biol. Bull.,* 117: 347–355.

Provasoli, L. K., Shiraishi, and J. R. Lance. 1959. Nutritional idiosyncrasies of *Artemia* and *Tigriopus* in monoxenic culture. *Ann. N. Y. Acad. Sci.,* 77: 250–261.

Raush, R. L., and V. L. Jentoft. 1957. Studies on the helminth fauna of Alaska. XXXI. Observations on the propagation of the larval *Echinococcus multilocularis* Leuckart, 1863, in vitro. *J. Parasitol.,* 43: 1–8.

Reagan, M. J. 1931. "The effect of sterile food on the bacterial flora of the intestines in guinea pigs, B.S. Thesis. Univ. Notre Dame, Notre Dame, Indiana.

Reback, J. F. 1942. "Studies on the intestinal flora of the white rat," M.S. Thesis. Univ. Notre Dame, Notre Dame, Indiana.

Reddish, G. F. 1954. "Antiseptics, Disinfectants, Fungicides, and Chemical and Physical Sterilization," 975 pp. Lea & Febiger, Philadelphia, Pennsylvania.

Rees, C. W. 1955. "Problems in Amoebiasis." Thomas, Springfield, Illinois.

Reid, M. E. 1958. Guinea pig nutrition. *Proc. Animal Care Panel,* 8: 23–33.

Reid, M. E., and G. M. Briggs. 1953. Development of a semi-synthetic diet for young guinea pigs. *J. Nutrition,* 51: 341–354.

Reyniers, J. A. 1930. "Micro-manipulation," M.S. Thesis. Univ. Notre Dame, Notre Dame, Indiana.

Reyniers, J. A. 1932. The use of germfree guinea pigs in bacteriology. *Proc. Indiana Acad. Sci.*, **42**: 35–37.

Reyniers, J. A. 1940a. Biological apparatus. U. S. Patent No. 2,185,711.

Reyniers, J. A. 1940b. Surgical operating device. U. S. Patent No. 2,219,564.

Reyniers, J. A. 1941b. Apparatus for and method of maintaining and working with biological specimens in a germfree controlled environment. Patent No. 2,244,082.

Reyniers, J. A. 1941b. Method and means for preventing cross infection. U. S. Patent No. 2,248,199.

Reyniers, J. A. 1942a. Rearing of a caesarian-born *M. rhesus* monkey under sterile conditions. A preliminary report. *J. Bacteriol.*, **43**: 778 (Abstr.).

Reyniers, J. A. 1942b. How to care for laboratory animals. *Modern Hosp.*, **58**(4): 62–63.

Reyniers, J. A. 1943. Introduction to the general problem of isolation and elimination of contamination. *In* "Micrurgical and Germ-Free Methods" (J. A. Reyniers, ed.), pp. 95–113. Thomas, Springfield, Illinois.

Reyniers, J. A. 1946a. Germ-free life applied to nutrition studies. *Lobund Rept.*, **1**: 87–120.

Reyniers, J. A. 1946b. Surgical operating device. U. S. Patent No. 2,403,400.

Reyniers, J. A. 1946c. Testing of germ-free animals for contamination. *J. Bacteriol.*, **52**: 399–400.

Reyniers, J. A. 1948. Germ-free animals are living test tubes. *Office Naval Research, Research Revs.*, pp. 8–12.

Reyniers, J. A. 1949. Some observations on rearing laboratory vertebrates germfree. *Proc. N. Y. State Assoc. Pub. Health Lab.*, **28**(2): 60–69.

Reyniers, J. A. 1950. Biological apparatus. U. S. Patent No. 2,516,419. (French Patent No. 839,219 and British Patent No. 501,110.)

Reyniers, J. A. 1951a. Germ-free animals and their use. *In* "Science Marches On" (J. Stokley, ed.), pp. 144–147. Ives Washburn Inc., New York.

Reyniers, J. A. 1951b. Germ-free life. *Sci. Counselor*, **14**: 79–81.

Reyniers, J. A. 1952. Introductory remarks and a critical analysis of the mode of action of antibiotics in producing growth stimulation in higher animals and a suggested experimental approach. *In* "Studies on the Growth Effect of Antibiotics in Germ-free Animals," a Colloquium. Univ. Notre Dame, Notre Dame, Indiana.

Reyniers, J. A. 1953. The significance of germfree life methodology (Gnotobiotics) to experimental biology and medicine. *M. S. C. Veterinarian*, **13**: 178–185.

Reyniers, J. A. 1956. Germfree life methodology (gnotobiotics) and experimental nutrition. *Proc. 3rd Intern. Congr. Biochem., Brussels*, pp. 458–466.

Reyniers, J. A. 1957a. Life in a germ-free world. *Cincinnati J. Med.*, **38**: 417–424.

Reyniers, J. A. 1957c. The control of contamination in colonies of laboratory animals by the use of germfree techniques. *Proc. Animal Care Panel*, **7**: 9–29.

Reyniers, J. A. 1957d. The production and use of germ-free animals in experimental biology and medicine. *Am. J. Vet. Research*, **18**: 678–687.

Reyniers, J. A. 1958. Rearing laboratory animals germ-free. *In* "U. F. A. W.

Handbook of Laboratory Animals" (A. N. Worden and W. Lane-Petter, eds.), 964 pp. U. F. A. W. Publ., London.

Reyniers, J. A. 1959a. Design and operation of apparatus for rearing germfree animals. *Ann. N. Y. Acad. Sci.*, **78**: 47–79.

Reyniers, J. A. 1959b. The germfree life program of Lobund Institute, University of Notre Dame: a summation from 1928–1958. Symposium V. *In* "Recent Progress in Microbiology" (G. Tunevall, ed.), pp. 261–287. Almquist & Wiksell, Stockholm.

Reyniers, J. A. 1959c. The pure-culture concept and gnotobiotics. *Ann. N. Y. Acad. Sci.*, **78**: 3–16.

Reyniers, J. A., and M. R. Sacksteder. 1958a. Apparatus and methods for shipping germ-free and disease-free animals via public transportation. *Appl. Microbiol.*, **6**: 146–152.

Reyniers, J. A., and M. R. Sacksteder. 1958b. Observations on the survival of germfree C₃H mice and their resistance to a contaminated environment. *Proc. Animal Care Panel*, **8**: 41–53.

Reyniers, J. A., and M. R. Sacksteder. 1958c. The use of germ-free animals and techniques in the search for unknown etiological agents. *Ann. N. Y. Acad. Sci.*, **73**: 344–356.

Reyniers, J. A., and M. R. Sacksteder. 1959a. Simplified techniques for the production, study and use of germfree animals. *Proc. Animal Care Panel*, **9**: 97–118.

Reyniers, J. A., and M. R. Sacksteder. 1959b. Tumorigenesis and the germfree chicken: a preliminary report. *Ann. N. Y. Acad. Sci.*, **78**: 328–353.

Reyniers, J. A., and M. R. Sacksteder. 1960a. Raising Japanese quail under germfree and conventional conditions and their use in cancer research. *J. Natl. Cancer Inst.*, **24**: 1405–1421.

Reyniers, J. A., and M. B. Sacksteder. 1960b. An explosion instrument for disrupting tissues and cells. *J. Natl. Cancer Inst.*, **25**: 663–681.

Reyniers, J. A., and P. C. Trexler. 1943a. The design of micrurgical machines for use in bacteriology. *In* "Micrurgical and Germ-Free Methods" (J. A. Reyniers, ed.), pp. 5–25. Thomas, Springfield, Illinois.

Reyniers, J. A., and P. C. Trexler. 1943b. The germ-free technique and its application to rearing animals free from contamination. *In* "Micrurgical and Germ-Free Methods" (J. A. Reyniers, ed.), pp. 114–143. Thomas, Springfield, Illinois.

Reyniers, J. A., and P. C. Trexler. 1955. Germfree research: a basic study in host-contaminant relationship. I. General and theoretical aspects of the problem. *Bull. N. Y. Acad. Med.*, **31**: 231–235.

Reyniers, J. A., P. C. Trexler, and R. F. Ervin. 1946. Rearing germ-free albino rats. *Lobund Rept.*, **1**: 1–84.

Reyniers, J. A., P. C. Trexler, R. F. Ervin, M. Wagner, T. D. Luckey, and H. A. Gordon. 1949a. A complete life-cycle in the 'germ-free' Bantam chicken. *Nature*, **163**: 67–68.

Reyniers, J. A., P. C. Trexler, R. F. Ervin, M. Wagner, T. D. Luckey, and H. A. Gordon. 1949b. Rearing germ-free chickens. *Lobund Rept.*, **2**: 1–116.

Reyniers, J. A., T. D. Luckey, P. C. Trexler, R. F. Ervin, M. Wagner, H. A. Gordon, R. A. Brown, G. J. Mannering, and C. J. Campbell. 1949c. Germ-free chick nutrition: development on synthetic-type diets. *Federation Proc.,* **8:** 392–393.

Reyniers, J. A., P. C. Trexler, R. F. Ervin, M. Wagner, T. D. Luckey, and H. A. Gordon. 1949d. Some observations on germ-free Bantam chickens. *Lobund Rept.,* **2:** 119–148.

Reyniers, J. A., P. C. Trexler, R. F. Ervin, M. Wagner, T. D. Luckey, and H. A. Gordon. 1949e. The need for a unified terminology in germ-free life studies. *Lobund Rept.,* **2:** 151–162.

Reyniers, J. A., P. C. Trexler, R. F. Ervin, M. Wagner, H. A. Gordon, and T. D. Luckey, R. A. Brown, G. J. Mannering, and C. J. Campbell. 1950. Germ-free chicken nutrition. I. Gross development and vitamin utilization studies employing White Leghorn chicks. *J. Nutrition,* **41:** 31–49.

Reyniers, J. A., P. C. Trexler, W. Scruggs, M. Wagner, and H. A. Gordon. 1956. Observations on germfree and conventional albino rats after total-body x-radiation. *Radiation Research,* **5:** 591 (Abstr.).

Reyniers, J. A., M. Wagner, T. D. Luckey, and H. A. Gordon. 1960a. Survey of germ-free animals. The White Wyandotte Bantam and White Leghorn Chicken. *Lobund Rept.,* **3:** 7–171.

Reyniers, J. A., M. R. Sacksteder, and W. M. Neal. 1960b. Nutrition of germ-free and conventional *Cotornix coturnix* Japanica (Japanese quail). *Abstr. 5th Intern. Congr. Nutrition, Washington, D.C., 1960,* p. 25.

Riback, J., and J. A. Reyniers. 1949. Personal communication.

Richards, A. G., and M. A. Brooks. 1958. Internal symbiosis in insects. *Ann. Rev. Entomol.,* **3:** 37–56.

Richter, O. 1911. Die Ernährung der Algen. (Monograph.) *Intern. Rev. ges. Hydrobiol. Hydrog.,* **2:** 1–193.

Riker, N. D. 1936. Apparatus and process for killing human and animal vermin. U. S. Patent No. 3,033,357.

Robbins, W. J. 1922. Effect of autolized yeast and peptone on growth of excised corn root tips in the dark. *Botan. Gaz.,* **74:** 59–79.

Robinson, D. L. H. 1956. A routine method for the maintenance of *Schistosoma mansoni in vitro. J. Helminthol.,* **29:** 193–202.

Roe, J. H., and C. A. Kuether. 1943. The determination of ascorbic acid in whole blood and urine through the 2,4-dinitrophenylhydrazine derivative of dehydroascorbic acid. *J. Biol. Chem.,* **147:** 399–407.

Rohrbacher, G. H. 1957. Observations on the survival *in vitro* of bacteria-free adult common liver flukes, *Fasciola hepatica,* Linn., 1758. *J. Parasitol.,* **43:** 9–18.

Rosenthal, S. R., T. Ward, L. Lindholm, and W. Spurrier. 1961. "Antitoxin phenomena in burned or injured germfree rats and mice. *Federation Proc.,* **20:** 32.

Ruegamer, W. R., J. Bernstein, and J. D. Benjamin. 1954. Growth, food utilization and thyroid activity in the albino rat as a function of extra handling. *Science,* **120:** 184–185.

Ryther, J. H. 1959. Potential productivity of the sea. *Science,* **130:** 602–607.

Sacquet, E., R. Vargues, and H. Charlier. 1961. Études sur l'hypo-γ-globulinémie des animaux sans germe (germ-free). *Ann. inst. Pasteur,* **101:** 703–721.

Sagan, C. 1959. Biological contamination of the moon. *Science,* **130:** 1424–1425.

Saito, S. 1955. Studies on physiological functions of *E. coli* group bacteria in the intestinal canal. *J. Chiba Med. Soc.*, **31**: 108–116.

Salle, A. J. 1948. "Fundamental Principles of Bacteriology," p. 730. McGraw-Hill, New York.

Salomonsen, C. J. 1877. "Studier over Blodets Forraadnelse." pp. 172. Kjobenh.

Salzman, N. P. 1961. Animal cell cultures. *Science,* **133**: 1559–1565.

Sandberg, R. L., J. J. Landy, and R. S. Benham. 1961. The sterile plastic isolator as an incubator. *Bacteriol. Proc.*, **1961**: 101.

Sanford, K. K., W. R. Earle, and G. D. Likely. 1948. The growth *in vitro* of single isolated tissue cells. *J. Natl. Cancer Inst.*, **9**: 229–246.

Sang, J. H. 1956. The quantitative nutritional requirements of *Drosophila melanogaster. J. Exptl. Biol.*, **33**: 45–72.

Sang, J. H. 1957. Utilization of dietary purines and pyrimidines by *Drosophila melanogaster. Proc. Roy. Soc. Edinburgh,* **B66**: 339–359.

Sang, J. H. 1959. Circumstances affecting the nutritional requirements of *Drosophila melanogaster. Ann. N. Y. Acad. Sci.*, **77**: 352–365.

Sang, J. H., and R. C. King. 1961. Nutritional requirements of axenically cultured *Drosophila melanogaster* adults. *J. Exptl. Biol.*, **38**: 793–809.

Saussure, N. T. de. 1804. Recherches chimiques sur la végétation. *Recherche Chim.*, **1804**: 206.

Schieblich, M. 1932. Methoden bei Arbeiten über Zusammensetzung und Wirkung der Magendarmflora. *Handb. biol. Arbeitsmethoden (Abt. 4)* **6**: 2, 1894–1920.

Schlössing, T., and A. Munz. 1875. Recherches sur la nitrification par les ferments organisés. *Compt. rend. acad. sci.*, **86**: 892–895.

Schottelius, M. 1899. Die Bedeutung der Darmbacterien für die Ernährung. I. *Arch. Hyg.*, **34**: 210–243.

Schottelius, M. 1902. Die Bedeutung der Darmbacterien für die Ernährung. II. *Arch. Hyg.*, **42**: 48–70.

Schottelius, M. 1908a. Die Bedeutung der Darmbacterien für die Ernährung. III. *Arch. Hyg.*, **67**: 177–208.

Schottelius, M. 1908b. Zur bakteriologischen Technik. *Münch. med. Wochschr.*, **55**: 2186.

Schottelius, M. 1913. Die Bedeutung der Darmbacterien für die Ernährung. IV. *Arch. Hyg.*, **79**: 289–300.

Schröder, H., and T. Von Dusch. 1854. Über Filtration der Luft in Beziehung auf Fäulnis und Gährung. *Annalen der Chemie und Pharmacie.* **89**: 232–243.

Schultz, J., P. St. Lawrence, and D. Newmeyer. 1946. A chemically defined medium for the growth of *Drosophila melanogaster. Anat. Record,* **96**: 540.

Schweinburg, F. B., and E. M. Sylvester. 1953. Bacteriology of the healthy experimental animal. *Proc. Soc. Exptl. Biol. Med.*, **82**: 527–530.

Seaman, G. R. 1952. Replacement of protogen by lipoic acid in the growth of *Tetrahymena. Proc. Soc. Exptl. Biol. and Med.*, **79**: 158–159.

Sedee, P. D. J. W. 1952. Qualitative vitamin requirements for growth of larvae of *Calliphora erythrocephala* (Meig.). *Experientia,* **9**: 142–143.

Sedee, P. D. J. W. 1954. Qualitative amino acid requirements of larvae of *Calliphora erythrocephala* (Meigen). *Experientia,* **9**: 262–269.

Semmelweiss, I. P. 1861. Die Aetiologie, der Begriff und die Prophylaxis des

Kindbettfiebers. 543 pp. C. A. Hartleben's Verlags Expedition. Pest, Wien and Leipzig.

Senft, A. W., and T. H. Weller. 1956. Growth and regeneration of *Schistosoma mansoni in vitro. Proc. Soc. Exptl. Biol. Med.*, **93:** 16–19.

Shaw, E. 1957. Potentially simple technique for rearing "germ-free" fish. *Science,* **125:** 987–988.

Shaw, E. S., and L. R. Aronson. 1954. Oral incubation in *Tilapia macrocephala. Bull. Am. Museum Nat. Hist.*, **103:** 379–415.

Sherman, H. W. 1919. Antibodies in the chick. *J. Infectious Diseases,* **25:** 256–258.

Sieburth, J. M. 1959. Gastrointestinal microflora of Antarctic birds. *J. Bacteriol.*, **77:** 521–531.

Singh, K. R. P., and A. W. A. Brown. 1957. Nutritional requirements of *Aedes aeggptili. J. Inst. Physiol.*, **1:** 199–220.

Slarick, J. 1952. LOBUND: a dream fulfilled. *Notre Dame Scholastic,* **94:** 16–19, 24.

Slater, J. V. 1952. Comparative biological activity of α-lipoic acid and protogen in the growth of *Tetrahymena. Science,* **115:** 376–377.

Smibert, R. M., M. Forbes, J. E. Faber, A. R. Gabuten, and H. M. De Volt. 1959. Studies on "air-sac" infection in poultry. Infection of germ-free turkeys with *Mycoplasma gallinarum* (avian PPLO) from sinal exudate and broth cultures. *Poultry Sci.*, **38:** 676–684.

Smith, C. K., and P. C. Trexler. 1960. Nutrition and physiology of germ-free ruminants. *Abstr. 5th Intern. Congr. Nutrition, Washington, D.C., 1960,* p. 26.

Smith, D. G., and H. J. Robinson. 1945. The influence of streptomycin and streptothricin on the intestinal flora of mice. *J. Bacteriol.*, **50:** 613–621.

Smyth, J. D. 1946. Studies on tapeworm physiology. I. Cultivation of *Schistocephalus solidus in vitro. J. Exptl. Biol.*, **23:** 47–70.

Smyth, J. D. 1947. Studies on tapeworm physiology. III. Aseptic cultivation of larval Diphyllobothriidae *in vitro. J. Exptl. Biol.*, **24:** 374–386.

Smyth, J. D. 1950. Studies on tapeworm physiology. V. Further observations on the maturation of *Schistocephalus solidus* (Diphyllobothriidae) under sterile conditions *in vitro. J. Parasitol.*, **36:** 371–383.

Smyth, J. D. 1954. Studies on tapeworm physiology. VII. Fertilization of *Schistocephalus solidus in vitro. Exptl. Parasitol.*, **3:** 64–71.

Smyth, J. D. 1955. Problems relating to the *in vitro* cultivation of pseudophyllidean cestodes from egg to adult. *Rev. ibérica parasitol.*, **15:** 65–68.

Smyth, J. D. 1958. Cultivation and development of larval cestode fragments *in vitro. Nature,* **181:** 1119–1122.

Smyth, J. D. 1959. Maturation of larval pseudophyllidean cestodes and strigeid trematodes under axenic conditions: the significance of nutritional levels in Platyhelminth development. *Ann. N. Y. Acad. Sci.*, **77:** 102–125.

Smythe, C. V., and C. G. King. 1942. A study of ascorbic acid synthesis by animal tissue *in vitro. J. Biol. Chem.*, **142:** 529–541.

Snow, D. L., and J. L. S. Hickey. 1960. Organizing for germfree research. *Proc. 2nd Symposium on Gnotobiotic Technol., 1959,* pp. 127–144. Univ. Notre Dame Press, Notre Dame, Indiana.

Spallanzani, L. 1765. "Saggio di osservazioni microscopiche concernanti il sistema della generazione dei Sigi di Needham e Buffon." Modena (Taken from Bullock, 1938, p. 75).

Spector, W. S. 1956. "Handbook of Biological Data," 584 pp. Saunders, Philadelphia, Pennsylvania.

Spray, C. M. 1950. A study of some aspects of reproduction by means of chemical analysis. *Brit. J. Nutrition,* 4: 354–360.

Springer, G. F. 1956. Inhibition of blood-group agglutinins by substances occurring in plants. *J. Immunol.,* 76: 399–407.

Springer, G. F. 1959. Einige Aspekte der Möglichkeiten und Grenzen moderner "keimfreier" Methoden für die Wirbeltierimmunologie. *Z. Immunitätsforsch.,* 118: 228–245.

Springer, G. F. 1960. Zum Ursprung der Normalantikörper. *Klin. Wochschr.,* 38: 513–514.

Springer, G. F., R. E. Horton, and M. Forbes. 1958a. Immunogenic origin of anti-human blood group agglutinins in germfree chicks. *Federation Proc.,* 17: 535.

Springer, G. F., R. E. Horton, and M. Forbes. 1958b. Origin of anti-human blood group B agglutinins in White Leghorn Chicks. *Proc. 7th Intern. Congr. Soc. Blood Transf., Rome,* 34: 529–535.

Springer, G. F., R. E. Horton, and M. Forbes. 1959a. Origin of anti-human blood group B agglutinins in germ-free chicks. *Ann. N. Y. Acad. Sci.,* 78: 272–275.

Springer, G. F., R. E. Horton, and M. Forbes. 1959b. Origin of anti-human blood group B agglutinins in White Leghorn Chicks. *J. Exptl. Med.,* 110: 221–244.

Standen, A. 1952. What will scientists think of next? *In* "Science and Society," Symposium, 1950 (R. F. Ervin, ed.). Univ. Notre Dame Press, Notre Dame, Indiana.

Steeves, T. A., I. M. Sussex, and C. R. Partanen. 1955. *In vitro* studies on abnormal growth of prothalli of the bracken fern. *Am J. Botany,* 42: 232–245.

Steeves, T. A., H. P. Gabriel, and M. W. Steeves. 1957. Growth in sterile culture of excised leaves of flowering plants. *Science,* 126: 350–351.

Steinman, H. G., V. I. Oyama, and H. O. Schulze. 1954. Carbon dioxide, cocarboxylase, citrovorum factor, and coenzyme A as essential growth factors for a saprophytic treponeme (S-69). *J. Biol. Chem.,* 211: 327–335.

Stenquist, H. 1934. Die Zellenwanderung durch das Darmepithel. *Anat. Anz.,* 78: 68–79.

Sternberg, G. M. 1881. Methods of cultivating micro-organisms. *Rept. Am. Assoc. Advance Sci., Ann. Monthly Microscop.,* V(1884): 183–185.

Steinberg, R. A. 1941. Use of *Lemna* for nutrition studies on green plants. *J. Agr. Research,* 62: 423–430.

Steinberg, R. A. 1943. Use of *Lemna* as test organisms. *Chronica Botanica,* 7: 420.

Steinberg, R. A. 1949. Symptoms of amino acid action on tobacco seedlings in aseptic culture. *J. Agr. Research,* 78: 733–741.

Stoll, N. R. 1940. *In vitro* conditions favoring ecdysis at the end of the first parasitic stage of *Haemonchus contortus* (Nematoda). *Growth,* 4: 383–406.

Stoll, N. R. 1948. Axenic cultures of *Neoaplectana glaseri* Steiner in fluid media. *J. Parasitol.,* 34: 12.

Stoll, N. R. 1951. Axenic *Noeaplectana glaseri* in fluid cultures. Second report. *J. Parasitol.,* **37:** 18.

Stoll, N. R. 1953a. Axenic cultivation of the parasitic nematode. *Neoaplectana glaseri,* in a fluid medium containing raw liver extract. *J. Parasitol.,* **39:** 422–444.

Stoll, N. R. 1953b. Continued infectivity for Japanese beetle grubs of *Neoplectana glaseri* (Nematoda) after seven years axenic culture. *Lucknow,* Thapar Commemoration Vol., pp. 259–268.

Stoll, N. R. 1954. Improved yields in axenic fluid cultures of *Neoaplectana glaseri* (Nematoda). *J. Parasitol.,* **40:** 14.

Stoll, N. R. 1959. Conditions favoring the axenic culture of *Neoaplectana glaseri,* a nematode parasite of certain insect grubs. *Ann. N. Y. Acad. Sci.,* **77:** 126–136.

Stotsenburg, J. M. 1915. The growth of the fetus of the albino rat from the thirteenth to the twenty-second day of gestation. *Anat. Record,* **9:** 667–682.

Stuart, L. S., and E. H. McNally. 1943. *U. S. Egg and Poultry Magazine,* **49:** 28–31.

Tajima, M. 1955. Fundamental studies on the blood of germfree guinea pigs. *Nagoya Igakkai Zasshi,* **70:** 766–775.

Takeshita, S., and M. Okunda, 1925. On the cultivation of Bancroft's filarial larvae and animal inoculation experiments. *Igaku Chuo Zasshi,* **23.**

Tamiya, H. 1957. Mass culture of algae. *Ann. Rev. Plant Physiol.,* **8:** 309–334.

Tanami, J. 1959. Studies on germfree animals. *J. Chiba Med. Soc.,* **35:** 1–24.

Tanami, J. 1960. Infection and germfree animals. *Modern Media,* **6:** 287–299.

Tanami, J., J. Nakamura, K. Tomioka, and S. Saito. 1957. Studies on bactericidal activity of germfree chicks. *Sogo Iqaku,* **14:** 27–32.

Taylor, A. R. 1959. Theoretical and practical considerations of germfree animals in virology. *Ann. N. Y. Acad. Sci.,* **78:** 102–115.

Taylor, A. R., F. B. Brandon, and J. A. Reyniers. 1959. Fractionation studies of tumor tissues from germfree chickens. *Ann. N. Y. Acad. Sci.,* **78:** 354–370.

Taylor, C. V., and W. J. van Wagtendonk. 1941. Growth studies of *Colpoda duodenaria* in the absence of other living organisms. *J. Cellular Comp. Physiol.,* **17:** 349–353.

Taylor, M. J., J. R. Rooney, and G. P. Blundell. 1960. Experimental anthrax in the rats the relative lack of natural resistance in germfree (Lobund) hosts. *Bacteriol. Proc. (Soc. Am. Bacteriologists).* **13:** 129–130.

Taylor, M. J., J. R. Rooney, and G. P. Blundell. 1961. Experimental anthrax in the rat. II. The relative lack of natural resistance in germfree (Lobund) hosts. *Am. J. Pathol.,* **38:** 625–638.

Teah, B. A. 1959. Personal communication.

Teah, B. A. 1960. Germ-free animal production at Lobund Institute. *Proc. Second Symposium on Gnotobiotic Technol., 1959,* pp. 25–28. Univ. Notre Dame Press, Notre Dame, Indiana.

Thimann, K. V., and J. H. Edmondson. 1949. The biogenesis of the anthocyanins. I. *Arch. Biochem.,* **22:** 33–53.

Thompson, J. C. 1958. Apparatus for maintaining axenic cultures of protozoa. *Turtox News,* **36:** 252–253.

Thorbecke, G. J. 1959. Some histological and functional aspects of lymphoid tissue in germfree animals. I. Morphological studies. *Ann. N. Y. Acad. Sci.*, **78**: 237–246.

Thorbecke, G. J., and B. Benacerraf. 1959. Some histological and functional aspects of lymphoid tissue in germfree animals. II. Studies on phagocytosis *in vivo*. *Ann. N. Y. Acad. Sci.*, **78**: 247–253.

Thorbecke, G. J., H. A. Gordon, B. S. Wostman, M. Wagner, and J. A. Reyniers. 1957. Lymphoid tissue and serum gamma globulin in young germfree chickens. *J. Infectious Diseases*, **101**: 237–251.

Tiegel, E. 1874. Über coccobacteria septica (Billroth) im gesunden Wirbelthier körper. *Virchow's Pathol. Arch. Anat. Physiol.*, **60**: 453–470.

Togano, K. 1958. Studies on germicidal power of serum of germfree animals. *J. Chiba Med. Soc.* **34**: 392–405.

Tomioka, K. 1959. Infection with intestinal bacteria and morphologic changes of the lymph nodes in germfree guinea pigs. *J. Chiba Med. Soc.*, **35**: 347–356.

Trager, W. 1935. The culture of mosquito larvae free from living microorganisms. *Am. J. Hyg.*, **22**: 18–25.

Trager, W. 1941. The nutrition of the invertebrates. *Physiol. Revs.*, **21**: 1–35.

Trager, W. 1947. Insect nutrition. *Biol. Revs., Cambridge Phil. Soc.*, **22**: 148–167.

Trager, W. 1948. Biotin and fat-soluble materials with biotin activity in the nutrition of mosquito larvae. *J. Biol. Chem.*, **176**: 1211–1223.

Treillard, M. 1924. Sur l'élevage en culture pure d'un crustacé cladocère. *Compt. rend. acad. sci.*, **179**: 1090–1092.

Treillard, M. 1925a. *Daphnia magna* Strauss, en culture pure. Perennité de la parthénogenèse; necessité de facteurs bactériens pour l'apparition des formes sexuees. *Compt. rend. soc. biol.*, **93**: 1354–1356.

Treillard, M. 1925b. *Daphnia magna* en culture pure; nutrition liquide et figurée; necessité de facteurs bactériens pour le métabolisme optimum. *Compt. rend. soc. biol.*, **93**: 1592–1594.

Trexler, P. C. 1951. Germ-free animals used in study of nutrition and disease at Notre Dame University. *Instrumentation*, **5**: 41–45.

Trexler, P. C. 1955. U. S. Patents No. 2,705,489; 2,779,331; and 2,786,464.

Trexler, P. C. 1956. Germicides as a step in the elimination of microbic contamination. *Chem. Specialties Mfrs. Assoc., Proc. 45th Ann. Meeting, 1955.*

Trexler, P. C. 1959a. Progress report on the use of plastics in germfree equipment. *Proc. Animal Care Panel*, **9**: 119–125.

Trexler, P. C. 1959b. The use of plastics in the design of isolator systems. *Ann. N. Y. Acad. Sci.*, **78**: 29–36.

Trexler, P. C. 1960a. Gnotobiotics in relation to space biology. *In* "Developments in Industrial Microbiology" (C. Koda, ed.), pp. 12–20. Plenum Press, New York.

Trexler, P. C. 1960b. Flexible-wall plastic film isolators. *Proc. 2nd Symposium on Gnotobiotic Technol., 1959*, pp. 55–60. Univ. Notre Dame Press, Notre Dame, Indiana.

Trexler, P. C. 1960c. Introduction to the symposium. *Proc. 2nd Symposium on Gnotobiotic Technol., 1959*, pp. 1–7. Univ. Notre Dame Press, Notre Dame, Indiana.

Trexler, P. C. 1960d. Sterile rooms. *Proc. 2nd Symposium on Gnotobiotic Technol., 1959*, pp. 121–125. Univ. Notre Dame Press, Notre Dame, Indiana.

Trexler, P. C. 1961. Report of the gnotobiotic workshop for laboratory animal breeders. *Proc. Animal Care Panel*, 11: 249–253.

Trexler, P. C., and E. D. Barry. 1958. Development of inexpensive germfree animal rearing equipment. *Proc. Animal Care Panel*, 8: 75–77.

Trexler, P. C., and L. I. Reynolds. 1957. Flexible film apparatus for the rearing and use of germfree animals. *Appl. Microbiol.*, 5: 406–412.

Underdahl, N. R., and G. W. Kelly. 1957. The enhancement of virus pneumonia of pigs by the migration of *Ascaris suum* larvae. *J. Am. Vet. Med. Assoc.*, 130: 173–176.

Underdahl, N. R., and G. A. Young. 1957a. An isolation brooder for raising disease-free pigs. *J. Am. Vet. Med. Assoc.*, 131: 279–283.

Underdahl, N. R., and G. A. Young. 1957b. An improved hood for swine hysterectomies. *J. Am. Vet. Med. Assoc.*, 131: 222–224.

Vago, F. J., and G. Meynadier. 1961. Culture of tissues from insects reared aseptically. *Compt. rend. acad. sci.*, 252: 2759–2761.

Vanderzant, E. S. 1957. Growth and reproduction of the pink bollworm on an amino acid medium. *J. Econ. Entomol.*, 50: 219–221.

Vanderzant, E. S., and T. B. Davich. 1958. Laboratory rearing of the boll weevil: a satisfactory larval diet and oviposition studies. *J. Econ. Entomol.*, 51: 288–291.

Van't Hoog, E. G. 1935. Aseptic culture of insects in vitamin research. I. *Z. Vitaminforsch.* 4: 300–324.

Van't Hoog, E. G. 1936. Aseptic culture of insects in vitamin research. II. *Z. Vitaminforsch.*, 5: 118–126.

Van Wagtendonk, W. J. 1955. The nutrition of ciliates. *In* "Biochemistry and Physiology of Protozoa" (S. H. Hutner and A. Lwoff, eds.), Vol. II, pp. 57–84. Academic Press, New York.

Ville, G. 1855. Chimie Vegetale—Rapport sur un travail de M. Georges Ville, dont l'object est de prouver que le gaz azoté de l'air s'assimile aux végétaux. (Commission composée de MM. Dumas, Regnault, Payen, Decaisne, Peligot, Chevreul, et rapporteur.) *Compt. rend. acad. sci. (Paris)*, 41: 757–778.

von Brand, T., and W. F. Simpson. 1945. Physiological observations upon larval *Eustrongylides*. IX. Influence of oxygen lack upon survival and glycogen consumption. *Proc. Soc. Exptl. Biol. Med.*, 60: 368–371.

Wagner, M. 1946. "The intestinal bacteriology following complete anal blockage of the adult rat," M.S. Thesis. Univ. Notre Dame, Notre Dame, Indiana.

Wagner, M. 1955. Germfree research: a basic study in host-contaminant relationship. II. Serologic observations in germfree animals. *Bull. N. Y. Acad. Med.*, 31: 236–239.

Wagner, M. 1958. Fecal indol and urinary indican in germfree and conventional (normal stock) animals. *Bacteriol. Proc. (Soc. Am. Bacteriologists)*, 11: 88–89.

Wagner, M. 1959a. Determination of germfree status. *Ann. N. Y. Acad. Sci.*, 78: 89–101.

Wagner, M. 1959b. Serologic aspects of germfree life. *Ann. N. Y. Acad. Sci.*, 78: 261–271.

Wagner, M. 1959c. Personal communication.

Wagner, M. 1960. Determination of germfree status. *Proc. 2nd Symposium on*

Gnotobiotic Technol., *1959*, pp. 83–95. Univ. Notre Dame Press, Notre Dame, Indiana.

Wagner, M., and J. A. Reyniers. 1946. Personal communication.

Wagner, M., and B. S. Wostmann. 1959. Studies on monocontaminated chickens (*Clostridium perfringes* or *Streptococcus faecalis*) fed penicillin. *Antibiotics Ann.*, **1958/59**: 1003.

Wagner, M., and B. S. Wostmann. 1961. Serum protein fractions and antibody studies in gnotobiotic animals reared germfree and monocontaminated. *Ann. N. Y. Acad. Sci.*, **94**: 210–217.

Walcher, D. N., J. Schaeffer, J. Draper, P. Beamer, and P. C. Trexler. 1960. Viral mono-contamination in the gnotobiotic (germfree) animal. *A.M.A. J. Diseases Children*, **100**: 642.

Walter, W. G. 1955. Symposium on methods for determining bacterial contamination on surfaces. *Bacteriol. Revs.*, **19**: 284–287.

Walton, G. N. 1958. "Glove Boxes and Shielded Cells for Handling Radioactive Materials." 515 pp. Academic Press, New York.

Ward, M. 1960. Callus tissues from the mosses *Polytrichum* and *Atrichum*. *Science*, **132**: 1401–1402.

Ward, T. G. 1959. Viruses in germ-free animals. Symposium V. *In* "Recent Progress in Microbiology" (G. Tunevall, ed.), p. 350. Almquist & Wiksell, Stockholm.

Ward, T. G. 1960. The technological problem of testing for viruses in germfree animals. *Proc. 2nd Symposium on Gnotobiotic Technol.*, *1959*, pp. 187–190. Univ. Notre Dame Press, Notre Dame, Indiana.

Ward, T. G. 1961. Spontaneous tumors in the germfree animal. *Federation Proc.*, **20**: 150.

Ward, T. G., and L. I. Lindholm. 1960. Experimental burns in the germ-free animal. *Federation Proc.*, **19**: 103.

Ward, T. G., and P. C. Trexler. 1958. Gnotobiotics: a new discipline in biological and medical research. *Perspectives in Biol. Med.* 1(4): 447–456.

Warren, K. S., and W. L. Newton. 1959. Portal and peripheral blood ammonia concentrations in germ-free and conventional guinea pigs. *Am. J. Physiol.*, **197**: 717–720.

Waterhouse, D. F. 1959. Axenic culture of wax moths for digestion studies. *Ann. N. Y. Acad. Sci.*, **77**: 283–289.

Waterhouse, D. F., and J. W. McKellar. 1961. The distribution of chitinase activity in the body of the American cockroach. *J. Insect Physiol.*, **6**: 185–195.

Weidel, W. 1959. "Virus." University of Michigan Press, Ann Arbor, Michigan. 159 pp.

Weinstein, P. P. 1953. The cultivation of the free-living stages of hookworms in the absence of living bacteria. *Am. J. Hyg.*, **58**: 352–376.

Weinstein, P. P., 1954. The cultivation of the free-living stages of *Nippostrongylus muris and Necator americanus* in the absence of living bacteria. *J. Parasitol.*, **40**: 14–15.

Weinstein, P. P., and M. F. Jones. 1956a. The *in vitro* cultivation of *Nippostrongylus muris* to the adult stage. *J. Parasitol.*, **42**: 215–236.

Weinstein, P. P., and M. F. Jones. 1956b. The effects of vitamins and protein hydrolysates on the growth *in vitro* of the free-living stages of *Nippostrongylus muric* under axenic conditions. *J. Parasitol.*, **42**: 14.

Weinstein, P. P., and M. F. Jones. 1957a. The axenic culture of *Strongyloides ratti* and *Strongyloides sp.* from the *Rhesus* monkey. *J. Parasitol.*, **43**: 45–46.

Weinstein, P. P., and M. F. Jones. 1957b. The development of a study on the axenic growth *in vitro* of *Nippostrongylus muris* to the adult stage. *Am. J. Trop. Med. Hyg.*, **6**: 480–484.

Weinstein, P. P., and M. F. Jones. 1959. Development *in vitro* of some parasitic nematodes of vertebrates. *Ann. N. Y. Acad. Sci.*, **77**: 137–162.

Weller, T. H. 1943. The development of the larvae of *Trichinella spiralis* in roller tube tissue cultures. *Am. J. Pathol.*, **19**: 503–515.

Wellman, C., and F. M. Johns. 1912. The artificial culture of filarial embryos. *J. Am. Med. Assoc.*, **59**: 1531–1532.

Went, F. W. 1957. "The Experimental Control of Plant Growth," 343 pp. Chronica Botanica Co., Waltham, Massachusetts.

Wetmore, R. H. 1953. Tissue and organ culture as a tool for studies in development. *Proc. Intern. Botan. Congr., 7th Congr., Stockholm, 1950*, 369–370.

Wetmore, R. H. 1959. Morphogenesis in plants—a new approach. *Am. Scientist*, **47**: 326–340.

White, C. F. 1937. Rearing maggots for surgical use. *In* "Culture Methods for Invertebrate Animals" (P. S. Galtsoff, ed.), pp. 418–427. Comstock, Ithaca, New York.

White, P. R. 1936. Plant tissue cultures. *Botan. Rev.*, **2**: 419–437.

White, P. R. 1939. Potentially unlimited growth of excised plant callus in an artificial nutrient. *Am. J. Botany* **26**: 59–64.

White, P. R. 1943. Germ-free plants and plant parts as material for physiological and pathological studies. *In* "Micrurgical and Germ-Free Methods" (J. A. Reyniers, ed.), pp. 188–204. Thomas, Springfield, Illinois.

White, P. R. 1946. Plant tissue cultures. II. *Botan. Rev.*, **12**: 521–529.

White, P. R. 1954. "The Cultivation of Animal and Plant Cells," 174 pp. Ronald Press Co., New York.

Whitehair, C. K. 1960. Application of disease-free techniques to livestock production. *Proc. 2nd Symposium on Gnotobiotic Technol., 1959*, pp. 163–169, Univ. Notre Dame Press, Notre Dame, Indiana.

Whitehair, C. K., and C. M. Thompson. 1956. Observations on raising "disease-free" swine. *J. Am. Vet. Med. Assoc.*, **128**: 94–98.

Williams, G. 1959. Virus Hunters, 497 pp. Knopf, New York.

Wilson, G. S., and A. A. Miles. 1955. "Topley and Wilson's Principles of Bacteriology and Immunity." Williams & Wilkins, Baltimore, Maryland.

Wilson, P. W. 1957. On the sources of nitrogen of vegetation, etc. *Bacteriol. Revs.*, **21**: 215–226.

Wilson, P. W., and R. H. Burris. 1960. Fixation of nitrogen by cell-free extracts of microorganisms. *Science*, **131**: 1321.

Wilson, R., and B. Piacsek. 1961. Differential response of germfree and conventional mice to lethal doses of whole body x-irradiation. *Bacteriol. Proc.*, **1961**: 144.

Windmueller, H. G., and R. W. Engel. 1956. Alterations in casein by exposure to ethylene oxide. *Federation Proc.,* **15**: 386.

Wolff, E., and E. Wolff. 1961. Culture de cancers humains sur du rein embryonnaire de poulet explanté "in vitro." *Presse méd.,* **69**(25): 1123–1126.

Wollman, E. 1911. Sur l'élevage des mouches stériles. Contribution à la connaissance du rôle des microbes dans les voies digestives. *Ann. inst. Pasteur,* **25**: 79–88.

Wollman, E. 1913. Sur l'élevage des têtards stériles. *Ann. inst. Pasteur,* **27**: 154–161.

Wollman, E. 1919. Elevage aseptique de larves de la mouche à viande (*Calliphora vomitoria*), sur milieu stérilisé à haute température. *Compt. rend. soc. biol.,* **82**: 593–594.

Wollman, E. 1921. La methode des élevages aseptiques en physiologie. *Arch. intern. physiol.,* **18**: 194–199.

Wollman, E. 1922. Biologie de la mouche domestique et des larves de mouches à viande, en élevages aseptiques. *Ann. inst. Pasteur,* **36**: 784–788.

Wollman, E., and Mme. E. Wollman. 1915. Les microbes dans l'alimentation des têtards. *Compt. rend. soc. biol.,* **78**: 195–197.

Wollman, E., A. Giroud, and R. Ratsimamanga, 1937. Synthèse de la vitamine C chez un insecte orthoptère (*Blattella germanica*) en élevage aseptique. *Compt. rend. soc. biol.,* **124**: 434–435.

Woolpert, O. C. 1936. Direct bacteriological experimentation on the living mammalian fetus. *Am. J. Pathol.,* **12**: 141–151.

Woolpert, O. C. 1952. Pure and mixed cultures. *In* "Science and Society," Symposium, 1950 (R. F. Ervin, ed.). Univ. Notre Dame Press, Notre Dame, Indiana.

Woolpert, O. C., and N. P. Hudson. 1943. The use of the mammalian fetus as an experimental animal in bacteriology, virology, and immunology. *In* "Micrurgical and Germfree Methods" (J. A. Reyniers, ed.), pp. 144–163. Thomas, Springfield, Illinois.

Woolpert, O. C., J. Stritar, I. S. Neiman, F. S. Markham, and N. P. Hudson. 1936. Bacteriologic experimentation on the guinea pig fetus. *Science,* **83**: 419–421.

Woolpert, O. C., F. W. Gallagher, L. Rubinstein, and N. P. Hudson, 1938. Propagation of the virus of human influenza in the guinea pig fetus. *J. Exptl. Med.,* **68**: 313–324.

Wostmann, B. S. 1959a. Nutrition of the germfree mammal. *Ann. N. Y. Acad. Sci.,* **78**: 175–182.

Wostmann, B. S. 1959b. Serum proteins in germfree vertebrates. *Ann. N. Y. Acad. Sci.,* **78**: 254–260.

Wostmann, B. S. 1961a. Recent studies on the serum proteins of germfree animals. *Ann. N. Y. Acad. Sci.,* **94**: 272–283.

Wostmann, B. S. 1961b. Histamine and serotonin in germfree animals. *Abstr. Intern. Congr. Biochem., 5th Congr., Moscow, 1961,* p. 425 (Pergamon Press, London).

Wostmann, B. S., and E. Bruckner-Kardoss. 1959. Development of cecal distension in germfree baby rats. *Am. J. Physiol.,* **197**: 1345–1346.

Wostmann, B. S., and H. A. Gordon. 1958. Electrophoretic studies on serum proteins of young germfree, conventional and antibiotic treated conventional chickens. *Proc. Soc. Exptl. Biol. Med.*, **97**: 832–835.

Wostmann, B. S., and H. A. Gordon. 1960. Electrophoretic studies on the serum protein pattern of the germfree rat and its changes upon exposure to a conventional bacterial flora. *J. Immunol.*, **84**: 27–31.

Wostmann, B. S., and P. L. Knight. 1961. Synthesis of thiamin in the digestive tract of the rat. *J. Nutrition*, **74**: 103–110.

Wostmann, B. S., and J. R. Pleasants. 1959. Rearing of germfree rabbits. *Proc. Animal Care Panel*, **9**: 47–54.

Wostmann, B. S., and N. L. Wiech. 1960. Serum cholesterol values in germfree, monocontaminated, and conventional rats and chickens. *Abstr. 5th Intern. Congr. Nutrition, Washington, D.C., 1960*, p. 14.

Wostmann, B. S., and N. L. Wiech. 1961. Total serum and liver cholesterol in germfree and conventional rats of various ages. Personal communication.

Wostmann, B. S., P. L. Knight, and J. A. Reyniers. 1958. The influence of orally administered penicillin upon growth and liver thiamin of growing germfree and normal stock rats fed a thiamin deficient diet. *J. Nutrition*, **66**: 577–586.

Wostmann, B. S., M. Wagner, and H. A. Gordon. 1960. Effects of procaine penicillin in chickens monocontaminated with *Clostridium perfringens* and with *Streptococcus faecalis*. *Antibiotics Ann.*, **1959/60**: 873–878.

Wright, W., B. P. Phillips, and W. L. Newton. 1959. Germ-free animal research at the National Institutes of Health. Symposium V. *In* "Recent Progress in Microbiology" (G. Tunevall, ed.), pp. 314–326. Almquist & Wiksell, Stockholm.

Wyatt, S. S. 1956. Culture *in vitro* of tissue from the silkworm (*Bombyx mori* L.) ·*J. Gen. Physiol.*, **39**: 841.

Yokogawa, M., T. Oshima, and M. Kihata. 1955. Studies to maintain excysted metacercariae of *Paragonimus westermani in vitro*. *J. Parasitol.*, **41**: 28.

Yokogawa, M., T. Oshima, and M. Kihata. 1958. Studies to maintain excysted metacercariae of *Paragonimus westermani in vitro*. II. Development of the excysted metacercariae maintained *in vitro* at 37° C. for 203 days. *Japan. J. Parasitol.*, **7**: 51–55.

Young, A. G. 1898. Disinfectants and disinfection. *Kennebec Journal Print* (*Augusta*).

Young, G. A., and N. R. Underdahl. 1953. Isolation units for growing baby pigs without colostrum. *Am. J. Vet. Research*, **14**: 571–574.

Young, G. A., N. R. Underdahl, and R. W. Hinz. 1955. Procurement of baby pigs by hysterectomy. *Am. J. Vet. Research*, **16**: 123–131.

Young, G. A., N. R. Underdahl, L. J. Sumption, E. R. Peo, Jr., L. S. Olsen, G. W. Kelly, Jr., D. B. Hudman, J. D. Caldwell, and C. H. Adams. 1959. Swine repopulation. I. Performance within a "Disease-Free" experiment station herd. *J. Am. Vet. Med. Assoc.*, **134**: 491–496.

Zimmerman, A. 1921. Recherches expérimentales sur l'élevage aseptique de l'anguillule du vinaigre. *Rev. suisse zool.*, **28**: 357–380.

Zorkendorfer. 1893. Über die im Hühnerei vorkommenden Bacterienarten nebst Vorschlägen zu rationellen Verfahren der Eikonservierung. *Arch. Hyg.*, **16**: 369–401.

Zweifach, B. W. 1959. Hemorrhagic shock in germfree rats. *Ann. N. Y. Acad. Sci.*, **78**: 315–320.

Zweifach, B. W., H. A. Gordon, M. Wagner, and J. A. Reyniers. 1958. Irreversible hemorrhagic shock in germfree rats. *J. Exptl. Med.*, **107**: 437–450.

Zwillenberg, L. O. 1956. Bacteriologically sterile planarians for tissue culture. *Nature*, **178**: 1183.

ADDITIONAL BIBLIOGRAPHY

1931. *Germ-free Review*, Lisbonne.

1946. *Notre Dame Scholastic*, March 29.

1948. Germ-free Technique. *Science*, **3**: 42 (July).

1949. Life without germs. *Life*, Sept. 26, pp. 107–113.

1949. Unique laboratories erected for University's tests. *The So. Bend Tribune*, Sept. 23, p. 10.

1950. Nutritional studies with germ-free chickens. *Nutrition Revs.* **8**: 212–214.

1951. Radiation sickness research begins in LOBUND Institute. *Notre Dame*, **UND4**: 14–15.

1951. Vitamin requirements of germ-free chicks. *Nutrition Revs.* **9**: 245–247.

1952. Life without germs. *Newsweek*, July 28, pp. 46–48.

1952. Pigs free of all ills. Report of SPF pigs reared by Dr. C. K. Witehair. *Cappers Farmer*, June.

1953. *Book of Popular Science*, pp. 2689–2693.

1953. Hood Pic. *J. Am. Med. Assoc.*, **151**: 41.

1955. Germ-free vs. mode of action of antibiotics. *Chem. Eng. News.*

1958. Germ-free Laboratory (at the University of Michigan), *Science*, **128**: 1563.

1958. They live in a germfree world. *Detroit Free Press*, Nov. 17, p. 14 (J. Pearson).

1958. University of Pennsylvania Project. Germ-free Animal Studies.

1959. Gnotobiotics. *Physicians Bull.* **24**: 3–6.

1959. New simplified germ-free laboratory. *Public Health Repts.* (*U.S.*), **74**(2): 180.

1959. Panel discussion. Germ-free vertebrates: Present status.

1959. Penicillin in germfree chicks. *Nutrition Revs.*, **17**: 236–38.

1959. The gnotobiotic future. *World Med. J.*, **6**: 119–120.

1960. *Arctic Bibliography*, Vol. 1–9. U.S. Govt. Printing Office, Washington, D.C.

1960. Germfree Animals in Medical Research, 16mm color sound movie. United World Films, Inc., New York.

1960. The germ-free animal. *Lancet*, **7119**: 322.

1960. Germ-free animals. *Lancet*, **279**: 86.

1960. Ethylene oxide treatment of diets. *Nutrition Revs.*, **18**: 314–316.

1960. Cecal enlargement in germfree animals. *Nutrition Revs.*, **18**: 313–314.

1961. W. Castle Co., C. E. S. tackles one of the toughest sterilization jobs of all time. *Science*, **133**: 1860.

1961. Clinical vistas for germ-free research. *Roche Medical Image*, **3**: 27–29.

Appendix I

Date	Name	Item
—	Sasruta	Advised cutting of nails and shortening of hair and wearing clean clothes in the operating room.
3000 B.C.	—	Arabs used clay filter-pots to cleanse water.
1300 B.C.	Moses	Leviticus 14: 44–46. ". . . and if disease has spread in the house; it is unclean. And he shall break down the house, its stones and timber and all the plaster of the house; and he shall carry them forth out of the city to an unclean place. Moreover he who enters the house while it is shut up shall be unclean until the evening." Leviticus 15: 3–12. Contamination from those with discharge.
350 B.C.	Aristotle	Systematic separation of species in a zoological garden.
1365	John of Burgundy	Purified air in rooms by fumes of burning sulfur.
1403		Venice established 30 to 40 day isolation hospital for certain travelers before they could enter the city.
1546	G. H. Fracastorius	Recognized a sub-vital element in infection and distinguished between tissue decomposition and contagious disease.
1569	A. Paré	Miasms in air, not pure air itself, contaminate wounds.
1573	J. A. Delacrois	Covered wounds (after the usual alcohol wash) with pitch and oil of turpentine.
1584	A. Paré	Pure air is beneficial to wounds, but air of sick rooms contains dangerous miasms.
1596	Wurtz	Shut doors while changing dressings as rapidly as possible—taught "air" contaminated wounds.
1616	Magatus	Seldom changed dressings since "air contaminated wounds," as in a punctured egg.
1658	A. Kircher	Reported seeing in 1646 "long worms" in blood of plague victims.
	C. Lang	Interpreted these "worms" as being infectious agents.
1675	A. van Leeuwenhoek	Described "little animacules" of the earth. The first clear picture of bacteria was seen.

APPENDIX I (*Continued*)

Date	Name	Item
1676	R. Boyle	Stated disease can best be understood by he who understands fermentation.
1681	D. Papin	Made a closed pressure digester to soften bones—the forerunner of the autoclave (and the steam engine).
1704	J. Colbatch	Fermentation leads to fatal symptoms.
1718	L. Joblot	Boil hay infusion 15 minutes: covered pot shows no growth, the uncovered pot grew abundant living creatures.
1739	P. A. Michele	Said fungi seed (spores) float in the air in "Nova Plantarum Genera."
1764	R. Bilguer	Washed wounds and protected them with cloth soaked in antiseptic instead of promiscuous amputation of wounded limbs.
1765	L. Spallanzani	No spontaneous generation occurs in properly boiled flasks.
1784	B. Bell	Used drainage of wounds and simple dressing to keep objectionable matters from the wound.
1811	F. Appert	Food preservation by heating in closed containers.
1813	H. Davey	Text concluded plants take nitrogen from the air.
1831	W. Henry	Heat inactivated infectious matter of cowpox.
1835	O. W. Holmes	Used lime chloride wash to prevent passing puerperal fever.
1836	H. Davey	Text suggested ammonia as chief form of nitrogen taken from the air by plants.
1837	T. Schwann	Clearly established the connection between putrefaction and microscopic life.
1837	Boussingault	Found plants gain N_2 as grown in "burnt" soil.
1838	Boussingault	Found plants gained 4 times more N_2 than was in the seed; concluded plants take N_2 from the air.
1840	J. Henle	Had the concept of the postulates of Koch.
1840	J. Liebig	Proposed plants need CO_2, H_2O, NH_3, and minerals.
1847–49	Semmelweis	Believed the contagion was "decomposing organic matter" on the hands of students coming from the autopsy room. Antiseptic procedures reduced puerperal fever death 10-fold.

APPENDIX I (*Continued*)

Date	Name	Item
1851	Boussingault	Peas and oats (in sterile sand) in an enclosure gained no N_2. In good soil they grew more luxurious than in the open air.
1853	M. G. Ville	Plants in washed sand gained 40 times more N_2 than was in the seed.
1854	Schroeder and Dusch	Used cotton in culture tubes and in air filtration.
1858	Boussingault	Sterile soil allows no N_2 uptake in plants; unsterile soil allows N_2 uptake.
1860	L. Pasteur	Heat at 110–112° C kills all organisms.
1861	J. B. Laws, J. R. Guilbert, and R. Pugh	Plants die on sterile soil.
1862	M. Jodin	When plants are grown in closed containers, N_2 disappears from the air.
1865–70	L. Pasteur	Developed the germ theory of disease.
1867	J. Lister	Wrote on the antiseptic principle in surgery.
1870	L. Pasteur	Disproved spontaneous generation by completely sterilizing apparatus with heat which neither Pouchet nor J. Wyman had done.
1870	W. Savary J. Lister	Used carbolic acid and Cl_2 to purify air and wounds. Prior to this, antibiosis was used. The wound was kept open to encourage "laudable pus" as the sign of benevolent infection to keep out disease.
1872	J. Schroeter	Made potato slice cultures—some were probably pure cultures.
1872	O. Brefeld	Outlined pure culture concept. Obtained pure cultures by diluting and blotting. Pioneered single cell and hanging drop methods.
1876	M. Nencki	Performed the first ultimate analysis of a ptomaine.
1876	M. Berthelot	Found N_2 was fixed by electricity. When the e.m.f. was lowered, N_2 was still fixed.
1877	M. Berthelot	Dextrin soaked paper increased N_2 fixation.
1877	Schloesing and Munitz	Showed appearance of nitrates in sand is due to living organisms (as predicted by Pasteur in 1862).
1878	J. Lister	Obtained pure cultures by dilution techniques to get single organisms.
1878	R. Koch	Obtained pure culture of *anthrax* by successive passage through animals. Specific germ theory and Koch's postulates.

APPENDIX I *(Continued)*

Date	Name	Item
1881	R. Koch	Put potato slice under glass for surface culture study.
1881	G. M. Sternburg	Grew pure cultures in "needle bulb" system.
1883	R. Koch	Developed pour plates and streak plates with nutrient gelatin to begin the science of pure culture technique of colonies from single cells.
1884	Chamberland	Developed autoclave after adaption of D. Papin's digester.
1885	M. Berthelot	Experiments indicated living organisms fix N_2.
1885	W. O. Atwater	Noted pea plants fix N_2 in closed chamber. He disregarded his data in lieu of the current belief of "authorities" of the day. He later developed whole animal respirometers, another closed system.
1885	E. Ducleaux	Confirmed older work that peas will not grow under sterile conditions. Sterile plants can not use complex sources of nutriment—bacteria are needed to break them down.
1885	L. Pasteur	Statement that he believed animal life would be impossible without intestinal bacteria. He suggested he would try to rear germfree chicks if he were younger.
1885	G. Ville	Studies prove N_2 is taken up by plants.
1886	Hellriegel and Wilforth	Showed cultivated soil caused nodules to form and "sterile" plants grew. Nodules teamed with bacteria. In such "sterile" experiments only legumes survived and had more N_2 than the original seeds.
1886	M. Nencki	Answered Pasteur—bacteria should not be necessary to life.
1887	R. J. Petri	Covered Koch jars to make Petri plates.
1894	A. C. Bernays	"In modern surgery the life of the patient and the result of the operation depends as much upon the precautions against infection as upon the operative skill on the part of the surgeon."
1895	J. Kijanizin	Isolated animals fed sterile food and water became sickly and lost N_2 from their body.
1895	Nuttall and Thierfelder	Obtained germfree guinea pigs. Could not raise them. Established basic techniques for germfree research at the University of Berlin.

APPENDIX I (*Continued*)

Date	Name	Item
1897	Nuttall and Thierfelder	Attempted to rear germfree chicks.
1897	M. Schottelius	Obtained germfree chicks; they did not grow. University of Freiburg.
1898	E. Bogdanow	Obtained germfree fly larvae to study fat synthesis.
1899–1912	M. Schottelius	Worked with chicks on the problem: "Is life possible without bacteria?"
1901	O. Metchnikoff	Germfree tadpoles grew very poorly.
1902	M. Schottelius	Inoculated germfree chicks with bacteria.
1905	O. Metchnikoff	Germfree tadpoles still grow poorly.
1905	E. Moro	Germfree tadpoles grow poorly.
1906–08	E. Bogdanow	Germfree meat fly larvae develop poorly.
1907	M. Cohendy	Began experiments with Schottelius at Freibourg.
1908	M. Schottelius	Inoculated chicks grow better than germfree chicks.
1908	E. Wollman	Germfree meat fly larvae grow poorly.
1910–1912	E. Metchnikoff	Believed animals with few intestinal microorganisms lived long.
1910	E. Küster	Began work as student and assistant to Schottelius at the University of Freibourg.
1911	E. Küster	Ran a pilot operation with germfree goat to show his proposed experiment was possible.
1911	E. Wollman	Germfree flies grow well.
1912	M. Cohendy	Obtained growth in germfree chicks.
1913	E. Guyenot	Meat fly larvae don't survive well in germfree state. Sterile yeast added to the diet reared them through two generations to 10,000 individuals.
1913	E. Küster	Reared a germfree goat 35 days at the University of Berlin.
1913	M. Schottelius	Criticized Cohendy apparatus.
1913	F. Wollman	Reared tadpoles to one month.
1914	M. Cohendy	Attempted to rear germfree guinea pigs with no success.
1914–17	E. Guyenot	Yeast extract can replace yeast. Germfree flies live longer than contaminated flies.
1916	J. Loeb and J. H. Northrop	Yeast helps germfree flies; evolution and nutrition theory.
1917	E. Küster	Reported on his germfree goats which were maintained for a shozt time.
1919	J. P. Baumberger	Germfree flies live longer than conventional flies.

APPENDIX I *(Continued)*

Date	Name	Item
1922	M. Cohendy and E. Wollman	Performed short experiments with germfree guinea pigs infected with virus.
1922	A. W. Bacot and A. Harden	Germfree flies need B vitamins.
1928	G. Glimstedt	Began germfree work with guinea pigs at the University of Lund.
1929	S. Matsumura	Began germfree studies at Chiba University.
1930	J. A. Reyniers	Began germfree work at the University of Notre Dame.
1931	F. F. Murdock and T. L. Smort	Reared sterile fly larvae for surgical use in cleansing tissue of debris.
1932	G. Glimstedt	Published his preliminary work with germfree guinea pigs.
1932	J. A. Reyniers	Obtained germfree guinea pigs.
1933	G. Glimstedt	Germfree guinea pigs survived 5 to 30 days.
1933	K. H. Lewis and E. M. McCoy	Studied root nodule formation of beans in tissue culture.
1934	P. C. Trexler	Began work with J. A. Reyniers at the University of Notre Dame.
1935	R. Kimura with R. Naito and E. Kobayashi	Germfree chicks reared at Kyoto University.
1936	G. Glimstedt	Monograph on lymphatic system of germfree guinea pigs. Reared guinea pigs to 60 days.
1937	—	Biology building at the University of Notre Dame occupied with rooms designed for germfree work.
1937	W. Trager	Sterile mosquito work.
1937	N. Balzam	Studied vitamin B deficiency and intestinal synthesis in germfree chicks. (University of Warsaw)
1937	A. W. Phillips	Began study with J. A. Reyniers at the University of Notre Dame.
1938	R. Glaser	Germfree houseflies grow well.
1940	S. Matsumura and K. Akazawa	Began rearing germfree chicks at Chiba University.
1940–1941	J. A. Reyniers	First patents on germfree apparatus.
1941	M. Wagner	Began study with J. A. Reyniers at the University of Notre Dame.
1942	J. A. Reyniers	Reported germfree monkey experiment.
1942	J. A. Baker and M. S. Ferguson	Grew germfree platyfish to 4 months.
1943	J. A. Reyniers	*Micrurgical and Germfree Methods* published. Details of operation presented.

APPENDIX I *(Continued)*

Date	Name	Item
1943	B. A. Teah	Began working with J. A. Reyniers at the University of Notre Dame.
1943	J. A. Reyniers and P. C. Trexler	Obtained germfree rats, rabbits, mice, and chicks.
1943	B. Gustafsson	Began germfree rat experiments under G. Glimstedt at the University of Lund, Sweden.
1944	J. Pleasants	Joined J. A. Reyniers at the University of Notre Dame.
1944	T. D. Luckey and B. Lakey	Germfree chick nutrition study begun at the University of Wisconsin.
1946	G. Glimstedt	Obtained germfree dogs (not worm-free).
1946	T. D. Luckey	Began work at the University of Notre Dame.
1946	B. Gustafsson	Reared germfree rats through weaning.
1946	H. A. Gordon	Began work at the University of Notre Dame.
1946	J. A. Reyniers, P. C. Trexler, and R. F. Ervin	Germfree rats weaned, Lobund Report 1.
1946	M. Miyakawa	Began germfree work on guinea pigs at Nagoya University. Developed the mechanical arm tank.
1948	Lobund* group	First germfree chicken layed eggs and one hatched.
1949	J. Reback	Returned to Lobund to work on virus problem.
1950	S. Saito and K. Tanikawa	Began systematic study of bacterial antagonisms in gnotophoric chicks, Chiba University.
1951	Lobund group*	First colony of germfree rats started.
1952	J. Tanami	Began rearing germfree chicks and guinea pigs at Chiba University.
1952	T. D. Luckey and B. A. Teah	Reared germfree rabbits to adult size.
1952	B. P. Phillips	Began study on germfree guinea pigs at Lobund.
1954	T. D. Luckey	Began germfree work at the University of Missouri.
1954	P. György and M. Forbes	Began the germfree research laboratory at Walter Reed Army Institute for the University of Pennsylvania.
1955	J. Pleasants	Germfree mice reared at Notre Dame University.

* This group was primarily J. A. Reyniers, H. A. Gordon, M. Wagner, and T. D. Luckey.

APPENDIX I *(Continued)*

Date	Name	Item
1955	A. W. Phillips	Syracuse University germfree laboratory started.
1956	B. Gustafsson	Reproduction in germfree rats, started a second colony.
1956	F. Daft and others	Germfree laboratory started at the National Institutes of Health; a special truck carried germfree rats from Notre Dame to NIH, U.S.P.H.S.
1957	T. Ward	Began study of viruses in germfree mammals.
1957	E. S. Shaw	Obtained germfree guppies.
1958	—	Breeding colony of mice shipped from the University of Notre Dame to National Institutes of Health.
1958	S. Levenson	Began work at Walter Reed Army Institute of Research.
1958	R. E. Horton with G. D. Abrams	Started germfree work at the University of Michigan.
1958	J. Pleasants	Second generation germfree mice survive to begin first mouse colony at the University of Notre Dame.
1959	J. A. Reyniers	Germfree laboratory started at Tampa University.
1959	B. A. Teah	Reproduction in germfree guinea pigs at the University of Notre Dame.
1959	W. L. Newton	Reproduction in germfree guinea pigs at the National Institutes of Health, U.S.P.H.S.
1959	M. Coates and M. Lev	Started germfree work with Gustaffson apparatus at Reading, England.
1959	D. N. Walcher	Germfree colony started at Indiana University Medical Center.
1960	J. Baker	Colony of wormfree dogs preparatory to attempts to obtain germfree and wormfree dogs.
1960	J. J. Landy with S. C. Bausor and T. G. Yerasimides	Germfree work at University of Arkansas to study shock, wound healing, organ transplantation in guinea pigs, experimental surgery, and irradiation.
1960	J. J. Landy and Sandberg	Obtained germfree pigs in June. Growth good.
1960	C. K. Whitehair, C. K. Smith, D. A. Schmidt, and G. L. Waxler	Begin studies on rearing germfree pigs and sheep, using plastic isolators at Michigan State University, the College of Veterinary Medicine.

APPENDIX I (*Continued*)

Date	Name	Item
1960	M. Merkenschlager	Reared germfree chicks at the University of Munich.
1960	E. Sacquet and M. Sabourdy	Ministry of Health, Centre de Selection des Animaux de Laboratoire, Gif-sur-Yvette, France. Received 6 germfree rats from Lobund, via air, to start a colony.
1960	Suter	Began germfree mice research at the University of Florida.
1961	Griesemer	Ohio State School of Veterinary Science begins work in germfree dogs and other mammals.
1961	J. J. Landy and S. Levenson (independently)	Major patient surgery performed in a bacteria-free environment (appendectomy, cholecystectomy, and orthopedics).
1961	B. Gustafsson	Germfree Research Laboratory established at the Karolinska Institutet, Stockholm.
1962	P. de Somer and H. Eyssen	Germfree suite occupied at Louvain University, Louvain, Belgium.
1962	M. Coates	Opened new building designed for research with germfree animals. Reading, England.
1962		Germfree animals became commercially available at the following farms:
		Carworth Farms, Inc. New City, Rockland Company, New York
		Manor Farms Staatsburg, New York
		National Laboratory Animals Creve Couer, Missouri
		Schmidt, C. O. 255 Wilson Mills Road Chesterland, Ohio
		The Charles River Breeding Laboratories Inc. 1018 Beacon Street Brookline 46, Massachusetts

Appendix II

Abiotic	Nonliving (Laboratory parlance).
Af	Antigen free.
Agnotobiotic	Xenic or bearing one or more organisms not known to the investigator. This should differ from the conventional animal in the sense that it may be reasonably expected to determine all living species in the association.
Alpha gnotobiote	An organism shown to be free of all living contaminants by thorough testing over a prolonged period of several generations. (Trexler and Reynolds, 1959).
Antigen free	The state of an organism, or material, which has had no contact with haptens or biologically distinct products of another species which will elicit antibody response.
Antigenostic	Free from unknown antigens excepting those from species known to be present. (From elision of *antigen* and *gnostic*.)
Aseptic	Used by Cohendy to mean free from germs. ("L'absence d'êtres microscopiques." *Duclaux*, 1885).
Axenic	Free from strangers (Baker and Ferguson, 1942). The term is defined to be equivalent to the word germfree rather than the term gnotobiotic. It has been used primarily for protozoa and invertebrates. Plant workers have used sterile in the same connotation.
Axenite	A germfree animal.
Axenity	The state of an axenic organism.
Axenize	To make germfree.
Axenobiosis	The state of germfreeness.
Bacteria free	Authors as Schottelius and Glimstedt used bacterienfrei. The term should mean exactly what it says; it is sometimes used loosely to be equivalent to germfree.
Beta gnotobiote	Designation for germfree animals with a pedigree of germfreeness for several years (Trexler and Reynolds, 1957). It also is applicable to other gnotobiotic states.
Bioincrassation	The concentration of material by taking greater quantities of other constituents from the mixture by a biological action or in a living organism.
Biologically pure	The state of an organism which exists with no direct contact with other living species or their biologically distinctive products. It is designated as Bp.
Bion	Equivalent to germfree animal as proposed by Just (1959). Monobiont, holobiont, and biontology are part of the system proposed.
Bp	Designation to indicate biologically pure, or a species in the monobiotic state. This is a more pure state than the germfree state.

486

Classic	A good term for the conventional (animal) (from *classique* by Sacquet *et al.*, 1961).
Conventional	A designation for polycontaminated organisms found in their usual environment, as the rats in a stock colony maintained with little regard to the total number of species of microorganisms associated with it. Herein designated as animals fed sterilized diets for comparison with gnotobiotic animals. It is designated as Cv. Classic means the same.
Cv	Designates conventional animals; = Bc, or Cn (Reyniers, 1959).
Db	Designation to indicate dibiote or dibiotic.
Dibiote	An organism in the dibiotic state. It can be either species; both species must be identified.
Dibiotic	The state of an organism which exists in intimate contact with only one species other than its own.
Disease free	Organisms which have not been exposed to, or affected by, microorganisms or other infectious agents capable of causing clinical illness. Pathogen free or specific pathogen free are preferred terms since even some germfree animals have diseases.
Gamma gnotobiote	Designation equivalent to germfree with only a short period for examination for contaminants.
Germfree	The condition of existence in the absence of all demonstrable living microorganisms. This word has been used historically as germ free, or germ-free and is equivalent to sterile as used in plant work, pure culture as used by microbiologists, and axenic used in invertebrate work. Nuttall and Thierfelder used *leben ohne Bakterien*. Pasteur expressed the concept with *pure* (aliments purs). Metchnikoff used *privé de microbes* and *privé de germes*. Küster used the word, *Keimfrei*. It developed from germ free (Reyniers) and germfree in the American literature. Other words as monoxenic, *aseptique*, monognotobiotic, biont or holobiont (T. Just), metrobic (A. W. Phillips), bioistic (J. Pleasants), isobiotic (J. F. Reback), have been proposed but are not presented that will soon be adopted. It is designated as Gf.
Gf	Designation to indicate germfree [Phillips and Smith (1959)].
Gnotobiota	Known flora and fauna: The base for related or derived terms.
Gnotobiote	An organism living free from contamination or in association with known organisms. Prefixes to this word such as *monognotobiote* have been suggested; they seem long.
Gnotobiotic	The designation of an organism free from contamination or in association with only organisms known to the investigator. It is designated as Gn.
Gnotobiotics	The field of investigation concerned with organisms which exist free from all others or in association with only other known species.

Gnotobiosis	The condition of existence either with no other species, i.e., germfree, or with only organisms known to the investigator.
Gnotobiology	The study of organisms living by themselves or in association with other known species in the absence of all other demonstrable living organisms.
Gnotophore	An organism in the gnotophoric state. Taken from the Greek: *gnosis* = knowledge and *phorein* = to bear.
Gnotophoresis	The state of existence of an organism bearing one or more known species in intimate contact with it and no other demonstrable viable organism.
Gnotophoric	Designation of an organism which exists in intimate contact with one more known species and no other demonstrable viable microorganisms or infestation of metazoans.
Holobiota	All living organisms. From the Greek: *holos* = entire, and *bioto* = life; or the new Latin term *biota* meaning fauna and flora.
Hormoligosis	Stimulation by small amounts of any agent which is harmful in larger quantities.
Hormology	The study of stimulants and excitation.
Lobund	Designation for *L*aboratories *o*f *B*acteriology, *U*niversity of *N*otre *D*ame which were devoted to germfree research.
Mb	A monobiote or the monobiotic state.
Mf	Monoflora.
Monobiote	The state of an organism which exists in the complete absence of all demonstrable living organisms of other species. This term is more vigorous than that of germfree in the sense that germfree is defined in terms of microorganisms. Germfree guinea pigs have been fed living plants and germfree dogs are not always worm-free; these are dibiotic rather than monobiotic systems. This is one of the few positive terms suggested for the pure culture concept of metazoa; germfree and axenic are negative terms. It is designated as Mb.
Monobiotize	To make equivalent to a pure culture.
Monocontaminated	Organism(s) accidentally exposed to intimate contact with one other species.
Monoflora	Metazoans living in intimate contact with a single species of demonstrable bacteria, mold, fungus, or other plant.
Monofauna	As monoflora with respect to animal species.
Monoxenic	An organism associated with only one other known species. Dixenic, trixenic, and polyxenic are other synxenic states (Dougherty, 1953).
Pathogen free	Free from infectious agents which cause disease. It is similar to disease free.
Pb	Designation of a polybiote or the polybiotic state.
Polybiote	An organism in the polybiotic state, often a conventional animal.
Polybiotic	The condition of existence in which an organism is in direct contact with two or more other species.

Polycontaminated	A host harboring more than one organism which was not purposely added. The host may or may not have been germ-free before contamination.
Pure culture	Only one species present, often progeny of a single cell or clone.
Specific pathogen free	An organism which has been shown by test or past history to be free of specified pathogens.
SPF	Specific pathogen free.
Sterile	Equivalent to germfree but more applicable to inanimate objects.
Syntype	Synthetic type.
Tribiote	An organism which exists in intimate contact with members of two species other than its own. Members of each of the three species would be tribiotes.
Tribiotic	The state of existence in which an organism is in direct contact with members of two other species known to the investigator and no others.
Vf	Designated to indicate virus free.
Virus free	The state in which an organism exists in the complete absence of viruses (symptomatic and asymptomatic). Germ-free animals are not necessarily virus free and virus-free animals need not be bacteria free. Designated as Vf.
Xb	Designated to indicate xenote, xenobiote, or xenic.
Xenbiote	An organism in the xenic state.
Xenbiotic or Xenic	The state of an organism existing with many kinds of organisms, some of which are not known to the investigator. This state is designated Xb.

Appendix III

Diets for Germfree Animals

Syntype Germfree Chick Diets

	L-137 (Luckey)	L-165 (Luckey)	L-240 (Luckey)
Casein, extracted (gm)	25	25	25
Salts II (gm)	5	6	5
Celluflour (gm)	—	—	6
Corn oil (gm)	6	6	7
Starch, corn (gm)	44	45	53
Vitamin A (I.U.)	400	400	600
Vitamin C (mg)	200	200	100
Vitamin D_3 (I.U.)	50	50	100
Vitamin E (mg)	25	25	10
Vitamin K (mg)	5	5	1
Thiamine (mg)	6	6	5
Riboflavin (mg)	3	3	2
Pyridoxine HCl (mg)	2	2	2
Calcium pantothenate (mg)	20	20	10
Nicotinamide (mg)	5	5	10
Choline Cl (mg)	200	200	200
Inositol (mg)	100	100	100
Biotin (mg)	0.04	0.04	0.05
Folic acid (mg)	1	1	2
Vitamin B_{12} (mg)	—	—	0.002
L-Cystine (gm)	0.2	0.2	0.4
Glycine (gm)	—	—	0.5
L-Arginine (gm)	—	—	0.3
Gelatin (gm)	10	10	—
Lactose (gm)	4	4	—
Dried yeast extract (gm)	2	2	—
Liver powder (gm)	2	2	—

PRACTICAL DIETS FOR GERMFREE POULTRY

Components (gm, except where otherwise indicated)	L-124-Chicks (Luckey)	L-289-Chicks (Luckey)	L-318-Turkeys (Luckey)
Corn, cracked	18	49.0	34.2
Soya meal(s)	3.3	23.2	23.2
Alfalfa leaf meal	3.3	2.8	3.7
Wheat	20	9.3	4.65
Milk powder, whole	3.3	—	—
Fish meal	3.3	2.3	8.4
Oats, ground	10	—	2.8
Liver meal	1	—	—
Meat scrap	3.3	2.3	4.65
Salt (iodized)	0.4	0.47	0.37
Viadex (4000 IU Vit. A; 1000 IU Vit. D)	0.4[a]	0.23	0.16
$CaCO_3$	2	1.67	0.74
$CaHPO_4$	—	1.49	0.74
Na_2HPO_4	1	—	—
$MnSO_4 \cdot H_2O$	0.006	0.024	0.026
K_2HPO_4	1	—	—
Corn gluten meal	—	—	3.7
Brewer's yeast, dried	1	—	4.65
Fish solubles	—	—	1.86
Casein	12	—	—
Starch, corn	16	—	—
Riboflavin (mg)	0.5	—	—
Niacin (mg)	2.5	—	—
Choline Cl (mg)	50	—	—
Ca pantothenate (mg)	3.5	—	—
Biotin (mg)	0.005	—	—
Folic acid (mg)	0.25	—	—

[a] Cod Liver Oil.

DIETS USED FOR GERMFREE GUINEA PIGS

Ingredients (gm)	L-412-D[a] (Phillips)	L-445-S[b] (Phillips)	L-463-S[b] (Phillips)	NG-36 (Miyakawa)	No. 1 (Landy)
Purina Lab Chow[c]	200	100	—	70[e]	—
Oats, rolled	100	100	100	—	—
Dextrose	12	10	10	9[f]	—
Grass powder	6	—	—	12[g]	—
Sodium chloride	—	5	5	—	—
Calcium carbonate	3	—	—	—	—
Ascorbic acid (mg)	10/day	10/day	10/day	25/2 days	75
Water	—	1000	1000	—	1000
Alphacel	15	—	—	—	—
Calcium chloride	3	—	—	—	—
Mixed tocopherols	2	—	—	—	—
Liver extract	—	—	—	0.025	—
Whole dry yeast	—	15	—	0.5	—
Inositol	—	—	—	0.1	—
Wheat germ	—	—	100	—	—
Homogenized cow's milk	—	—	—	—	750
Mineral mixture[d]	—	—	—	7[h]	4
Thiamine HCl (mg)	—	5	—	9	12.5
Riboflavin (mg)	—	—	—	2	3
Pyridoxine HCl (mg)	—	—	—	2	1.5
D-Pantothenyl alcohol (mg)	—	—	—	10	15
Biotin (mg)	—	—	—	0.1	—
Nicotinamide (mg)	—	—	—	—	50
Folic acid (mg)	—	—	—	2.5	—
Choline (mg)	—	—	—	300	—
Vitamin B_{12} (mg)	—	—	—	—	0.025
Vitamin K (mg)	—	—	—	2.5	+
p-Aminobenzoic acid (mg)	—	—	—	5	—

[a] D = Dry
[b] S = Semisolid.
[c] Purina Mills, Buffalo, N.Y.
[d] Mineral mix: $FeSO_4 \cdot 7H_2O$ (49.8 gm)
               $MnSO_4 \cdot H_2O$ (3.2 gm)
               $CuSO_4 \cdot 5H_2O$ (3.9 gm)
               KI   (0.26 gm)
               Water   (to 1 liter)
[e] Roasted soybean flour.
[f] Sucrose.
[g] Gum arabic
[h] Composition not given. Additional vitamin preparations were given.

MILK FORMULA FOR RATS[a]

Constituent	24N (Reyniers et al.)	Diet L-102 (Luckey)	L-135 (Luckey)	1-185 (Luckey)	L-220 (Luckey)
Cream (20%)	75.8 gm	75.8	—	75.8 gm	50 gm
Casein	17.75 gm	8 gm	8 gm	8 gm	8 gm
β-Lactose	—	—	3 gm	—	—
HMW Salts-F	0.8 gm	0.8 gm	1 gm	0.8 gm	0.8 gm
Lactalbumin	0.6 gm	0.6 gm	0.6 gm	—	0.5 gm
Butter (sweet)	—	—	13 gm	—	17 gm
Lecithin	—	—	0.1 gm	—	—
Vitamin A	—	—	300 I.U.	2000 I.U.	—
Vitamin D_3	—	—	100 I.U.	165 I.U.	—
Vitamin E	—	—	50 mg	—	—
Vitamin K_3	—	—	0.5 mg	—	—
Thiamine chloride	—	—	1 mg	—	1 mg
Riboflavin	—	—	1.2 mg	—	1.2 mg
Pyridoxine HCl	—	—	1.2 mg	—	1.2 mg
Nicotinamide	—	—	1.2 mg	—	1.2 mg
Choline chloride	—	—	30 mg	50 mg	30 mg
Biotin	—	—	0.01 mg	0.005 mg	0.010 mg
Calcium pantothenate	—	—	2.5 mg	0.5 mg	2.5 mg
Folic acid	—	—	0.1 mg	0.1 mg	0.1 mg
Water (+ca. 0.5 cc 0.9% NaOH; 6 ml)	—	15 ml	74 ml	15 ml	19 ml
$MnSO_4 \cdot H_2O$	—	—	—	0.6 mg	—
Cocoanut-lard	—	—	—	—	5 gm

[a] All diets supplemented with 4 mg ascorbic acid and 6.25 mg of $NaKHPO_4$.

COMPOSITION OF DIETS FOR GERMFREE RATS

Constituent	Unit	L-103 (Luckey)	L-109 (Luckey)	L-128a (Luckey)	L-120 (Luckey)	L-356b (Luckey)	L-283 (Luckey)	K-deficient (Gustafsson)	D-7 (Gustafsson)	L-462 (Wostmann)	L-222 (Luckey)
Casein, vitamin-free	gm	25	25	20	25	20	25	22	22	5	15
Corn starch	gm	58	54	0.5	59	—	59	—	—	0.1	75
Corn oil	gm	5	6.8	1	6.8	2	5	10[c]	10	2	8
Cellophane spangles	gm	—	2	3	2	5	2	—	—	—	—
Salts II	gm	6	2	5	6	5	6	4.0[d]	4.0[d]	1.9[e]	2
Vitamin A	I.U.	400	800	800	800	800	800	2100	2100	800	800
Vitamin D_3	I.U.	50	100	100	100	100	100	450	450	100	—
Ascorbic acid	mg	200	200	200	200	200	2000	100	100	—	200
α-Tocopherol	mg	25	50	50	50	50	50	50	50	37.5	—
Vitamin K_3	mg	5	10	10	10	10	—	—	1	10	—
Thiamine HCl	mg	1.5	6	6	6	6	5	5	5	3	1
Riboflavin	mg	1	3	3	3	3	3	2	2	1.5	1
Nicotinamide	mg	5	5	5	5	5	5	20	20	2.5	—
Nicotinic acid	mg	5	—	—	5	5	5	—	—	2.5	—
Calcium pantothenate	mg	20	30	30	30	30	30	10	10	15	4
Inositol	mg	100	100	—	100	100	—	100	100	—	—
Choline chloride	mg	200	200	200	200	200	200	200	200	100	50
Pyridoxine HCl	mg	1	2	2	2	2	2	2	2	1	0.5
Biotin	mg	0.1	0.1	0.1	0.1	0.1	—	0.1	0.1	0.05	—
Folic acid	mg	1	1	1	1	1	—	2	2	0.5	—
Vitamin B_{12}	μg	—	—	—	—	2.5	—	2	2	0.001	—
p-Amino benzoic acid	mg	5	5	5	5	5	5	30	30	2.5	—
Pyridoxamine HCl	mg	0.3	0.4	0.4	0.4	0.4	0.4	—	—	0.2	—
β-Pyracin	mg		1	1	1	1					
Wheat starch	gm	—	—	—	—	—	—	63	63	—	—
Yeast extract	gm	2	2.5	2	2	2	—	—	—	2	—
Liver extract	gm	3	2.5	2	—	2	—	—	—	—	—
Rice (polished)	gm	—	—	62	—	58[f]	—	—	—	—	—
Hydrogenated oil	gm	—	—	5	—	5	—	—	—	—	—
Flour, wheat	gm	—	—	—	—	—	—	—	—	30	—
Corn meal	gm	—	—	—	—	—	—	—	—	32	—
Lactalbumin	gm	—	—	—	—	—	—	—	—	10	—
Milk powder	gm	—	—	—	—	—	—	—	—	10	—
Alfalfa leaf meal	gm	—	—	—	—	—	—	—	—	2	—

[a] Plus 5% sugar water ad libitum. Diet L-III is identical without cellophane.
[b] Also used for mice and rabbits.
[c] Peanut oil.
[d] HMW salts.
[e] Salts L-17 are the trace minerals of salts L-11 + 0.3% NaCl and 0.6% $CaCO_3$.
[f] Rice flour.

MILK FORMULAS FOR GERMFREE RATS, MICE,[a] AND RABBITS

Components	420 (Pleasants)	449-G-E-1 (Wostmann-Pleasants)	449 C (Pleasants-Wostmann)
Cow's milk (whole) (ml)	50	25	50
Light cream (18%) (ml)	50	75	50
Vi-syneral (ml)[b]	0.1	0.2	0.2
Mixed tocopherols (mg)	1.7	6.6	3.3
Vitamin K (mg)	0.17	0.33	0.33
DL-Methionine (gm)	—	0.2	0.2
L-Tryptophan (gm)	—	0.06	0.06
Skim milk protein (gm)	—	6.00	4
L(—)-Cystine (gm)	—	0.1	—
Choline hydrogen citrate (gm)	—	0.1	—
Salts (Fe^{++}, Cu^{++}, Mn^{++})	+	+	+

[a] Mice diets were fortified with 0.05% quercetin.

[b] Vi-syneral aqueous vitamin drops (U.S. Vitamin Corporation, New York, New York).

MISCELLANEOUS DIETS

Constituent	Units	Lamb[a] Diet U-3 (Luckey)	Rabbits[b] L-461B-E1 (Wostmann and Pleasants)	Pigs Diet-1 (Landy)	Rats (Himsworth)
Casein	gm	30	7	—	—
Corn oil	gm	8	0.7	—	7.0[c]
Glucose	gm	48	—	—	—
Alpha cell	gm	3	—	—	—
Cellophane	gm	3	—	—	—
Salts L-I	gm	8	—	0.4	3.0[d]
Vitamin A	I.U.	10,000	280	—	—
Vitamin D$_3$	I.U.	2,000	35	—	—
Ascorbic acid	mg	1,000	35	7.5	—
α-Tocopherol	mg	10	52.5	—	—
Vitamin K$_3$	mg	1	3.5	—	0.2
Thiamine HCl	mg	2	1.75	1.25	4.0
Riboflavin	mg	2	0.7	0.3	0.4
Niacinamide	mg	10	3.5	5.0	—
Calcium pantothenate	mg	5	3.5	1.5	2.0
Inositol	mg	200	35	—	—
Choline chloride	mg	200	70	—	—
Pyridoxine HCl	mg	2	0.7	0.15	0.3
Biotin	mg	0.1	0.018	—	—
Folic acid	mg	2	0.7	—	—
Vitamin B$_{12}$	mg	0.05	0.0007	0.0025	0.02
Rabbit chow	gm	—	62	—	—
Bran, ground	gm	—	30	—	—
Starch, Corn	gm	—	0.2	—	79.5
Milk[a]	ml	—	—	85.0	—
Yeast, Brewer's		—	—	—	18

[a] The goats of Küster, the monkeys of Reyniers, the pigs of Walker, and the lamb of Smith and Trexler were fed milk as the basic diet with trace elements and other supplements.

[b] The rabbits of Luckey and Teah were fed diet L-109.

[c] Peanut oil 5.8 gm and cod liver oil, 1.2 gm.

[d] Salts USP III.

SALT MIXES
(gm/100 gm diet)

Compound	L-I	L-II	L-15	HMW[a]
$CaCO_3$	1.8	1.80	1.2	54.3
$CaHPO_4$	1.35	0.33	0.22	—
K_2HPO_4	—	1.35	0.90	—
Na_2HPO_4	1.20	1.20	0.80	—
NaCl	0.3	0.30	0.20	6.9
KI	0.0045	0.005	0.003	0.008
$MnSO_4 \cdot 4H_2O$	0.075	0.075	0.05	0.035
$MgSO_4 \cdot 7H_2O$	0.45	0.45	0.30	1.6 anhydrous
Fe(citrate)(ic)	0.45	0.45	0.30	—
$CuSO_4 \cdot 5H_2O$	0.023	0.023	0.015	0.09 anhydrous
$CoCl_2 \cdot 6H_2O$	0.003	0.003	0.002	—
$ZnSO_4 \cdot 7H_2O$	0.006	0.006	0.004	—
$Na_2B_4O_7 \cdot 10H_2O$	0.003	0.003	0.002	—
$AlK(SO_4)_2 \cdot 12H_2O$	0.0045	0.005	0.003	0.017
$MgCO_3$	—	—	—	2.5
NaF	—	—	0.001	0.1
$FePO_4 \cdot 4H_2O$	—	—	—	2.05
KH_2PO_4	—	—	—	21.2
KCl	—	—	—	11.2
MgO	.4	—	—	—
K-acetate	2.0	—	—	—
$Na_2B_4O_7 \cdot 10H_2O$	0.003	0.003	0.002	—
$Na_2MoO_3 \cdot 2H_2O$	0.03	—	0.002	—

[a] According to Hubbel, Mendel, and Wakeman (1937).

Index

A

Abdomen, 288, 289
Abnormalities, 381–388
Absorption, 234, 251, 253, 341
ACTH, 360
Actidione, 48
Adapter, 205
Adrenal gland, 259, 260, 367, 427
Adrenal necrosis, 265
Aedes aegypti, 56
Aerobacter aerogenes, 85, 404, 419, 423
Af, *see* Antigen free, 30
Agammaglobulinemia, 20
Agar, 66, 380
Agent, transmissable, 197
Agglutinin, 370, 407, 417
Aging, 14, 355, 389
Agria affinis, 58, 59
Air, 61, 64, 100, 110, 111, 130, 141, 156, 157, 159, 160, 283
  exhaust, 21, 123, 156
Albumin, serum, 329
Alcaligenes, 402
Alcohol, 66, 144, 147, 148
Algae, 39, 67, 170
Alkylating compounds, 147
Antagonism, *in vivo,* 409–413
Alopecia, 239, 266
Alpha gnotobiote, 31
Amino acid, 44
Ammonia, 149, 150, 203, 357
  blood, 329
  urine, 357
Amnion, 187
Amoeba histolytica, 195
Amoebiasis, 422
Amoebic lesion, 423
Amphibia, 68, 173, 285
Amylase, 343, 351
Anal block, 207, 385

Ancyclostoma braziliense, 52
  caninum, 52, 424
  duodenal, 52
Anesthesia, 177
Animal, antigen free, 12, 31, 218, 399
  arctic, 7
  biologically impure, 17
  conventional, classic, 17, 31, 283
  dibiotic, 26, 402
  experimental, 17, 127
  gnotobiotic, 96, 171
  gnotophoric, 26
  inoculated, 26, 107
  monobiotic, 218
  monoinoculated, 27
  triflora, 26
  virus free, 20
Animal cell, culture, 42
Annelida, 52
Anorexia, 260, 382
Anoxia, 382
Antibiotic sterilization, 223
Antibiotics, 27, 40, 42–45, 58, 163, 209, 224, 269, 278–280, 387
Antibody, 186, 197, 198, 370, 371, 373, 374, 380, 408
  formation, 20, 253
  plant, 42
Antigen, 163, 193, 373
Antigen free, 9, 12, 20, 25, 30, 99, 399
Antigenic reaction, 9
Appearance of animals, 286
Appetite, 78
Application, practical, 21
Arm, mechanical, 101, 121
Armadillo, 24
Arthropoda, 53, 196
Ascaris lumbricoides, 425
Ascorbic acid, *see* Vitamin C
Aschelminthes, 48
Aseptic procedure, 23, 40, 48, 170, 209

Asexual propagation, 40
Ash, *see* specific tissues
Aspergillus niger, 351
Autolysis, 390
Autopsy, 205
Aves, 70
Axenic state, 28, 43, 284
Axone, 41

B

Bacillus anthracis, 418
  coli (gallinorium), 56, 73
  megatherium, 209
  proteus, 56, 419
  pseudonthracis, 53
  putrificus, 56
  stereothermopholus, 223
  subtilus, 10, 201, 402, 413, 417, 419, 423
Bacteria, 7, 425
  harmful, 69
  in germfree feces, 179, 427
Bacteremia, 387
Bacteria-host gnotobiotes, 402
Bacterial fermentation residue, 276
Bacterophogous strongyles, 49
Balance study, 251, 252, 265, 266
Barbiturate, 226
Barrier, 10
  bacterial, 172
  biological, 172
  isolation, 6, 106
  microbial, 99
  physical, 100
Basophil, 326
Bath, germicidal, 110
Beak, 291, 332, 359
Bean sprout, 245
Bedding, 11
Bell, diving, 109
  jar, *see* Jar, bell
Beri beri, 79
Beta globulin, 417
Beta gnotobiote, 31
Beta propriolactone, 147
Bile, 355
  chemical analysis, 355, 356
Biochemistry, *see* specific tissues

Bioincrassation, 193, 253, 254, 348
Biological value, 218
  individuality, 14
Biologically pure, 29
Biosynthetic potential, 213
Biotin, 265, *see also* specific tissues
  deficiency, 265, 266
Biotron, 23, 221
Birds, 70, 173, 287
Blanket, insulation, 153
Blatella germanica, 59
Blood, 45, 53, 61, 186, 187, 193, 195, 284, 409
  chemical composition, 327
  cells, red, 267, 325
  clearance, 380
  clotting, 274, 327
  morphology, 320–327
  vessels, 311, 388
  volume, 325
Bone, 240, 270, 271, 294, 295, 296
  alveolar, 384
  ash, 239, 255, 256
  chemical composition, 239, 258, 271, 294
Bone marrow, 268
Boric acid, 69, 173
Bouillon, 41, 185
Brachionus variabilis, 48
Brain, 230, 260, 271, 359
Brain heart infusion agar, 187
Bread, 68, 69
Breathing, 389
Bromine water, 40
Bronchi, 260, 332
Broth, infusion, 66
Building, germfree, 133
Burn, 387
Bursa fabricius, 265, 363
Butyric acid, 234
B-vitamin, 253

C

Caenorhabditis briggsae, 49
Cages, 99, 138
  breeding, 139
  control, 284

holding, 138
ideal germfree, 100
metabolism, 139
space, 140
sterilization, 150
transfer, 138
Calcium, 256
  chloride, 158
  hypochlorite, 40
Calculus, oral, 383
Capillary formation, 388
Carbohydrate utilization, 218
Carbon, 380
  dioxide, 149, 161
Carborundum, 111
Carcinoma, mammary, 379, 420
Caries, dental, 384, 418
Carmelization, 220
Carnitine, 56, 310, 353
Carrot root, 42
Casein hydrolyzate, 85
Cataract, 239
Cathepsin, 390
Cautery, 177
Cecal contents, 346
  B-vitamins in, 265, 403–405, 415
Cecal wall, 346, 416
Cecum, 193, 343, 344, 427
  distension, 14, 65, 81, 83 85, 86, 89,
      241, 247, 248, 252, 254, 277,
      286, 288, 289, 345, 346, 384,
      387, 416, 427
Cell,
  dead, 2, 399
  mesenchymal, 389
  red blood, 325, 422
  reticulo-endothelial, see Reticulo-
      endothelial cells
  white blood, 325, 422
Cell theory of biology, 2
Cellfree filtrates, 402
Cellulose, 213, 350
  digestion, 214
Cesarean entry, 137
Cesarean operation, 15, 23, 85, 88, 93,
    96, 121, 170, 171, 174, 177, 195,
    382, 420, 421
Cestoidea, 46

Chamberland candle, 173
Characteristics of germfree animals,
    283, 286
Chemical hood, 21, 24
Chick, 13, 70–81, 241, 265, 271, 291–
    389
  monocontaminated, 73, 79, 402
  paralysis, 265
Chilo suppressalis, 57
Chitinase, 59
Chloramine-T, 45
Chlorella, 39, 48
Chlorella pyrenoidosa, 48
Chloromycetin, 209
Chlorophyceae, 39
Chlorotetracycline, 48
Cholera vibrio, 402
Cholesterol, 351, 353
  adrenal, 260, 367
  serum, 328, 367
Cholic acid, 351
Choline, 221, 269
Choristoneura fumiferana, 58
Cilia, 369
Circulatory system, 311
Citrovorum factor, 268
Claws, 291
Clay, 249
Clorine, 147, 218
Clostridium bifermentans, 407
  perfringens (welchii), 217, 351, 405,
      407, 408, 417, 418
  sporogenes, 408
  welchii, see Cl. perfringens
Clotting time, 260, 274
Cobalt source, 144
Cold trap, 156
Colon, 343
Colostrum, 235, 249
Colostrum factor, 227, 229
Comb, 291
Complement, 371, 377
Composition, body, 289, 290, 292, 293
  see specific tissues
Connective tissue, 340
Contaminant, 15, 16, 18, 195, 201 see
    also Detection
Contamination, 6, 10, 14, 15, 66, 148,

187, 189, 199, 201, 202, 206, 213, 345
planets and celestial vehicles, 5, 22, 24
Control, 16, 399
Conventionalization, 425, 426
Corn root tip, 41
Corpus luteum, 368
Cortisone, 360
Cotton, 168
Creatine, 269
Cresol, 147, 247
Crop, 337
Crowding, 58, 248
Crustacea, 53
Culture,
    continuous suspension, 43
    tissue and organs, 41, 42, 43, 199
Cysteine, 148, 423
Cysts, 196
Cystococcus, 39
Cytopathogenic agent, 197

D

Death, 389
Decontamination, 5, 15, 17, 22, 23, 60, 172, 206, 208, 401
Defecation, 383
Defense mechanisms, 14, 20, 27, 42, 172, 368
Dental caries 27, 418
Dermatitis, 266
Detection,
    of microbial contamination, 3, 6, 15, 58, 65, 66, 67, 69, 104, 142, 143, 179–188, 192, 205, 398, 401
Detergent, 168, 169, 201, 203
Deuterium, 269
Diaprene chloride, 131, 149, 169, 178
Diarrhea, 257, 266, 409, 413
Diatoms, 40
Dibiotic system, 26, 30, 48, 400–426
Diet, 242
    antigen free, 12, 164, 216
    bacteria free, 12
    bacteria in, 278
    biotin deficient, 265
    browning reaction, 218

cariogenic, 418
changes during sterilization, 218
chemically defined, 24, 59, 245
chicken, 242
cream base, 237
dead microorganisms in, 216
egg yolk, 237
fish, 242
folic acid low, 266
guinea pigs, 245
high fat, 237
holidic, 49
marginal, 207
mice, 248
monkey, 249
pig, 249
preparation, 205
quail, 245
rabbit, 248
radiation sterilized, 223
rat, 247
riboflavin deficiency, 265
ruminants, 248
sterilization, 16, 161, 162, 219, 221
synthetic, 163, 216
thiamine deficient, 279
turkey, 245
Digestion, 214, 251
Digestive system, 337
Dinoflagellates, 40
Dirofilaria immitis, 52
Disease, 381
    free colony, 6, 15, 19
    free stock, 14, 21, 31, 40, 96
    physiological, 12, 20, 389
Disposable isolators, 133
Dissociation, 399
Dog, germfree, 7, 90, 195
Dreft, 173
Drosophila ampelophilla, 56
Drosophila melanogaster, 53, 57
Dry boxes, 21, 24, 106
Dry weight, see specific tissue, 221, 289, 294
Dugesia orotocephalia, 45
Dunk tank, 11
Duodenum, 343
Dutchman, 205

E

Ear, 357, 360
Ecology, 5, 6
Eggs, 6, 14, 20, 23, 45, 53, 58, 61, 68,
    169, 171, 424
    albumin, 68, 361, 379
    production, 81, 368
    sterilization, 45, 48, 49, 168, 173,
        200
Electricity, 141
Electron beam sterilization, 144, 163,
    221, 223
Electrophoretic pattern, of serum pro-
    tein, 330, 416
Elimination, 225
Embryo, 6, 14, 15, 61
Enchytraeus fragmentosus, 52
Endamoeba histolytica, 422, 423
Endocarditis, 27
Endocrine glands, 366
Energy, 217, 254
Enlarged ceca, *see* Cecum
Enteritis, 409
Entry, sterile, 136, 137, 154
Envelope, plastic, 105
Environment, 283
    sterile, 4, 48, 209
Enzyme, *see also* specific enzymes
    digestive, 63, 390
Eosinophil, 325, 326
Epidermis, regenerating, 388
Epididymus, 367
Epithelium, ciliated, 363
Ergothionine, 328
Escherichia coli, 7, 48, 52, 79, 81, 351,
    376, 380, 381, 402, 408, 409, 411,
    412, 416, 417, 418, 423, 425
Estrous cycle, 367
Ether, 66, 146, 170, 177, 226
Ethyl sulfate, 357
Ethylene amine, 147
Ethylene oxide, 45, 121, 147, 149, 154,
    163, 223, 254
Euglenaphyceae, 39
Euglobulin, 329
Eumycophyta, 35
Evans blue, 380

Ewes, 178
Examination unit, 111, 136
Excretion, 251
Excretory system, 356
Exemplar, 100, 101, 203
Exhaust, free flow, 143
Eye, 359

F

Fat, 63, 94, 213, 221, 231, 235, 253,
    295, 388
    (*see* specific tissue)
Fatty acid, 44
Fatty alcohol, 57
Fatty liver, 231
Feathers, 291
Fecal smears, 186, 193
Feces, 252, 343, 349
Feed, 250
Femur, 294
Fetal guinea pig, 413
Fetus, 6, 23, 413, 414
Fiber, 241, 277, 345, 350
Fibroblast, 41
Fibrosarcoma, 386
Filter, 111, 138, 160
    Cambridge low pressure, 130, 160
    cotton, 156
    electrostatic, 145
    forced air, 138
    free flow, 138
    glass wool, 156, 187
Filtration, 163
Fish, 66, 172, 242, 284
Flame, 40
Fleming nodule, 362
Flora,
    fixed, 207
    intestinal, 18, 57, 60, 64, 284
    locked, 16, 22
    microbial, 19
    uncontrolled, 19
Fluorine, 305
Folic acid, 56, 221, 223, 268, *see* spe-
    cific tissue
    deficiency, 262, 263, 266–268

Food, 11, 61, 64, 161, 217
  efficiency, 251
  restriction, 241
Formaldehyde, 52, 58, 67, 121, 127,
    147–150, 158, 168, 382
Foster mother, 15, 248
Foster suckling, 420
Fracture, spontaneous, 239, 240
Freon, 149, 204
Frog, 68, 173
Fungi, 35, 42
Fur, 291

G

Gall bladder, 260, 355
Gamma globulin, 20, 373, 407, 408,
    411, 416, 417
Gamma gnotobiote, 31
Gamma radiation sterilization, 163, 221,
    see also Ray, gamma
Gaskets, 142
Gelatin, 185
Genetics, 23
Geotropism, 43
Germfree,
  in gnotobiotic monitoring, 183
  inoculation, 16
  cage, 100
  concept, 9, 10, 15
  conditions in nature, 4
  culture of tissue, 41
  humans, 5, 22, 25
  invertebrates, 43
  mammals, first colony, 225
  status, 172
  tank, 101
  transition to classic, 426, 427
Germicidal entry, 11
Germicide, 102, 144, 147, 166
Germ theory of disease, 34
Gf, 28, *see also* Germfree
Gilts, 178
Gizzard, 338
Glass wool, 110, 130, 152, 156
Globule leucocyte, 340
Globulin, 329, 417, 427, *see also* α-,
  β-, and γ-,

Gloves, 65, 110, 140
  protector, 139
Glucose,
  blood, 328
Gnotobiology, 25
Gnotobiosis, philosophic goal, 184
Gnotobiota, 8
Gnotobiote, 14, 26, 399
  bacteria-host, 402
  invertebrate-host, 424
  protozoa-host, 422
  virus-host, 419
Gnotobiotic colony, 400
Gnotobiotic state, 15
Gnotobiotization, 206
Gnotobiotope, 25
Gnotophore, 26
Gnotophoresis, 26, 398
Gnotophoric animals, 26, 398
Goat, 93, 94, 108, 170, 213, 225
  diet, 249
Gonads, 367
Granulocyte, 325
Growth, 288
Growth promotants, 408
Growth rate, 83, 86, 88, 92, 93, 94,
    227–229, 243, 244, 246, 247, 289
Growth stimulation, 278
Guinea pig, 62, 64, 81, 170, 171, 225,
    268, 277, 285, 288–388
  diet, 245

H

Haemonchus contortus, 52
Hamster, 225
Handfeeding, 15, 225
Hatchability, 168
Heart, 259, 265, 270, 311, 388, 389,
    402
Heart disease, 402
Heat, 154
  dry, 145, 166
  intermittent, 146
Heligmosomum skrjabini, 52
Hellman reaction centers, 369
Helminthes, 7
Hemagglutinin, 371
Hematology, 276

Hemorrhagic hypotension, 387
Heparin, 332
Hepatic necrosis, 259
Hepatitis, 420
Heteroagglutinin, 371
Heterophil, 326
Hexamethylenetetramine, 150
Hexaresorcinol, 150
Himsworth diet, 273
Histamine, 311, 333, 338, 343, 357
Histidine, 290, 294
Historical development, 34, 109
Homogenization, 221
Honey guide, 57
Hood, plastic, 121
Hormoligosis, 278
Hospital, 132
Humidity, 142, 165, 287
Hungry crazy, 82
Hydrochloric acid, 166
Hydrogen peroxide, 45, 56, 69, 147
Hylemya antiqua, 56, 57
Hymenolopis nana, 425

I

Ileocecal junction, 364
Ileocecal tonsil, 361, 370
Ileum, 341, 343, 407, 408
Immunity, 379
  inate, 20
Incinerator, 111
Incubation, 14, 191
Incubator, 204
Indican, 357
Indole, 13, 61, 351, 357
Infection, 4, 6, 19, 21, 27, 42, 391
Infectivity, 10
Inflammation, 20, 384
Ingesta, 252, 253, 344
Inoculation, 9, 15, 22, 73, 195, 206, 398, 400
Inoculum, 73, 284
Insecta, 53–60
Instinct, motherly, 242
Interrelationship between host and microorganisms, 21
Intestinal, content, 253
  flora, 20, 206

microorganisms, 214, 278
mucosa, 340, 342
synthesis theory, 19, 27, 214
tract, 7, 8, 11, 13, 16, 196, 209, 370, 416, 427
wall, 43, 419
Intestine, 252, 260
  large, 349
Invertase, 343, 351
Invertebrate, 43, 45–60, 284
Invertebrate-host gnotobiote, 424
Iodine, 66, 147, 150, 170, 178, 218
Isolation, 6, 8, 39
  biological, 1, 14, 35, 99
  single cell, 35
Isolators, 99, 110–130
  bubble, 123
  dispensable plastic, 133
  doughnut, 121
  Fisher-Horton, 141

J

Jar, 104
  bell, 24, 36, 40, 64, 109
  churn, 102, 105, 109, 138, 207
Jejunum, 343

K

Kahn reaction, 371
Kenophobia, 425
Kidney, 49, 187, 356
Kupffer cell, 380
Kurloff cell, 327

L

Lactation, 242
Lactobacillus, 209, 376
Lactobacillus acidophillus, 26, 408, 411, 416, 417
  var. bifidus, 5, 411, 412
  casei, 417
  lactis, 407, 408
Lamb, 95, 96
Lamina propria, 341, 407, 408
Larva, 53, 56, 67, 196, 213
Larynx, 337
Leaks, 201, 203, 204
Leaves, excised, 42

Lecane inermis, 48
Leucocytes, 41, 357, 368, 380
Leucotoxine-like substances, 389
Lieberkuhn crypt, 341, 385
Life, 2, 3, 4, 8, 30
　origin, 5, 22, 25
Light, 283
Limits of knowledge, 183
Lipid, 353
Lipase, 343
Lithocolletis, 8
Liver, 45, 258, 265, 271, 276, 351–355,
　381, 416
　vitamins, 231, 264, 267, 273, 403–
　　405, 415
　cirrhosis, 269, 388
　necrosis, 273, 388
Lock, sterile, 101, 110, 136, 153, 205
Lordosis, 345
Lung, 332
　consolidation, 198, 332, 386, 421
Lupine, 37
Lymph node, 193, 360, 362, 410, 419,
　427
Lymphatic system, 9, 14, 20, 337, 360,
　362, 369, 373, 411
Lymphocyte, 325, 340, 362, 370, 380,
　407, 427
Lymphomatosis, 421
Lysine, 221
Lysol, 129, 149

M

Maggots, 53, 57
Maintenance, 123, 201
Malnutrition, 382
Maltase, 343
Mammalia, 81–96, 174
Mammary gland, 259
Maturation, 355
Maturity of the young, 225
Mazzini reaction, 371
Meat, 69
Mechanical, arms, 101, 103
Media, 57, 66, 191
Melanoma, 379
Menadione sulfate, 276
Mende "overfeeding" technique, 239

Meningeal proliferation, 421
Mercuric chloride, 10, 40, 53, 129, 136,
　140, 144, 148, 158, 166, 168, 169,
　173
Mercuric iodine, 209
Merthiolate, 150, 170
Metaphen, 168
Metazoa, pure culture, 45
Methylcholanthrene, 386, 420
Methyl groups, 269
Methyl indole, 351
Microbes, effect of the dead, 9, 399
Microbial flooding, 391
Microbial gnotobiotes, 398
Microbiological monitoring, *see* Detec-
　tion
Micrococcus aureus, 56
　epidermis, 419
Micromanipulation, 35
Microorganisms, in nutrition, 216
Microsomal particle, 421
Milk, 65, 69, 82, 85, 93, 94, 161, 222,
　230–236, 249, 250
Mineral, 254, 256
　requirement of the rat, 220
Mixed culture, 30
Mitochondria, 325
Mobility, 143, 204
Monkey, 90, 170, 225
　diets, 249
Monoamine oxidase, 353, 407
Monobiote, 9, 30, 138
Monocyte, 327
Monoflora studies, 16, 26, 423
Morphological survey, 285
Morphology, gross, 78
Mosquito, 56
Moth, 57
Mouse, 87, 171, 225, 277, 294–387
　diets, 223, 248
Mouth, 337
Mummification, 390
Musca domestica, 56, 57, 58
Muscle, 256
　chemical composition, 256, 257, 271,
　　305
　tonus, 340, 345
Musculature, 305

Mycobacterium smegmatus, 254, 349
Mycoplasma gallinarum, 402
Myxomycophata, 35

N

Narcosis, natural, 171
Necator americanus, 52
Necrosis, 413
Nematoda, 49, 67
Nematospiroides dubius, 424
Neoaplectana glaseri, 49, 67
Nepticula, 8
Nervous system, 359
Neutrophil, 326
Niacin, 221, 264, 265, *see also* specific
    tissues
    deficiency, 262, 263, 265
Nippostrongylus muris, 49, 424
Nitrogen, 213, 231, *see also* specific
    tissues
    balance, 64
    fixation, 36, 60, 110
Nodule, 38, 360, 364, 365, 410
Nomenclature, 27, 184
Nose, 357, 332
Nuclear reactor, 145
Nucleic acids, 44, 56, 57
Nutrient,
    agar, 41
    essential, 217
    loss of, 221
Nutrition, 15, 19, 73, 213, 217
    plant, 36, 42
Nutritional deficiencies, 20
    inadequacies, 213
    requirements, 44, 250

O

Oatmeal, 82, 249
Observation, 192
Odor, 185, 287
Oesophagus, 337
Oligo-1, 6-glucosidase, 343
Omentum, 351
Onion, 57
Ontogenetic law, 1

Operation,
    Caesarean, 65
    surgical, 123, 133
Operator, effect of upon animal, 9
Opisthotonus, 260
Oral, abnormalities, 383
    cavity, 337
    vaccination, 216
Orchid, 42
Orchinol, 42
Orexis, 383
Ova, 196
Ovary, 57, 260, 367, 388
Ovum, 6
Oxygen, 147, 161, 218
Ozone, 145

P

Pancreas, 259, 338, 343
Panthotenic acid, 163, 221, 223, 265,
    267, *see also* specific tissue
    deficiency, 265
Paracolobactrum aerogenoides, 373
Paralysis, 265
Paramecia, 44
Parasite, 6, 10, 16, 44, 100, 189, 198,
    423, 424
    detection, 180, 195
    intracellular, 2
Parathyroid, 260
Parturition, 64, 171, 174
Pathogen free, 31
Pathology, 195
Peas, 36
Pectinophora gossypiella, 57
Pedigree, 192, 199
Pellobates fuscus, 68
Penicillin, 48, 265, 279, 407, 420
Penis, 367
Peptone, 41
Peracetic acid, 45, 121, 131, 147, 153,
    154, 174, 178
Periodontal disease, 384
Perioral gland, 337
Periplaneta americana, 59
Peristalsis, 345
Perosis, 270
Peyer's patches, 360, 361, 413, 427

pH, 222, 338, 343, 344, 350
Phaenica regina, 56
Phaeophyceae, 40
Phage, 21, 401
Phagocyte, 14, 20, 193, 369, 411
Phagocytic index, 380
Phagocytosis, 4, 380, 388, 412
Pharynx, 337
Phenol, 147, 357
Philodina acerticornis, 49
Phormia regina, 56, 57
Phosphorous, 221, 256, 295, 353
Physarum polycephalum, 2
Pig, 96, 179, 225
    diet, 249
Pigment, loss, 45
Pisces, 66
Pituitary, 260, 367
Placental, broth, 186
Plant,
    commercial, 40
    culture, 40
    feeding live, 277
    inoculated, 60
    sterile, 26, 36, 39, 41
    virus free, 40
Plasma cell, 361, 363, 364, 427
Platyfish, 66
Platyhelminthes, 45
Platypoecilus maculatus, 66
Pleuro-pneumonia like organism, 198
Plexiglass cages, 123
Pneumonia, 420, 421
    aseptic, 382
Post mortem changes, 389
Polybiote, 30
Polysaccharides, 63
Potassium, 343
    chloride, 156
    dichromate, 44
    hydroxide, 156
    mercuric iodide, 170
Potato, 56
Precipitron, 145
Pressure,
    negative, 21, 114
    positive, 107, 199
Pre-sterilization, radiation, 166

Pre-sterilized material, 205
Procurement of germfree material, 36
Production, 201
Properdin, 378
Prostate, 260, 367
Protein, 221, 254, 295, 357
    serum, 329, 330
    supplement, 244
Proteolytic activity, 341
P. Aurelia, 44
P. gregaria, 49
P. multimicronucleatum, 44
Proteus vulgari, 416
Prothrombin, 274
Protozoa, 7, 43
    detection, 193
Protozoa-host gnotobiotes, 422
Proventricules, 337
Provirus, 197
Pseudosarcophaga affinis, 58
Ptomaine, 61
Pups, *see* Dog
Pure culture, 34, 36
    concept, 1, 25, 39
Putrification changes, 390
Pyridoxine, 221

Q

Quail, 70, 81
    diets, 245
Quaternary ammonium compounds, 137,
    140, 149
Quercetin, 248
Quinosol, 158

R

Rabbits, 63, 89, 171, 225, 241, 277,
    289
    diets, 248
Radiation, 5, 121, 163, 166, 205
    damage, 386
    sickness, 20
    sterilization, 144, 221, 223
Rads, 145
Rana temporaria, 68, 69
Rat, 85, 170, 225, 251, 268, 274, 277
    diet, 238, 247

growth and survival, 226, 237–239, 291–387
milk, 230, 235, 236
Rays,
 beta, 144
 gamma, 144, 163, 220, 221
 ultraviolet, 144
 X-, 144
Rectal content, 349
Rectum, 349
Refrigeration, 205
Related concepts, 13
Relative humidity, *see* Humidity
Renal calcification, 258
Repair, 201
Reparative processes, 388
Reproduction, 14, 56, 81, 83, 87, 88, 90, 247, 248, 288, 345, 367
Respiratory system, 332
Reticulo-endothelial cells, 340, 407
 system, 408
Rib, 270
Riboflavin, 221, 223
 deficiency, 262–265, *see also* specific tissues
Rickettsia, 7, 196
Rigor mortis, 390
Roccal, 149, 169, 209
Rodophyceae, 40
Room,
 bubble, 105, 130
 germfree, 105, 127, 129, 134, 135, 142
 sterilizing, 130, 153
Roughage requirement, 254
Rous sarcoma, 420
Ruminant, 14, 27, 92

S

Sabouraud's agar, 186
Sacrifice, 286
Salmonella pullorum, 15, 374
Salmonella typhi, 370
Sample, 181, 189
Sampling procedure, 188
Sarcoma, 379
Scenedesmus, 39

Schistosoma mansoni, 425
Schollen leucocytes, 407
Seminal vesicles, 260
Senescence, 389
Sensory organs, 357
Separation, 24
Serological reaction, 186, 199
Serology, 370
Serum, 48, 405
 bactericidal power, 370, 411, 414
 cholesterol, 328, 417
 dog, 52
 embryo, 49
 hepatitis, 420
 protein, 330, 416, 417, 427
Sheep, 225
Shigella flexneri, 370, 412, 419
Shock, 387
Sibs, identical, 23
Sinus maxillaris, 363
Skatole, 13, 61, 357
Skeletal system, 294, 296
Skin, 237, 259, 291, 369
 abnormalities, 291
 culture, 41
 wound, 388
Skull, 294, 295
Small intestine, 337, 338
Snail, 52, 425
Snood, 291
Soap, 147, 203
Sodium, 343
 chloride, 147
 laurel sulfate, 149
 perborate, 68
 thioglycollate, 423
Sound, 283
Space, 204, 283
 floor, 140
 vehicles, 5, 24
Specific pathogen free animals, 15
Sperm, 367
Spermatocyte, 367
SPF, specific pathogen free, 31
Spleen, 260, 265, 268, 363, 365, 419
Sponge, sterile, 389
Spontaneous generation, 60
Standardization, 16, 23

Staphylococcus, 81, 82, 201
  albus, 402
  aureus, 380, 381, 419
  mesentericus, 402
Starch, 220
Starvation, 251, 383
Statistical treatment, 286
Steam, 141, 150, 218
  proportioning control, 136, 174
  sterilization, 254
Sterile,
  plants, 35
  techniques, 123
  tissue, 19
Sterility, *see also* Detection
  bacteriological, 7
  test, 184
Sterilization, 24, 65, 109, 143, 152, 153,
    154, 156, 166, 205
  food, 161, 222–224
  incomplete, 201
Sterol, 56
Stictococcus, 20
Stomach, 337
Storage, 205
Streptobacillus, Shaffer-Frye, 423
Streptococcus faecalis, 26, 351, 376,
    402, 404, 405, 408, 411, 417, 418
  liquefaciens, 407, 418
Streptomycin, 48, 209, 420
Stress, 20, 426
Strongyloides ratti, 52
Sucrose, 220
Sugar, 94, 249, 253, 350
Suit, sterile, 101, 131, 132
Sulfhydryl molecule, 148
Sulfuric acid, 156
Suppliers, commercial, *see* Chronology
Surface area, small intestine, 341
Surfactant, 153
Surgery, 123, 133, 209
Surgical technique, 112
  sterile, 19, 22
Symbionts, 20, 40, 59
Synthesis, abiotic, 24
System, dibiotic, 26

T

Tadpole, 13, 68–70, 173, 213
Tail length, 283
Tank, *see* Isolator
Tape worm, 48
Taste, 288
Taurocholic acid, 351
Technique, migration-dilution, 44
Teeth, 294, 337, 383, 418
  plaque, 193
Temperature, 141, 154, 155, 226
Tenebrio, 57
Tent, plastic, 178
  sterile, 170
Terminology, 27
Test, bacteriological, *see also* Detection
  cultural, 16
Testicle, 260, 367
Tetrahymena, 44
Thalamyd, 207
Theorical biology, 19
Theory of germfree life and gnotobi-
  ology, 1
Thermocouple, 141
Thermometer, 142
Thiamine, 163, 221, 225, 260, 406, *see
    also* specific tissues
  deficiency, 79, 261–264, 404
  metabolism, 264
Thiobacillus thiooxidans, 5
Thioglycolate, 148, 186, 187
Thorium dioxide, 380
Thymidine, 49
Thymocyte, 366, 427
Thymus, 265, 362, 364, 366, 427
Thyroid, 260, 366
Tilapia microcephala, 67
Time, parturition, 174
Tinea, 8
Tissue,
  bacteriologically sterile, 4, 19
  cultures, 26, 35, 41, 43, 187
Toad, 68
Tongue, 357
Tonsils, 193
Torula, 273
Toxocara canis, 424

Trachea, 332
Transfer, 11, 14
  aseptic, 23, 171
  system, 133
Trap,
  condensation, 141
  germicidal, 11, 101, 136, 137, 152, 174
Trauma, 389
Trematodes, 46
Treponema microdentium, 414
Triaryl phosphate, 160
Tribiote, 30
Trichomonas vaginalis, 424
Trifolium, 36
Trimethylamine, 269
Trypanosoma cruzi, 422
Trypsin, 53, 343, 351
Tryptophan, 221
Tuberculosis, 83
Tumor, 197, 386, 420, 421
  sterile plant, 42
Turbatrix aceti, 49
Turkeys, 70, 81, 169, 241, 278, 291
  diet, 245
Typhoid vaccine, 379

U

Ulcer, 412
Unknown factors in nutrition, 276–278
Urate, 349
Urea, 357
Urease, 357
Uremic poisoning, 225
Urine, 357
Urobilinogens, 351
Urobilins, 418
Uterus, 177, 388
Utilization, food, 251–254

V

Vf (*see* virus free), 30
V-tube, 43, 44
Vaccination, oral, 179, 214
Vacuum, *see* Pressure, negative
Vagina, 260, 367
Valvular insufficiency, 402

Variables,
  biological, 15
  unwanted, 284
Vertebrates, 60
Vibrio cholerae, 82, 412
Villi, intestinal, 341
Vipporus japonicus, 52
Virus, free, 25, 99, 146
  plants, 40
Virus, 1, 2, 7, 10, 26, 29, 163, 179, 180, 184, 185, 187, 197, 199, 386, 401, 419
  asymptomatic, inapparent, occult, 2, 15, 21, 28, 29, 419
  disease, 21, 172
  symptomatic, 28, 29
Virus-host gnotobiote, 419
Visitor, inoculation, 17, 284
Visual stimuli, 283
Vitamins, 163, 221, 257
Vitamin,
  A, 221, 257
    deficiency, 257–260
  B, 56, 73, 79, 260, 289, 403, 405
    metabolism, 273
    (*see* specific tissue)
  B12, 221, 267, 268
  C, 79, 85, 163, 221, 230, 247, 265, 268, 269, 270, 310, 353, 427
    deficiency, 270, 421
    metabolism, 230
    required for rat, 230–232
  D, deficiency, 270–272
    destruction, 244
  E, 221, 273
  K, 273–276
Volvulus, intestinal, 345, 347, 389

W

Wasting disease, 421
Water, 142, 160, 250, 251, 283, *see also* specific tissues
  biological, 165
  sterilization, 165
Waves,
  electromagnetic, 144

ultra-sonic, 145
White cell count, 193
Worm free, 7
Worms, 195, 424
Wound healing, 20

X

Xenbiot, 31

Y

Yeast, 41, 44, 45, 52, 56, 79, 207, 213, 276, 425
Yolk, 67

Z

Zepherine chloride, 177
Zinc sulfate, 195, 196